Mechanically
Assisted
Manual
Techniques:
Distraction
Procedures

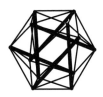

Mechanically Assisted
Manual Techniques:
Distraction Procedures

Thomas F. Bergmann, DC, FICC
Professor, Chiropractic Methods Department
Faculty Clinician
Northwestern College of Chiropractic
Bloomington, Minnesota

P. Thomas Davis, MUP, DC, DACBOH
Associate Professor of Research
Northwestern College of Chiropractic
Bloomington, Minnesota

Photographs by Arne Krogsveen
Illustrations by Ken Shipper

with 348 illustrations and photographs

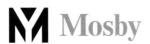 Mosby

St. Louis Baltimore Boston Carlsbad Chicago Naples New York Philadelphia Portland
London Madrid Mexico City Singapore Sydney Tokyo Toronto Wiesbaden

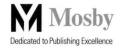
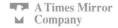

Vice President and Publisher: Don Ladig
Executive Editor: Martha Sasser
Developmental Editor: Amy Christopher
Project Manager: Mark Spann
Production Editor: Beth Hayes
Book Design Manager: Judi Lang
Composition Specialist: Terri Knapp
Manufacturing Supervisor: Karen Boehme

Printed in the United States of America
Composition by Mosby Electronic Production, St. Louis
Lithography film by Top Graphics
Printing/binding by Maple-Vail Book Mfg. Group

Mosby–Year Book, Inc.
11830 Westline Industrial Drive
St. Louis, MO 63146

The authors have made every effort to ensure the accuracy of the information herein, particularly with regard to technique and procedure. However, appropriate information sources should be consulted, especially for new or unfamiliar procedures or equipment. It is the responsibility of every practitioner to evaluate the appropriateness of a particular technique or type of equipment in the context of actual clinical situations and with due consideration to new developments. Authors, editors, and the publisher cannot be held responsible for any typographical or other errors found in this book.

Library of Congress Cataloging–in–Publication Data
Bergmann, Thomas F.
  Mechanically Assisted Manual Techniques: Distraction Procedures / Thomas F. Bergmann, P. Thomas Davis.
      p.   cm.
  Includes index,
  ISBN 0-8151-0900-8
    1. Manipulation (Therapeutics)   2. Chiropractic.   3. Orthopedic traction.
  I. Davis, P. Thomas.   II. Title.
    [DNLM: 1. Manipulation, Orthopedic--methods.   2. Chiropractic.
  3. Traction.   WB 905.9 B499d 1998]
  RZ255.B474   1998
  615.5'34—dc21
  DNLM/DLC
  for Library of Congress   96-40215
                                                                 CIP

98 99 00 01 02 / 10 9 8 7 6 5 4 3 2 1

Author Biographies

Thomas F. Bergmann, DC, FICC, began his chiropractic teaching career in 1978 as a lecturer for the International College of Chiropractic (now The Royal Melbourne Institute of Technology, School of Chiropractic) in Melbourne, Australia. Since 1982 he has been on the faculty at Northwestern College of Chiropractic, currently at the rank of professor. In 1993 the students honored him as Teacher of the Year. Dr. Bergmann is also a faculty clinician in the Center for Clinical Studies, where he maintains a private practice and participates in the care of clinical research patients. Dr. Bergmann is the founding editor of the journal *Chiropractic Technique*, serving as the editor-in-chief for 8 years. He is a member of the editorial review board of *Topics in Clinical Chiropractic*. Dr. Bergmann is a co-author of the textbook *Chiropractic Technique Principles and Procedures*, has contributed chapters to five other books, and authored many papers published in the scientific literature. He was a participant in the first Low Back Manipulation Consensus Panel, sponsored by the RAND Corporation in 1990. Dr. Bergmann is the chiropractic consultant to MetraHealth Medicare and serves as a site team member for the Council on Chiropractic Education Accreditation Committee. Dr. Bergmann received his B.S. degree in biology from Northern Illinois University in 1969 and his D.C. degree from National College of Chiropractic in 1977.

P. Thomas Davis, MUP, DC, DACBOH, is an Associate Professor of Research in the Wolf-Harris Center for Clinical Studies at Northwestern College of Chiropractic. Dr. Davis is the principal investigator for a randomized clinical trial of the chiropractic/allopathic treatment of carpal tunnel syndrome. He was in clinical practice in both Alaska and in Indiana before joining Northwestern. Dr. Davis holds a diplomate in occupational health and provides consulting in this field. He has written several articles for professional journals and is preparing an article for publication on the carpal tunnel syndrome clinical trial. His research continues in the areas of the application of distraction techniques in the extremities and in the lumbar spine, specifically for radiculopathy. Dr. Davis holds a BA from Southern Illinois University and an MUP from the University of Illinois, as well as a DC from Palmer College of Chiropractic. He has been in practice since 1977. Dr. Davis was involved with Thomas Hill in the development of Hill's GAIT Technique before Hill's untimely death and was encouraged by him to continue with its development. He has used flexion-distraction in his practice since 1979.

Foreword

All chiropractors and all students of chiropractic are going to love *Mechanically Assisted Manual Techniques: Distraction Procedures*. Dr. Tom Bergmann, in partnership with Dr. Tom Davis, has produced a magnificent work on technique. This is the first text to look comprehensively at the specialized field of motion-assisted techniques and equipment.

Whether you are large or small, male or female, youthful or less robust than you once were, Dr. Bergmann and Dr. Davis explain what mechanical motion equipment is available to assist your technique. They also address what your technique might be. And, because they are experienced clinicians interested in all equipment but beholden to none, you get reliable comparative information shorn of promotion hype and bias.

I was drawn particularly to Chapter 1, which reviews the history and evolution of tables and other equipment that provide motion assistance. Through this history and the excellent illustrations I can now pretend to be an expert on spring-loading, drop pieces, and worm drive. The following chapters review all aspects of motion-assisted technique, and the ways in which individual tables and other equipment in current use are adapted for use at each region of the spine and extremities. This book is a clinical gold mine with easy extraction of ore, because it is beautifully planned, concise, and unusually readable.

If you have any enthusiasm for the art and science of the chiropractic adjustment or any desire to follow in the footsteps of the founders, with more finesse and less wear on your frame, this book is for you. Read, learn, and enjoy.

David A. Chapman-Smith LLB (Hons)
Editor, The Chiropractic Report
Secretary-General, World Federation of Chiropractic

Foreword

The treatment of patients with spine-related complaints is confounded by many uncertainties and equally many options. Inspection of the volumes of literature on spine disorders and their treatment leaves the reader struck by the breadth of clinical options and the extraordinary weakness of the collective scientific foundations. Few remedies have attained the scientific support that manipulation of the spine has achieved.[1]

Fortunately, the natural history for symptomatic episodes is favorable for the majority of cases and the effects are rarely disabling in the long term.[2] Popular support of spinal manipulation has waxed and waned over the course of centuries, with the clinical wisdom of the times. With recent scientific emphasis on spinal research, the preponderance of evidence for manipulation of the spine as a preferred mode of treatment in the acute episode has been favorable.[1] Even for patients in the subacute and chronic stages, some recent evidence exists that there may be a positive effect on the patient's experience of pain and speed of functional return.[3,4] In contrast with other treatment methods, manipulation has stood the tests of time and scientific query rather well. Yet, we still have only vague notions about highly relevant matters affecting practice daily, including thresholds of response to treatment, optimal dosage, and duration of care, as well as the influence of combining treatments.[5]

Why is it so difficult to settle the questions of clinical effectiveness of treatment for spinal disorders? With the long history, why do we have over 90 named systems of manipulation technique, all empirically derived, with no clear evidence as to indications, contraindications, or relative effectiveness of their use? What an irony for experts in spine care to face!

The answers to these questions come from a far-reaching range of influences. They reflect the social priorities in research funding, scientific ambiguities as to the basis for spinal symptoms, naiveté as to the clinical and scientific effects of manipulation, and the biased contest between proponents and opponents of the various systems. A major contribution to these many elements of complexity is the absence of a cogent, authoritative source of information for the practitioner. Without common lexicon and procedures, no effort to resolve and improve on the clinical outcomes from treatment can be expected.

The contribution of this volume is based on its effort to anchor the clinical practice of treatment into a common language, with available scientific evidence as a foundation. Focusing on the specific styles of treatment that incorporate distraction or tensile loading of the spine as a structure, the clinical methods are clearly described. The empirical foundations are merged with the physiologic and biomechanical science, forming the hypotheses for clinical practice.

As a consolidation and clarification of what is practiced with these methods, with this book the authors have served the chiropractic profession well. The material found in this book gives an excellent means of learning for the novice. At the same time, it sets the stage for more highly competent research in manipulation biomechanics. Information on the physical performance of technique is integrated with the intended purpose and supported, where available, by research results. Armed with this reference, the clinical scientist is benefited in the design of future biomechanical and clinical work to develop the full potential of these methods. Who are the patients who will have the greatest benefit? What specific procedures are best matched to presenting clinical characteristics? How often and for what duration is treatment necessary to achieve desired results? What are the physiologic and biomechanical consequences of successful use of these procedures?

A rich and fulfilling future awaits us by resolving these questions. I am grateful for the step toward its fulfillment afforded by the work presented in the pages that follow.

John J. Triano, DC, MA

Director, Texas Back Institute Chiropractic Division

Plano, TX

REFERENCES

1. Bigos S et al. *Clinical practice Guideline No. 14: Acute Low Back Problems in Adults*, Agency for Health Care Policy and Research; 1994. US DHHS Public Health Service publication 95-0642.
2. Andersson GRJ. The epidemiology of spinal disorders. In: Frymoyer JW, ed. *The Adult Spine: Principles and Practice*, 2nd ed. New York: Raven Press; 1997.
3. Triano J, McGregor M, Hondras M, Brennan P. Manipulation therapy vs. education programs in chronic low back pain. *Spine*. 1995;20(8):948-955.
4. Triano J, McGregor M, Skogsbergh D. Use of chiropractic manipulation in lumbar rehabilitation. *J Rehabil*, 1997 (in press).
5. Triano J. Standards of care: manipulative procedures. In: White A, Anderson R, eds. *Conservative Care of Low Back Pain*. Baltimore: Williams & Wilkins; 1991.

Preface

The history of man's CREATIVE effort is the story of his struggle to control "direction" by the ELIMINATION of known RESISTANCE.

R. Buckminster Fuller

The primary impetus for developing this book came from two directions. First, one of the authors, P. Thomas Davis, long before experience with chiropractic, became intrigued with structural and functional icosahedrons through university course work with Buckminster Fuller. These unique structures, which are used in design and architecture, represent an unusual balance between compression members and tension members to maintain their shape and form. When external forces are applied, they distort, adapt, and return to their original form. Secondly, both authors were introduced to an adjusting table like no other. Thomas Hill, DC, developed and began manufacturing a table that had a controlled linear distraction movement of the pelvic section, produced by a motor. The pelvic section could be set in a sloping up or down position, allowing linear distraction with flexion or extension prestress. This piece of equipment produces a form of mechanically assisted distractive manipulation. Thinking of the spine and extremities as tension/compression integrity systems that must adapt to the gravitational loads, the use of linear distraction in the y axis of the body makes sense and is an exciting concept that should be explored further.

The use of manual procedures as a part of alternative or complimentary health care is growing in popularity and acceptance. This acceptance of spinal manipulation by other health care professions, industry, and the general population continues to grow despite controversies in clinical practice and lack of appropriate validation. Right or wrong, this demonstrates how an empirically discovered method of treatment can become a part of science through perseverance and systematic analysis. Manual procedures are advocated for the treatment of functional disturbances in the spine and extremity joints. However, a wide variety of manipulative procedures exist that affect different aspects of joint function. A common factor with these methods is the application of external forces to the body for the purpose of affecting the flexibility and comfort of the spine and its contiguous tissues. In spite of these common factors, the assumption that all forms of manual therapy are equivalent must be avoided, because many significant differences exist, as well. Studies designed to compare the effectiveness and efficiency of the many technique systems have not been done. Other texts have been written describing those manual techniques that use a thrust. These have been authored by chiropractic, physical therapy, and medical manipulators. This book is intended for those individuals who seek knowledge of the applications of manual procedures. It discusses and describes the use of manual distractive techniques that are applied with the assistance of a mechanical component of the treatment table.

Manual distractive techniques apply forces that are designed to stretch soft tissues and to separate joint surfaces. These procedures have been used for many years in the treatment of painful conditions of the spine and extremities. They have been applied in several ways, using variation in direction and amount and form of applied traction force. Distractive techniques especially influence movement in the long axis of the joint (y axis). This is a commonly used vector in the extremity procedures but is not often discussed in techniques applied to the spine. The field of manipulative mechanics is beginning to develop, with the information available being applied to explain what may happen when joint surfaces and contiguous soft tissues are separated, stretched, and mobilized. To our knowledge, no one has investigated these methods, discussed their differences, nor formulated a collective hypothetic and/or theoretic basis for the usage. The purpose of this book is to bring together the information relative to the pathomechanics of joint structures and the principles of application of the various forms of distractive and/or traction techniques. Specific attention is given to how the forces are developed and the direction in which the body part being treated is placed (flexion, extension, lateral flexion, long axis translation, and so on). Although there has been renewed interest in manipulative procedures referred to as *high-velocity, low-amplitude thrust techniques*, there has been very little written about patient tolerance for these procedures or what to do when the procedures cannot be applied. Distractive techniques are thought to be more easily tolerated by the patient while imposing less physical demand on the practitioner.

Chapter 1 presents a brief history of manual therapy in general and distraction/traction techniques specifically. Also, the development or evolution of the equipment used to administer manipulative therapy is provided. Chapter 2 discusses biomechanical considerations necessary to appreciate the fundamental principles of joint function and dysfunction relative to manipulative therapy. Clinical models are discussed that delineate similarity and difference between structural and pathologic processes. However, detailed discussion of the diagnosis and treatment of specific pathologies is beyond the scope and purpose of this book. An overview of manual procedures is presented in Chapter 3 that includes the clinical effects and forms of manipulation. Also discussed are the evaluative procedures used to identify the dysfunctional joint and characteristics that might suggest a specific technique approach. Chapters 4 and 5 describe the application of distraction to the spine and extremities. Specific information is given on the use of McManis, Cox, Jensen, Leander, and Hill techniques in an unbiased and straightforward method. Chapter 6 presents the relatively new concept of motion-assisted thrust technique, thought to be capable of providing some assistance in developing the critical force required to produce joint separation. Because of the variation in patient characteristics and clinician size and capabilities, sometimes it is difficult to produce this critical force. Therefore the addition of a manual and motorized mechanical device is considered. Chapter 7 discusses adjunctive approaches to traction, including the VAX-D, LTX 3000, inversion, continuous passive motion (CPM), and sustained traction. Finally, Chapter 8 covers the use of outcome measures that are necessary to determine the effectiveness and efficiency of any therapeutic procedure, along with research perspectives for distractive techniques. Also included are a sampling of case reports to consider the clinical application of distraction techniques.

Which is the best technique for any given problem? This is not presently known. There is no research that would withstand the scrutiny of peer review that relates to comparison of chiropractic techniques nor are there any clinical trials involving specific technique testing. This book presents information on the use and clinical trials involving specific technique testing. This book presents information on the use and clinical utility of mechanically assisted forms of manual therapy and suggests the need for further study.

Thomas F. Bergmann, DC, FICC
P. Thomas Davis, MUP, DC, DACBOH

Acknowledgments

This book acknowledges the contribution made by Thomas Hill, DC, and the work he started, both with the technique that he described and the table that he developed in defining linear axial distraction with motion-assist. Although he experienced an early departure from this life, Hill made a major contribution through his devotion and perseverance.

There are also those outside chiropractic who helped define the characteristics of life, its components, and how it all works. From the cell to the planets, we have people who labored, sometimes long ago, to find the pieces of the puzzle and to fit them together so that we could use the product of their efforts.

Those who labored to define in more detail the practice of chiropractic through study and research must also be recognized for their contribution to the profession and to the relief of human suffering. It is hoped that this effort will add to the knowledge base of chiropractic as a manual procedure for the spine and other body articulations. And finally, recognition must be given to the efforts of the designers and manufacturers of the many pieces of equipment that have improved the practice of the discipline for both the delivery of the adjustment to the patient and for the protection of the physical form of the clinician.

A special appreciation is offered to John Triano, DC, of the Texas Back Institute, who reviewed a portion of the book concerned with biomechanics and was kind enough to write a Foreword. Additional appreciation is offered for David Chapman-Smith, the Executive Director of the World Federation of Chiropractic, for his contribution of a Foreword.

Appreciation is due the manufacturers of equipment and publishers of books and other publications for providing photographs for reproduction and approvals for using their figures in this book. Finally, the efforts of both the photographer, Arne Krogsveen, and the illustrator, Ken Shipper, are acknowledged, as are those of an engineer, Michael Schwartz, PhD, of St. Thomas University, in an attempt to create body figures. A special thank-you is provided for the several chiropractic students who posed for the photographs of the tables and the application of the various techniques.

A special gratitude is due to the wives of both authors, Evelyn Bergmann and Barbara Davis for their patience during the writing of the book and the period of its review. Without this support the effort would not be possible.

Thomas F. Bergmann, DC, FICC
P. Thomas Davis, MUP, DC, DACBOH

Contents

Mechanically
Assisted
Manual
Techniques:
Distraction
Procedures

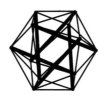

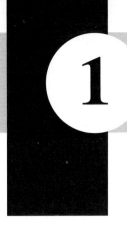

The History of Manipulation and the Evolution of Manipulative Equipment

Much has been written about the historic and philosophic roots of manipulation and the profession of chiropractic. To understand chiropractic and its application today, it is important to understand other healing philosophies that existed in the United States during the early years of the profession. These philosophies include Hahnemann's homeopathy, Still's osteopathy, and the eclectics. The primary instrument of chiropractic treatment is the hands of the practitioner; the next instrument of importance is the table on which the manipulations and adjustments are applied.

The focus of the following chapters is the way in which techniques may be applied and enhanced through the use of traction. Techniques involving traction and distraction are examined, with emphasis on methods of performing the techniques and vehicles (in most cases, tables) used in applying them. Explanation is provided that presents an approach to the method as supported by the literature rather than rigid adherence to the method as promoted by the founder of the technique.

EARLY MANIPULATION

Many cultures have used manipulation of joints, especially the spine, in the treatment of physical problems affecting the human body. Drawings from various parts of the eastern and western world demonstrate the application of this treatment form from the time of the ancient Greeks through the Middle Ages. Although early equipment was primitive, it demonstrated many of the characteristics of equipment today, such as traction, assistive devices, and multiple postures in which the forces can be applied. The early equipment and methods used were different from those of contemporary chiropractic. The tables were not adjustable and manipulation was primarily nonspecific and indirect.

Early spinal manipulation, as identified by Ambroise Pare (1510-1590), was commonly practiced. Pare gave the same instructions on manipulation as were given in the *Corpus Hippocraeteum* (circa 400 BC). After the seventeenth century, however, there is no further evidence of medical physicians having performed manipulation. During this period, physicians became aware of the danger of applying force to bone affected by tuberculosis (known as tuberculous joints). Anderson[1] notes that Pott indicated in testimony that spinal caries was a widespread vertebral disorder and that manipulation of a weakened tubercular joint could have disastrous consequences.

In the sixteenth and seventeenth centuries, fear of injury to bone damaged by tuberculosis caused bonesetting, as manipulation was called at that time, to become known as a "folk art" instead of a medical technique.

THE ORIGINS OF HOMEOPATHY, OSTEOPATHY, AND CHIROPRACTIC

Common endemic illnesses of the nineteenth century included malaria, dysentery, pneumonia, and tuberculosis. Gaucher-Peslherbe[2] notes that the illnesses included epidemics "...of cholera, with outbreaks like those in New Orleans in 1832 and New York in 1854, and yellow fever...occurring every year between 1800 and 1879." Most of the techniques used to combat these scourges were ineffectual but were used in the belief that even if they did not help, they would do no harm.

Many of the early methods of medical treatment were employed into the late nineteenth century. For example, the recommended treatment for a particular type of torticollis in the neck and a type of sprain in the lumbar region included, "rest and immobilization by means of a fixed appliance, while pain was recommended to be treated with opium, leeches and cupping."[3] Although this seems a questionable treatment by today's standards, similar treatments were used for many other problems.

Bonesetting was often practiced by families. It evolved from the peasant revival of manipulation in the seventeenth century. D.D. Palmer (the founder of chiropractic) and Andrew Taylor Still (the founder of osteopathy) became acquainted with bonesetting techniques. They also practiced magnetic healing, a reflex therapy that occasionally included vigorous paraspinal massage.[4] Bonesetting and magnetic healing were instrumental in the founding of chiropractic and osteopathy.

By the midnineteenth century, medical practice included many approaches to treatment. Significant among these was the European method of homeopathy, which used microdoses of drugs. The practitioners of this approach initially were trained by a German physician, Samuel Christian Hahnemann. Hahnemann also trained some of the American homeopaths. In the United States, homeopathy was considered a specialty of medicine, because only physicians could become homeopaths. The practice was not, however, well received by the medical establishment.

The basic premise of homeopathy is its doctrine of similars, which is treatment with a drug that produces symptoms in a healthy person identical to those experienced by a sick person. This approach assists the body in achieving its natural response to illness.[5] Although no longer in use in the United States by the early twentieth century, this treatment is still practiced in Europe. The United States is presently experiencing a resurgence of homeopathy.

An eclectic approach to treatment that drew from many philosophies of healing grew out of the thinking of the midnineteenth century. Gaucher-Peslherbe[2] wrote,

> ...in principle, eclecticism was not a system like all the rest, but a philosophical method that ....when applied to the medical sciences, seeks to extract from all the doctrines professed up to the present time what is reasonable and true in them, and with this to build a body of knowledge founded on the wise and just use of experience.

Andrew Taylor Still, an unorthodox medical practitioner, founded a significant method of treatment (incorporating manipulation) in the late nineteenth century, which he named osteopathy. From its founding, osteopathy focused on the blood-vascular system, using the "rule of the artery" and its primary role in good circulation for the health of the individual.[3]

Chiropractic, founded in 1895 by D.D. Palmer, focuses primarily on the nervous system. Osteopathy and chiropractic are similar in that both promote the theory that the human body has an innate ability to maintain good health. Both disciplines also teach the use of manipulation of bones. Much has been written about the relationship between D.D. Palmer and A.T. Still and their influence on each other. An allegation was made that Palmer stole osteopathy and transformed it into chiropractic.

> Did D.D. Palmer "steal" the manipulative techniques of A.T. Still? The most probable answer is no. As noted by Brantingham, "Palmer was not the first to manipulate, but, neither was Still. Still was the first to develop bonesetting into a general system of health care. Palmer followed with chiropractic."[4]

On the other hand, as Brantingham[4] continues, "Why did osteopathy expand to include allopathic medicine?" One reason he cites is that Still, desiring to see his new profession licensed, allowed some "medicalization" at Kirksville. Palmer, however, would not compromise and did not allow "medicalization" of any chiropractic college with which he was directly involved.

It is not known whether there was significant contact between the proponents of the two manipulative disciplines during these early years. The osteopath J.V. McManis, through the chiropractor James Cox, provided a contemporary osteopathic influence on chiropractic. Much of Cox's initial work in flexion/distraction was similar to the work of McManis. The design of the early Cox table, especially as in the Barnes table, is a direct descendant of the McManis table of the early 1900s.[7, 8, 9]

PHILOSOPHIC ROOTS

Judah[6] notes that spiritualism, which developed in the United States in the 1840s, spawned many interrelated religious, healing, and paranormal investigative groups. A common ground for these philosophies is possible because of the brief span between 1840 and 1875 in which they developed. Their foundation was the extreme liberalism of American transcendentalism, which began in the 1830s and produced the philosophy of Ralph Waldo Emerson. His concept of an innate and educated dual mind follows a similar theosophic belief.[10] D.D. Palmer believed the innate mind to be an essential focus of early chiropractic thinking. He stated that "spirit and body" comprise a dualistic system and that "innate and educated mentalities" look after the body and its environment.[11] This idea of innate intelligence is critical to the 1956 work by B.J. Palmer[12] which states that "Innate is the ONE eternal, internal, stable, permanent factor that is a fixed and reliable entity, does not fluctuate up and down scales to meet idiosyncrasies...."

This concept persists in the chiropractic philosophy of mind-body connection. However, from the early days of chiropractic, scientists and vitalists (who believe that the principles that govern life are different from the principles of inanimate matter) have held divergent philosophic views. Waagen and Strang[13] note that D.D. Palmer believed that both philosophies are important and have a place in the concept of innate intelligence.

Many of the early conceptualizers of chiropractic were dogmatic in their beliefs; others, however allowed progression of thought and connection with contemporary scientific thought. Osteopaths followed the allopaths and became absorbed into medicine; chiropractors stayed apart to form a separate health care system. Chiropractic's approach is by hand and is a "specific type of health care characterized not by ailment treated, but by method of treatment."[13]

TERMINOLOGY

Criticism leveled at the Palmers for not using accepted terminology led to a critique of chiropractic and chiropractors by medical practitioners. John Howard, D.C., (founder of the National College of Chiropractic) wrote that Palmer turned away from medical terms such as "diagnosis" and "treatment" primarily for legal reasons. Although this separated Palmer and chiropractic from mainstream practice, it created a new health care discipline with its own terminology.[6] The separation raised a barrier to cooperation with the medical establishment, resulting in the opposition of many publications to chiropractic. The AMA/Wilk case settled in 1990 provided an opportunity for the opposition to take a formal stance against chiropractic.[14]

Although this separation persists as a negative barrier, it has produced an environment for independent development of ideas and chiropractic equipment. Chiropractic provides a noninvasive approach to health care with a direct effect on the nervous system. The approach employed by the chiropractor is manipulation or adjustment of the human frame, including the articulations of the spine and extremities. Over the years, terminology used by manipulators, adjusters, and manual therapists has been indiscriminately mixed. *Manipulation* is a broad term for the therapeutic application of manual

force, such as in mobilizing, applying traction, massaging, and so on; *adjustment* is a more specific term referring to the articular movement of the spine by dynamic thrust. These terms are defined in the context of current practice by Gatterman and Hansen[15] as follows:

> Manipulation: A manual procedure that involves a directed thrust to move a joint past the physiological range-of-motion without exceeding the anatomical limit.
> Adjustment: Any chiropractic therapeutic procedure that utilizes controlled force, leverage, direction, amplitude and velocity, which is directed at specific joints or anatomical regions. Chiropractors commonly use such procedures to influence joint and neurophysiological function.

Manual therapy may be the best description of chiropractic treatment. Although disagreement occurs within the profession on the use of the word *therapy*, it may be the most-understood term in this era of new forms for "health care delivery." Use of the term *manual therapy* may aid in chiropractic's early integration into the mainstream allied health care.

ANCIENT DEVICES

Illustrations (in some cases from ancient books) show early practitioners with several assistants using a traction table with tensioning cords to perform adjustments. While applying tension, the operators applied force with an instrument of leverage similar to a large wooden board placed in a specific location(s) along the spine to press on a specific vertebra (Fig. 1-1).

Tables were developed for the practice of osteopathy and chiropractic. Many were designed to allow concentration of energy into certain parts of the spine, providing the clinician with the ability to apply a controlled force to a specific spinal area. The early practices of health care did not change significantly for hundreds of years. This is evident in modification of the Hippocrates table in the sixteenth century (Fig. 1-2).

THE OLD WOOD TABLES OF CHIROPRACTIC

The first table used in chiropractic was a flat wooden table with turned legs such as on a piano. It was approximately two feet tall, with minimal covering and no face

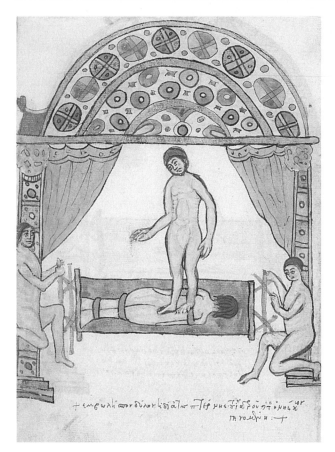

Fig. 1-1 Hippocrates' table. *(Courtesy Piccarda Quilici, Lucia Parmiggiani, and Jean-Paul Jolivet, Biblioteca Universitaria, Archiginnasio de Bologna, Bologna, Italy.)*

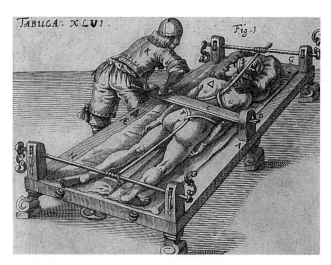

Fig. 1-2 Modifications to Hippocrates' table in the sixteenth century. *(Courtesy Bibliotheque Interuniversitaire de Medicine, Paris.)*

opening. The flat surface offered no softening material to absorb force. Little provision was made for the comfort or positioning of the patient for delivery of a better adjustment (Fig. 1-3). The adjustment was the high-velocity, low-amplitude thrust, which delivers a force sufficient to generate the click, or crack, sound familiar to chiropractors and patients. The face hole and split headpiece with adjustable sides were not yet available. Eventually, other disciplines, including osteopathy and physical therapy, influenced the design of modern chiropractic tables.

Complaints of painful adjustments and a desire to facilitate the giving of the adjustment led D.D. Palmer and his son, B.J. Palmer, to experiment with improvements to the table. The first improvement was a board sloping from the forward end of the table toward the floor at approximately a 45-degree angle. The patient was placed on the table in the prone position, with the head and neck bent downward over the sloping board and the nose and chin facing the board. This position

required less exertion of force by the adjuster but did not improve patient comfort.[16]

Adjustments were considered more difficult to perform in the dorsal region than in the cervical region and required more force. In 1943, Widmoyer designed a pad for the adjusting table. The pad was a thoracic hump that became known as the *dorsal roll*.[17] The dorsal portion of the table was padded with firm pillows, raising the dorsal piece. A great deal of experimentation was involved, because soft pillows absorbed much of the force of the adjustment and various angle combinations provided differences in the comfort level of the patient.[17]

As new tables were developed, attention was paid to patient positioning and the location of the clinician, providing for increased leverage and an advantageous adjacent stance. The patient was helped on and off the table with the use of the hy-lo table, which moved the patient from standing to prone and back to standing. This allowed patients with acute low-back pain to get on and off the table more easily. This was an important advance in a field in which practitioners had little access to the technology of the day (with the exception of radiology, the only significant technology available to the chiropractor in the early period of practice) (see Fig. 1-8).

Improvements were made to the table and attention paid to patient placement for the delivery of the adjustment. Placement included positioning the patient with the head in a particular position, often using the split headpiece to center the head and releasing the headpiece for specific angling of the head and neck. Other posi-

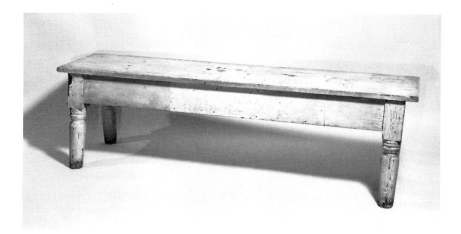

Fig. I-3 Early flat table. *(Courtesy Palmer College of Chiropractic Archives, Davenport, Iowa.)*

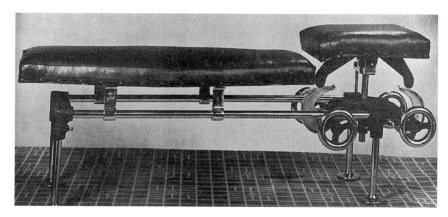

Fig. I-4 Side-posture table. *(Courtesy Palmer College of Chiropractic Archives, Davenport, Iowa.)*

tioning included releasing the center, or chestpiece, of the table to allow the thoracic spine to drop and decrease resistance to this area, making the adjustment easier. The drop headpiece table, a significant change in equipment design, allowed side-posture treatment of the cervical spine and the application of a mechanically assisted device for chiropractors. This was the first significant mechanical assist since the much earlier innovation of traction. The technique that arose from this device was known as the *hole-in-one*, made famous by B.J. Palmer. The position used in this technique provided support for the side of the head with a slight elevation, higher than the lower shoulder. The table had a rapid-drop mechanism that created additional leverage for the chiropractor through increased speed of the adjustment.

The hole-in-one approach originated with Carver's use of the side-posture table in 1908, although the Palmer hole-in-one technique was announced in 1935. In the early 1900s the Palmer recoil technique was widely used. The development of Palmer recoil was followed by several side-posture approaches to adjusting. Different table configurations accommodated placement of the head to make delivery of the adjustment easier on clinician and patient.[17] This position led to the design of a low, flat table with light cushioning over the portion supporting the body. The headpiece was raised to support the head and maintain a neutral position for the head and neck. The internal drop mechanism of the headpiece released when force was applied to the patient's cervical spine. The table had contours for the head and neck but provided a flat surface for the body (Fig. 1-4). The focus of this technique was limited to the cervical spine, and treatment was applied to only the articulations of the occiput, C1 and C2.

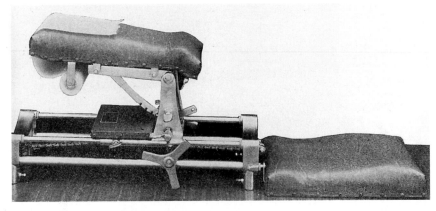

Fig. 1-5 Knee-chest table. *(Courtesy Palmer College of Chiropractic Archives, Davenport, Iowa.)*

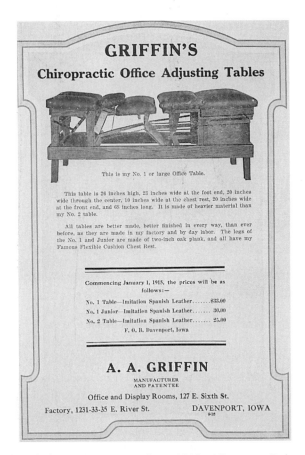

Fig. 1-6 Griffin table, circa 1915. *(Courtesy Palmer College of Chiropractic Archives, Davenport, Iowa.)*

Adjustment of the lumbar spine posed new problems, and various methods of suspending the abdomen were attempted. This led to the development of the knee-chest table, which positioned the body with the knees flexed in a kneeling position and the head and chest suspended on the upper section of the table. This posture allowed the clinician easy access to the lumbar spine and placed the patient in a relaxed position (Fig. 1-5).

Some early tables included a slot for the nose and a cutout in the pelvic piece for positioning of the male genitalia. A dorsal-lumbar piece was added in 1911, and between 1912 and 1914 springs were added to provide tension and give partial support for the pregnant or obese patient.[17]

The Griffin Table Company in Davenport, Iowa, produced a wood table on which the contemporary table is based. (Fig. 1-6) This unit had a split, adjustable headpiece, an adjustable drop abdominal section, and a padded top; a spring mechanism provided resistance.

The Palmer Hy-lo (or Hi-lo) was the first mechanical table (Fig. 1-7). The table assisted the patient from standing to prone or supine, with minimal patient effort. Evins and Stiles created the spring-loaded hy-lo and, later, a motor-powered lift (Fig. 1-8). The Griffin Company obtained a patent for these spring-loaded hy-los in 1913. No significant improvements were made in the hy-lo table from 1915 until the invention of the drop mechanism in the early 1950s.[17]

TRACTION TABLES

The manual traction table was a fifteenth- and sixteenth-century modified version of the fifth-century BC Hippocrates table. The early description of traction dates to Hippocrates. The two types of traction are axial and intersegmental. The traction method involved binding the patient at the head, pelvis, knees, and ankles and stretching. The most effective method added downward

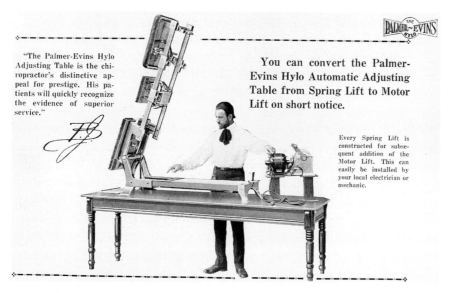

Fig. I-7 B.J. Palmer's Hy-lo table. *(Courtesy Palmer College of Chiropractic Archives, Davenport, Iowa.)*

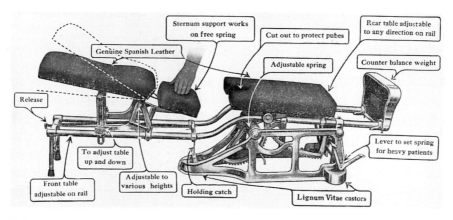

Fig. I-8 Hy-lo table. *(Courtesy Palmer College of Chiropractic Archives, Davenport, Iowa.)*

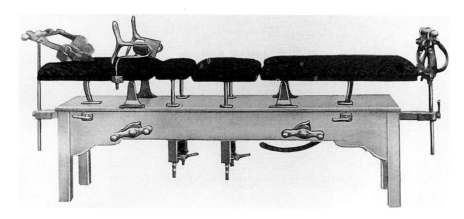

Fig. I-9 Cropp table. *(Courtesy Palmer College of Chiropractic Archives, Davenport, Iowa.)*

force to a padded stout beam across the back of a prone patient while traction was maintained.

About 1937, with the establishment of the Spinalator Co., Ollie Donahoe, an osteopath, began production of the intersegmental traction table.[18]

In 1923 the Cropp all-in-one table was marketed to the medical community (Fig. 1-9). The traction method described by Hippocrates allowed practitioners to use tension therapy in treatment of disease and injuries, correction of deformities, and so on. This table allowed fastening of the patient at the armpits for application of tractive force with cranks and gears within the table. The patient was strapped around the waist with a harness and traction generated by manual turning of the cranks.[18]

MCMANIS TABLE

Early tables were designed to articulate from the neck to the upper trunk to the lower extremities, to place the patient in a positon advantageous for patient and practitioner in delivering the appropriate thrust. Tables were produced with drop pieces for various spinal areas. These drop pieces were designed to move very rapidly and stop abruptly, thus facilitating movement of a specific vertebra and reducing the amount of force required. Further innovations were incorporated in the manual flexion-distraction tables, modifications of the McManis table of osteopathic design and use.

The McManis table was designed to provide vertical lift, flexion-distraction, rotation, and a split headpiece on a padded metal table. The table contained many features not available in other tables being manufactured at the time. McManis, an osteopath, patented his table in 1909. It was the basis for the table in the later work on flexion-distraction by James Cox, a chiropractor. The McManis table provided traction and functioned using a universal joint that provided multidirectional movements to the segments of the spine and sacroiliac joints (Fig. 1-10).[18]

The table designed by McManis was ahead of its time and incorporated features that would be duplicated only in much later models. A hydraulic mechanism, similar to that of a barber chair, with a cast iron base trimmed with cast brass, raised and lowered the table. A handle (later a foot pedal) was used to raise and lower the whole unit. The table had a split facepiece and a flexion/extension lower section that also laterally flexed. A coil-spring mechanism provided tensioning for the flexion/extension motion and could be adjusted by crank to accommodate the height or weight of the patient. Ankle straps were used to increase traction.

The McManis table was one of the first to allow positioning of the patient for various types of adjustments. The table provided the clinician advantages in the horizontal and vertical planes. This is probably the first table in which the concept of "incremental manipulation" was possible. Before this time, techniques were applied in an "all or nothing" manner, in which the thrust was given with a push by the practitioner, after careful positioning of the patient. On the McManis table, the patient was

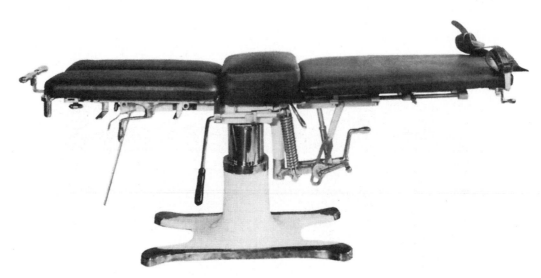

Fig. 1-10   McManis table. *(From McManis JV. McManis Table Technic: Technic Instructions and General Information. Hannibal, Mo: Standard Printing Co; 1938.)*

easily positioned, with various accentuated angles and tilts possible. This allowed the treating physician to be positioned to best advantage and with enough leverage to achieve the desired effect.

In performing the various manipulations, the practitioner could stand adjacent to the patient and move the table into a position that would enhance the manipulation and allow it to be performed incrementally or in stages. This allowed the clinician to put slight-to-moderate pressure on the patient without thrusting, thus testing the patient's capability of withstanding the force. This approach is useful with the elderly, the frail (often with osteoporosis), and the acute patient in splinting muscle spasms (and marked pain). Incremental application of force allows accommodation of patient tolerance.

MODERN TABLES

Williams Manufacturing Company is one of the oldest table manufacturers still in operation (1916). Williams has produced many mechanically enhanced tables, including the spring assisted Hy-lo version, the electric "worm

drive," the electric hydraulic (Fig. 1-11, *A*), Verti-Lift tables, the Zenith-Cox flexion-distraction table, and the most recent, the Zenith ACS table. Clinician and technique demands were the impetus for changes in table design. Various practitioners, including Gonstead, Thompson, Pierce, and Cox designed modifications for the table. The drop mechanism allowed for one of the most significant innovations in adjusting technique. Major credit for the drop mechanism goes to J.C. Thompson, who invented it in the early 1950s.[18] Newer models of the Williams' tables have a vertical lift mechanism to accommodate the height of the clinician. The latest Williams' table is a sculptured model with shaped sectional pieces and a sophisticated control mechanism for positioning.[20] It incorporates the features of the Hy-lo for patient positioning, a vertical height adjustment, and drop pieces corresponding to sections of the body (Fig. 1-11, *B*).

In the 1960s, Lloyd Steffensmeier developed equipment for DeJarnette's SOT technique and eventually designed and produced several electric-hydraulic tables.[18] Some of Steffensmeier's contemporary models incorporate capabilities for flexion-distraction using a pneumatic mechanism for balancing the weight of the

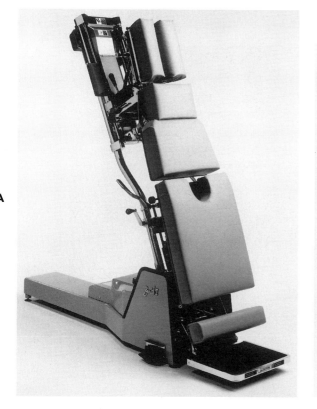
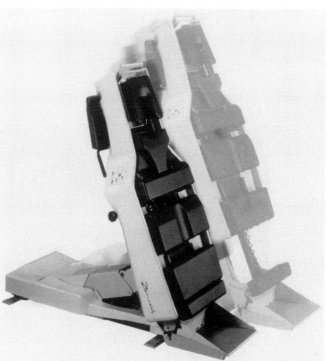

A

B

Fig. 1-11 **A**, Williams Hi-lo and **B**, Zenith ACS tables. (*Courtesy Williams Healthcare Systems, Elgin, Ill.*)

patient on the table and an electric mechanism for producing linear distractions (see Fig. 4-1).

THE FLEXION-DISTRACTION TABLES

Barnes, a manufacturing company, developed the Chiro-Manis table for Cox. This table was a simplified version of the original McManis table. It had many of the characteristics of the original McManis table with the coil spring flexion/distraction mechanism. Later designs included a motorized lift, an improvement over the early fixed-height models. The table had a center post, split into upper and lower sections, for support. The table rotated on the center post and was stabilized by a heavy steel base. The original version of this table had a fixed-angle head portion that provided a slot for the face. The lower section could be flexed and locked into position or extended slightly. Lateral flexion was also possible but could not be locked in place. In later models, position-locking was possible, as was a rotational position in the lower section, which was used by Cox in the treatment of scoliosis. Flexion and extension were performed manually, with the hand of the clinician on the lower section of the table applying downward force to produce flexion movement. The clinician's other hand was placed on the

patient, providing resistance to the pull of the lower section and creating traction force at a specific spinal segment. The primary action was in the saggital plane.

Cox collaborated with Williams on the second-generation model, after the design of the Barnes table. Variations in the design of the table reflected innovations in the spring mechanism and ease of operation, with positive locks in all positions. The lower section (which performed distraction) of the early distraction tables tended to gradually release when weight was placed on the section. A friction lock was used as a braking mechanism. With wear, the friction lock would slowly release with the patient's weight on the lower section. The positive-lock mechanism in later tables improved this characteristic.

The latest Zenith-Cox table has a headpiece for distraction of the cervical spine (Fig. 1-12). This multipositional neck-traction unit is purported to do for the cervical spine what the flexion-distraction table does for the lower and middle back. Several years ago, Barnes developed a cervical headpiece with positional capability. Both of these units are in the early stages of development and testing of the related technique. Adjustment using a specific distraction headpiece has not been performed on the cervical region to the extent that it has on the lower back. Barnes and Willams have incorporated drop pieces in their design and have added power elevation units to the table.

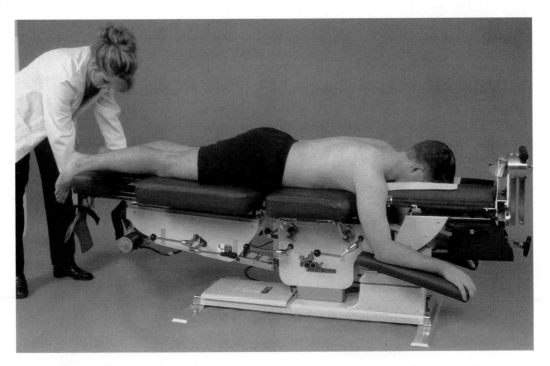

Fig. 1-12 Zenith-Cox table with cervical distraction component. *(Williams Healthcare Systems, Elgin, Ill.)*

The Chattanooga Group developed the Spinalator Ergostyle table to perform flexion/distraction manually and provide a drop mechanism for sections of the spine (Fig. 1-13). This table incorporates characteristics of other tables that provide for flexion/distraction in combination with vertical lift capability, drop mechanisms, and an adjustable headpiece.

Chattanooga Corporation developed the Ergostyle table and equipped it with the full range of mechanically assisted devices, such as adjustable headpiece with drop, drops on the thoracic and lumbar sections, manual flexion-distraction and a motorized vertical height adjustment. The newest table, which is still in the prototype stage, is the Ergotrak table. It will add motorized linear distraction capabilities to an already well-equipped vehicle for the chiropractic adjustment/manipulation procedures. It is anticipated that the table will incorporate a Δ elevation for application of the Thomas Hill GAIT technique. A new feature on this table is the drop mechanisms that can be applied while the table is in linear motion and while the various flexion-extension and/or lateral flexion movements are applied (Fig. 1-14).

The table has the same characteristics as the Ergostyle table, with the same headpiece and the various-level drops with manual flexion-extension capabilities for use in applying the Cox approach. In addition the table will incorporate mechanized linear distraction. All of these capabilities can be used singly or in combination. A tethered control is being developed that will allow the clinician to stand away from the table and perform the starting and stopping operation and adjust some of the table settings. This will relieve the clinician from constantly bending over the table, thus reducing stress. This table will incorporate the features of the Thomas Hill Intertrac table, with other features giving the table expanded capabilities beyond those of most tables presently available. The final prototype should be available soon and production will follow.

Leander Health Technologies manufactures a table based on the design of Leander Eckard. This table has power capabilities, or motorized motion-assistance, for creating flexion-distraction (Fig. 1-15). Leander also produces a manual unit similar to the Barnes or Zenith-Cox tables. This table incorporates many of the design features of previous tables, such as flexion, slight extension, and lateral flexion. It has two characteristics that the others do not, that is, lateral flexion is accomplished using the cephalad section of the table (as opposed to Zenith-Cox and Barnes units, which use the caudal section), and the abdominal section of the table can be released to enhance lumbar curvature (lordosis). Flexion-extension is possible using the motor-driven lower unit, which has variable-speed control and is adjustable for the amount of flexion or extension applied. The table is also adjustable in height and has a movable headpiece but no distraction capabilities for the cervical spine as demonstrated on the Barnes or Zenith-Cox tables.

Other tables have distraction functions similar to those described but have incorporated minor design innovations. Firms manufacturing these tables include Titan Health Care Manufacturing, Spinalight Corporation, Lloyd Table Company, and Omni Technologies. Each of these tables can be used in distraction and incorporate most of the characteristics of the

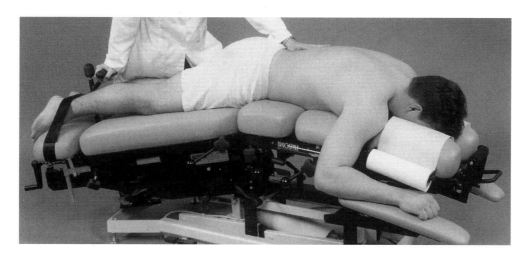

Fig. 1-13 Chattanooga Spinalator Ergostyle table. *(Chattanooga Group Inc., Hixon, Tenn.)*

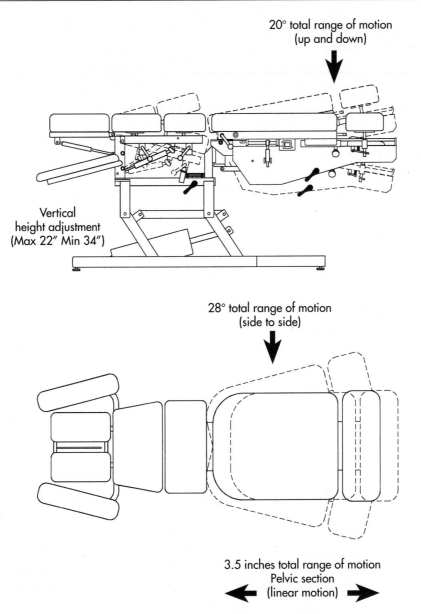

20° total range of motion
(up and down)

Vertical
height adjustment
(Max 22″ Min 34″)

28° total range of motion
(side to side)

3.5 inches total range of motion
Pelvic section
(linear motion)

Fig. I-14 Chattanooga Ergotrak table. The table has full capabilities of the Chattanooga Ergostyle table. Additions to the table include motorized axial distraction with speed and trajectory controlled by the clinician. The unit can tilt, with the lower section elevating (Δ positive) for applying Thomas Hill's GAIT technique.

basic tables of Barnes and Zenith-Cox but do not provide motion-assisted (motorized) movement; some, however, incorporate power elevation or allow adjustments to accomodate patient size.

Robert Jensen designed the Jensen table, which is motion-assisted and powered to provide flexion-distraction with full circumduction on a patient in a kneeling position (Fig. 1-16). This table, manufactured by Annova Enterprises, Inc., differs significantly from others that provide for distraction in that it is positional. It is similar to the knee-chest table, giving full support to the chest

and abdomen. The power unit of the Annova table allows full circumduction of the kneeling patient and lateral flexion of the cervicothoracic section, with a variable-speed control for the circumductive movement. This table, however, allows only prone positioning of the patient, with kneeling as the only option.

The Intertrac table of Thomas Hill provides a platform for accomplishing linear distraction along the long axis of the body (Fig. 1-17). The table is positioned parallel to the floor and tractions the body without flexion or by introducing flexion, extension, or lateral flexion in the process.

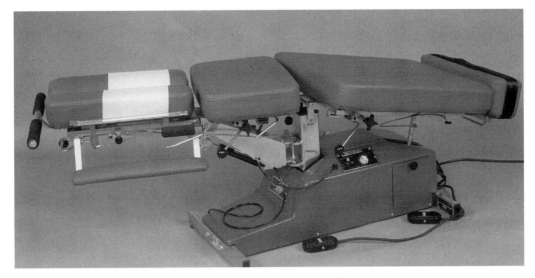

Fig. 1-15 Leander table. *(Leander Health Technologies Corporation, Port Orchard, Wash.)*

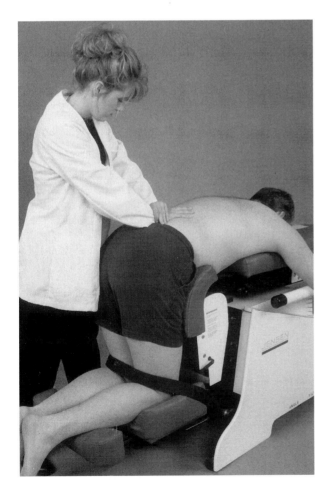

Fig. 1-16 Jensen table. *(Annova, Alexandria, Minn.)*

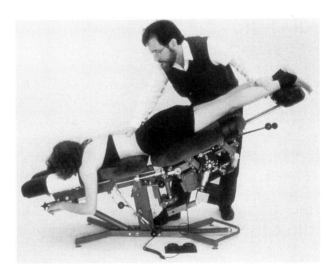

Fig. 1-17 Hill Intertrac table. *(Courtesy Hill Table Co., Lakefield, Ontario.)*

The table is capable of flexion, extension, lateral flexion, and a 30-degree tilt of the table cephalad. The Intertrac uses several electric motors for motion-assisted distraction for flexion-extension and for the vertical lift or tilt of the table. The speed of the caudal section can be adjusted, but the distance of movement, or excursion, of the section is fixed. The facepiece is split but cannot be tilted, and there are no provisions for drop pieces on the table. Cervical traction can be performed manually on a supine patient, with the lower unit providing the tractive force as the patient's neck and head are held in the clinician's hands.

The VAX-D table (which stands for *vertebral axial distraction*) developed by the medical profession offers many of the functions of the linear-axial-distraction, motion-assisted table. However, this table, which is computer-controlled and monitored, provides only linear sustained traction via a harness. Except for operation of the computer, a clinician is not required with this table. A harness is worn by the patient, and linear traction is applied with a power-assist, with the patient in the prone position and holding handles on the cephalad end of the table. Traction is sustained for a given period, with the patient holding the handles. There is no deviation from the straight long axis of the body. The clinician is discouraged from providing any manipulation while traction is being delivered. (See Fig. 7-4).

CONSIDERATIONS FOR THE FUTURE

The design of tables has changed with the development of the chiropractic profession. Initially, the population of practitioners was male. In the past few years, many women have moved into the profession, as evidenced by increased enrollment in chiropractic colleges. Techniques developed for and by men are not always appropriate for the build and strength of some women. The latest tables address this with improvements such as enhancing upper-body strength with mechanically-assisted and motion-assisted motorized tables. As more women become involved in the development of techniques and tables, alternatives will increase. Equipment design for the future must consider the many techniques practiced by chiropractors of various sizes and builds. As with contemporary office furniture, which is designed to accomodate men and women of all sizes, chiropractic equipment must accommodate the size, strength, and reach of all practitioners.

Managed care systems have made the efficient delivery of services in the office a critical issue. More than ever before, it is necessary that a clinician's table function effectively and efficiently, with power-assist options to conserve the clinician's energy.

The following chapters discuss distraction techniques and use of the major tables. The discussion provides student and clinician an overview of commonly used approaches. On this basis, an informed decision on technique may be made.

REFERENCES

1. Anderson RT. On doctors and bonesetters in the 16th and 17th centuries. *Chiropr Hist.* 1983;3:10-15.
2. Gaucher-Peslherbe P-L. *Chiropractic: Early Concepts in Their Original Historical Setting.* Lombard, Ill: National College of Chiropractic; 1993.
3. Duplay S, Reclus P. *Traite Chirugie.* Paris: Denoel; 1891.
4. Brantingham JW. Still and Palmer: the impact of the first osteopath and the first chiropractor. *Chiropr Hist.* 1986;6:20.
5. Wardwell WI. *Chiropractic: History and Evolution of a New Profession.* St Louis: Mosby; 1992.
6. Judah JS. *The History of the Metaphysical Movements in America.* Philadelphia: Westminster Press; 1967.
7. Cox JM. *Low Back Pain, Mechanism, Diagnosis, Treatment.* Baltimore: Williams & Wilkins; 1985.
8. Taylor H. The McManis table, professional papers. *ACA J Chiropr.* 1978;12:100.
9. McManis JV. *McManis Table Technic: Technic Instructions and General Information.* Kirksville, Mo: McManis Table Co; 1938.
10. Donahue RJ. D.D. Palmer and inate intelligence. Development, division, and derision. *Chiropr Hist.* 1986;6:31.
11. Palmer DD. *The Chiropractor's Adjuster, Textbook of the Science: Art and Philosophy of Chiropractic for Students and Practitioners.* Portland, Ore: Portland Printing House Co; 1910.
12. Palmer BJ, Jensen C, eds. *History in the Making.* Davenport, Iowa: Palmer School of Chiropractic; 1957:35.
13. Waagen G, Strang V. Origin and development of traditional chiropractic philosophy. In Haldeman S, ed. *Principles and Practice of Chiropractic.* Norwalk, Conn: Appleton and Lange; 1992.
14. Special communication. Wilk v AMA. *JAMA.* 1988;259:81.
15. Gatterman MI, Hansen D. Development of chiropractic nomenclature through consensus. *J Manipulative Physiol Ther.* 1994;17:302.
16. Dye A. *The Evolution of Chiropractic.* Redmond Hill, NY: Richmond Hall; 1969.
17. Wells D. From workbench to high tech: the evaluation of the adjustment table. *Chiropr Hist.* 1987;7:35.
18. Cropp DB. *Cropp All-in-One Table.* Pandiculator Co; c 1925.
19. Taylor H. The McManis Table, professional papers. *ACA J Chiropr.* 1978;12:87.
20. Williams Manufacturing Company brochure, the ACS table. Elgin, Ill; 1995.

2

Biomechanical Considerations

The chiropractic profession maintains that the most specialized and important therapy involves the adjustment of the articulations of the human body, particularly the spinal column. An adjustment may be performed manually or with mechanical assistance to restore normal articular relationship and function while reestablishing neurologic integrity to influence physiologic processes. This chapter identifies general concepts of the mechanical properties of joint systems and discusses the ways in which these systems become dysfunctional. These concepts are then applied to develop a rationale for the application of various forms of manipulative therapy.

The principles of mechanics that determine which functions the body is able to perform are the same for athletic, recreational, and occupational activities and the activities of daily living. It is interesting to note that the musculoskeletal system accounts for over half the body's mass yet clinically is the most overlooked system in the body.

The assessment and treatment of mechanical problems of the joints should be based on a clear understanding of normal biomechanics. Knowledge of biomechanics and the ability to detect changes in joint mechanics are essential for the successful management of mechanical dysfunction of the joints. Manipulative therapy is applied to restore normal joint alignment, create free movement between articular surfaces, and establish functional balance of the joint's contiguous soft tissues. Because manipulative techniques may not be indicated in all cases, a thorough clinical investigation is necessary to clarify the nature and the extent of the lesion. If joint manipulation is appropriate, suitable techniques must be selected and applied based on the direction and extent of joint malposition, restriction of joint movement, and the nature of the soft tissues involved.

Trying to understand biomechanics is often overwhelming because of its mathematic and engineering emphases. Other works present thorough explanations of the these concepts.[1-6] However, an understanding of certain clinically useful biomechanical concepts is necessary for description and interpretation of changes in joint function.

BASIC CONCEPTS

Biomechanics is the application of the laws of mechanics to living structures, specifically to the locomotor system of the human body. Clinical biomechanics is the study of the interrelationship of the bones, muscles, nerves, and joints. In mechanics, a lever, one of the simplest of all mechanical devices that can be called a machine, is used to its greatest advantage when a force moves the lever about a pivot point, or fulcrum. In the body, nerves produce energy for muscles to provide the forces necessary to move the bony levers around the joint, which forms a pivotal hinge (Fig. 2-1). The relationship of fulcrum to force to resistance distinguishes the different classes of levers (Table 2-1).

The usual approach in biomechanics is to observe the anatomy and try to establish its role in body stability and movement. Often, kinematics (movement without regard to forces) is studied without an understanding of kinetics (the forces affecting movement). Even less attention is paid to statics (the equilibrium of bodies at rest). The body exists as a structure that is stable and fixed in space; therefore it is logical to try to understand the statics before exploring the dynamics.[7] An alternative approach in biomechanics is envisioning the requirements necessary to perform a specific function and then trying to understand how the organism meets the requirements.

The efficiency of the musculoskeletal mechanical unit depends on the integrity of each joint and its surrounding soft tissues. Knowledge of the ways in which joint movement, muscular action, and osseous lever systems work

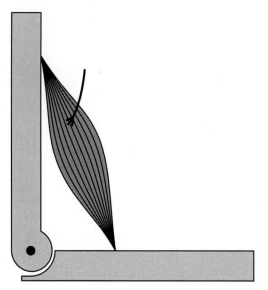

Fig. 2-1 Diagrammatic representation of a biomechanical lever system with the bones serving as levers, the joint and its capsular ligaments as the hinge, the muscle providing the force or load, and the nerve as the source of energy stimulation.

■ TABLE 2-1   Characteristics of Lever Classes

Lever Type	Fulcrum Position	Joint Example
First class lever	Fulcrum between force and resistance	Flexion/extension of spinal joints
Second class lever	Resistance between fulcrum and force	Opening the mouth against resistance
Third class lever	Force between fulcrum and resistance	Flexion of elbow

together to produce the composite activity of the joints of the spine and extremities is necessary to be able to identify abnormalities and then to apply corrective manipulative therapy. With this knowledge, the health care provider is able to evaluate musculoskeletal disorders and understand the anatomic and physiologic bases of their conservative management.

JOINT FUNCTION

Specific body planes of reference have been delineated and are used to describe the structural position and directions of functional movement for joint systems. The standard position of reference, or anatomic position, is the body facing forward; the hands at the sides of the body, with the palms facing forward; and the feet pointing straight ahead. The body planes are derived from dimensions in space and are oriented at right angles to one

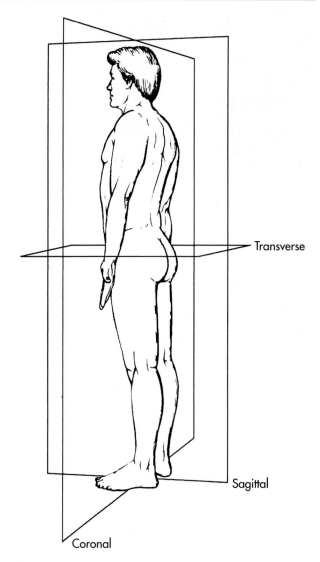

Fig. 2-2 The three cardinal planes of the body: sagittal, coronal, and transverse. *(Modified from Bergmann TF, Peterson DH, Lawrence DJ.* Chiropractic Technique. *New York: Churchill Livingstone; 1993.)*

another. The sagittal plane is vertical and extends from front to back, or from anterior to posterior, dividing the body into left and right components. The coronal plane is vertical and extends from side to side, dividing the body into anterior and posterior components. The transverse plane is a horizontal plane dividing the structure into upper and lower components (Fig. 2-2).

An intersection of any two planes produces an axis around which motion can occur. Three axes are formed in this way and also are oriented at right angles to one another. This configuration is expressed as a three-dimensional coordinate system with x, y, and z used to mark the axes (Fig. 2-3). This coordinate system defines, or locates, the extent of rotation or translation movement possible at each joint rotation and translation.[1] Specific motions or resultant positions are defined by the axis around which movement takes place and the plane through which movement occurs.[8] Therefore, movement of the body's articulations occurs around three axes and in three planes. The resultant types of movement that a joint can perform are rotation (movement around an axis) or translation (motion through a plane) (Fig. 2-4).

A force that produces a translational movement is called an *axial*, or *shear*, force; the load that produces a rotational movement is called *torsion*.

The rotational movements in the sagittal plane (around the x axis) are flexion and extension; the translational movements along the z axis consist of anterior-to-posterior and posterior-to-anterior glide (Fig. 2-5). Rotational movement in the transverse plane (around the y axis) is axial rotation; translational movement along the y axis is axial compression and distraction (Fig. 2-5). Rotational movements in the coronal plane (around the z axis) are lateral flexion movements; translational movement along the x axis is lateral glide (Fig. 2-5).

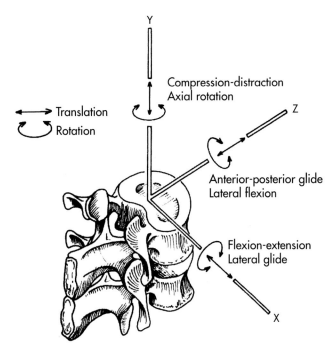

Fig. 2-3 The three axes of motion for a vertebral motion segment around or along which the six degrees of motion occur. (*From Bergmann TF, Peterson DH, Lawrence DJ:* Chiropractic Technique, *New York, 1993, Churchill Livingstone.*)

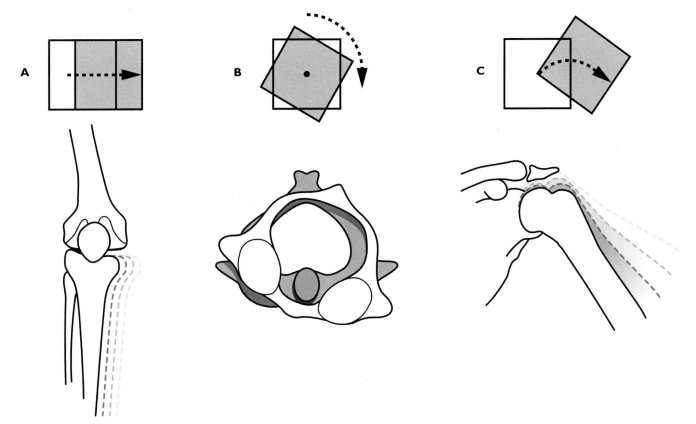

Fig. 2-4 Examples of **A**, translation movement (lateral-to-medial glide of the tibiofemoral joint); **B**, rotation movement (right axial rotation of the atlantoaxial joint); **C**, and a combination of the two, producing roll and slide (abduction of the glenohumeral joint).

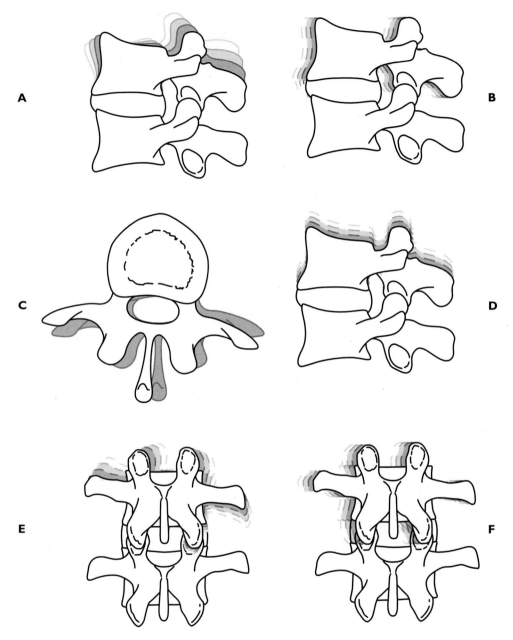

Fig. 2-5 Examples of movement in the six degrees of freedom in the spine: **A,** flexion/extension (x-axis rotation); **B,** anterior/posterior glide (z-axis translation); **C,** right and left axial rotation (y-axis rotation; **D,** distraction/compression (y-axis translation); **E,** right and left lateral flexion (z-axis rotation); **F,** right and left lateral glide (x-axis translation).

TABLE 2-2 Description of Joint Motion

Common Description	Anatomic System	Biomechanical System
Flexion	Anterior sagittal rotation	$+ \Theta$ X (rotation)
Extension	Posterior sagittal rotation	$- \Theta$ X (rotation)
Left lateral flexion	Left coronal rotation	$- \Theta$ Z (rotation)
Right lateral flexion	Right coronal rotation	$+ \Theta$ Z (rotation)
Left (axial) rotation	Left horizontal rotation	$+ \Theta$ Y (rotation)
Right (axial) rotation	Right horizontal rotation	$- \Theta$ Y (rotation)
Anterior glide	Anterior sagittal translation	+ Z (translation)
Posterior glide	Posterior sagittal translation	- Z (translation)
Axial distraction	Superior coronal translation	+ Y (translation)
Axial compression	Inferior coronal translation	- Y (translation)
Left lateral glide	Left horizontal translation	+ X (translation)
Right lateral glide	Right horizontal translation	- X (translation)

Movements are based on the joint anatomy and, specifically, the plane of the joint surface. Although true of all synovial joints, this is especially important in the spinal joints. Each synovial articulation in the body should therefore exhibit flexion, extension, right and left lateral flexion, right and left axial rotation, anterior-to-posterior glide, posterior-to-anterior glide, lateral-to-medial glide, medial-to-lateral glide, compression, and distraction.[8] These movement possibilities are called *the six degrees of freedom*. However, there are actually 12 movements from neutral: 6 positive and 6 negative (Table 2-2).[7]

LOADS APPLIED TO THE JOINTS

Biomechanical studies on the effects of loads on spinal structures have been performed on spinal motion segments. A motion segment includes two adjacent vertebrae and the associated intervertebral disc. The intervertebral disc and the two facet articulations form a three-joint complex. The motion segment and its three-joint complex is the smallest unit that exhibits all of the characteristics of the spine: support, mobility, and protection. A load is the application of a force and/or a moment (torque movement about an axis) to a structure. An external load results in deformations within the spinal struc-

tures and produces movements between the structures.[9] The resultant movements (moments) are the rotational and translational qualities listed in Table 2-2, which commonly occur in combination or coupled with one another. The other important load characteristics of compression, tension, shear, and torque affect the spine during various activities.[4]

COMPRESSION

Compression occurs when a load produces forces that push the material together, creating a deforming stress. The behavior of a structure in compression depends largely on its length and how far or long the load must be carried. Gordon[10] states that the structural loading coefficients used in engineering are inappropriate for measuring metabolic or structural efficiency in animals. Compressive forces are transmitted to the vertebral body and intervertebral disc in the spine. The nucleus pulposus is a semiliquid, or gel, with the characteristics of a fluid, or hydraulic, structure. It is incompressible and therefore must distort under compressive loads. The nucleus pulposus dissipates the compressive force by redirecting it radially. It is important clinically to note that mechanical failure occurs first in the cartilaginous endplate when compressive forces applied alone are too great. The result is nuclear herniation into the vertebral body, called a *Schmorl's node*. Failure may be modified when the spine is loaded in either flexion or extension. Compressive loads applied in flexion cause anterior collapse of the endplate or vertebral body, where the bony structure is weaker. With compressive loads applied in extension, much of the compressive load is transmitted through the facets, leading to capsular changes or bony failure. Compressive loads applied with torque around the y axis can produce circumferential tears in the disc annulus.

TENSION

The force known as tension occurs when a structure is stretched longitudinally. A tension force pulls a structure apart, causing the cross-sectional area of the structure to decrease. When a material is stretched in the direction of the pull, it contracts in the other two directions. When the primary stress is tensile, there will be secondary compressive stresses and vice versa. The tension elements of the body are the soft tissues (fascia, muscles, ligaments, and connective tissue). Although largely ignored as construction members of the body frame, the tension elements are an integral part of the construction, not just a secondary support. In the spine, the ligaments are loaded in tension.[9] Tensile forces also occur in the intervertebral disc during the rotational movements of flexion, extension, axial rotation, and lateral flexion. The nucleus bears most of the compressive load while the annular fibers bear most of the tensile loads.

SHEAR

Biomechanical effects would be easier to understand if the loads, stresses, and strains were all either tensile or compressive. Another force exists, however, that creates sliding or, more specifically, resists a tendency to slide. This force is called a *shear* force. Although the need for shear strength and shear stiffness causes trouble for engineers, living structures do not have the same major shear requirements. Shear forces in the spinal motion segment are resisted primarily by the facet joints and the fibers of the annulus fibrosus. Under normal physiologic conditions, the facets can resist shear forces. If, however, the disc space is narrowed by degeneration, with subsequent thinning of the disc, abnormally high stresses may be placed on the facet joints. The limit of resistance to such forces is not well documented.[11-12] Little provision for resisting shear stress is present; therefore the risk of disc failure is greater with tensile loading than with compression loading.[1] Most studies demonstrating the effects of shear forces on the lumbar spine have been performed on cadavers from which the posterior elements have been removed. The posterior element of the spinal motion segment is composed of the pedicles, lamina, spinous process, and articular facets. The lumbar facets are aligned mainly in the sagittal plane, with an interlocking mechanism that allows only a few degrees of rotation. In the lower lumbar segments, where shear force is the greatest, the facet joints provide resistance to shear.

TORQUE

Torque is a load produced by parallel forces directed in opposite directions about the long axis of a structure (the y axis in the spine). Torsion occurs when an object twists; the force that causes the twisting is referred to as *torque*. When a torque load is applied to a curved structure such as the spine, bending will occur. Farfan et al[13] estimate that approximately 90% of the torque strength of a motion segment is provided by its disc. This is particularly true of the annulus and the two facet joints. They further state that the annulus provides most of the torsional resistance in the lumbar spine and speculate that annular layers will tear with torsional injury, leading to disc degeneration. This concept is based on the theory

that when torsional forces are created in the spine, the annular fibers oriented in one direction will stretch and those oriented in the other direction will relax. Thus only half of the fibers are available to resist the force. Adams and Hutton,[14] however, demonstrate that the torsion of the lumbar spine is resisted primarily by the facets, and the compressed facet is the first structure to yield at the limit of torsion. Other experiments support the theory that the posterior elements of the spine, including the facet joints and ligaments, play a major role in resisting torsion.[15,16] In deference to the conclusions of Farfan et al, these authors suggest that torsion is unimportant in the etiology of disc degeneration and prolapse because rotation is produced by voluntary muscle activity, and the intervertebral disc experiences relatively small stresses and strains. Perhaps both concepts have merit, and neither can stand alone as the sole explanation of the torque and torsion effects on the spine.

EFFECTS OF LOADS

The disc and its annular fibers must support two types of stress: compressive, or perpendicular force, and shearing, or parallel force. With axial rotation of the disc, the incurred torsional force produces shear stress in the transverse and axial planes.[1] Most studies on the effects of torsion have focused on the lumbar spine because of the prevalence of low back pain. Many of the studies were performed on cadaver spine sections from which the posterior elements had been removed. Conclusions, especially any inference in application to the living being, must therefore be viewed with caution. Moreover, the effects of torsional forces on the cervical and thoracic segments have not been adequately studied. In these spinal regions the facets do not interlock as in the lumbar spine and therefore allow greater axial rotation and the potential for torsional effects. The thoracic spine has the rib cage attachments that limit movement in all directions, thereby reducing torsional effects. However, the cervical spine is the most mobile region of the spine, yet the incidence of disc herniation there is much less frequent than in the lumbar spine. This suggests that more than a torsional force is responsible for disruption of the intervertebral disc.

Using a theoretic disc model, Broberg[17] studied the response to compression, shear, bending, and axial rotation of an intervertebral disc. He reported that the stiffness of the intervertebral disc increases considerably with axial load. This finding implies that most experimental data obtained at zero axial load may reflect poorly on real situations in which axial loads are typical for upright posture. A further observation was made that within normal physiologic limits, bending, shear, or axial rotation do not appear to constitute a risk of fiber rupture, except in combination with very high axial loads. Moreover, at pure compression the likelihood of fiber rupture is small because endplate failure occurs earlier, before the rupture is manifest.[18]

Adams and Hutton[19] state that the physiologic range of rotational motion is about 10 to 15 degrees for the whole lumbar spine or about 2.5 degrees for each joint. With degeneration, the amount of rotational movement increases to about 7 degrees. This amount of movement casts doubt on the role of torsion in producing damage to the intervertebral joint. In a cadaveric model, torsion of the lumbar spine was resisted primarily by the apophyseal joint in compression, although the intervertebral disc played a major role. The capsular ligaments of the tension facet and the supraspinous and interspinous ligaments were uninvolved or unimportant. Adams and Hutton[19] concluded that torsion appeared to be unimportant in the etiology of disc degeneration and prolapse. These studies were, however, limited to the neutral and extension positions of the spine.

Adams and Hutton[19] also demonstrate that when a compressive force in the amount produced by the extensor muscles was applied to the lumbar spine while in flexion, the result was a prolapsed lumbar intervertebral disc. They conclude that slightly degenerated discs are more susceptible than healthy discs to prolapse.

ROLE OF THE SOFT TISSUES

The scientific and heath care communities have studied the mechanical properties of the soft tissues that provide support and flexibility. Previously, the strength and elastic behavior of soft tissues had been considered incidental to their growth mechanisms and metabolic functions.[10] However, the development of living things requires extensible tissues of sufficient strength to carry loads and sufficient flexibility for growth, evolution, and movement. Tension loads are usually carried by tendons, muscles, and membranes. A combination and balance of compression and tension structures is required to apply or resist localized forces. A system based entirely on soft tissues would be too flexible and imprecise.

The model for many biologic soft tissues is the surface of a liquid.[10] The elastic behavior of soft tissues at low and moderate strains resembles the behavior of the

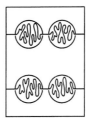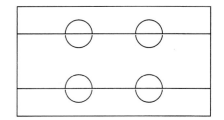

Fig. 2-6 Model of collagen and elastin demonstrating that at rest the fibers are folded on themselves and, with stretch, they straighten to allow lengthening to occur.

surface of a liquid. When forces are applied to the soft tissue, only a small amount of displacement occurs initially. As more force is applied, the displacement increases rapidly. The result is a J-shaped stress-strain curve. Most soft tissues are prestressed, giving them a resting tension. Because the mechanisms of soft tissues are quite complicated and can vary significantly, the subject of the functions of soft tissues is not free of controversy.

COLLAGEN

Collagen provides an extracellular framework of considerable tensile strength. It provides a rigid support and tensile strength to tendons, ligaments, cartilage, bone, and intervertebral discs. Collagen is combined with elastin to become important constituents in most soft tissues. The collagen serves to reinforce elastin and modify its properties. Collagen is the most abundant and most important extracellular fibrillar protein in the human body. Collagen is a fibrous material constructed of long polypeptide chains with a tension behavior much as a stringlike substance, producing passive elasticity (Fig. 2-6). When an external force produces tension in a collagen fiber, it will first extend fairly easily, but as the fiber contracts in diameter, it hardens and becomes stiff. When the load is removed the fiber returns to its original length and character. The distinct fibrillar structures of collagen take on various forms based on genetically derived types. By far the most commonly occurring form is type I collagen, which forms broad fibrils found in bone, skin, ligament, tendon, and the annulus fibrosus. The primary function of type I collagen is to resist tension, therefore the orientation of fibers and existence of cross-linking will vary according to the local environment. It is the strongest fiber in the body. Type II collagen forms fibrils that are thinner than type I and are found in cartilage (including facet joints and end plates of the disc), nucleus pulposus, and the vitreous body. The function of type II collagen is to resist intermittent pressure. Type III collagen forms reticular fibers that are small in diameter and predominate in pliable organs, such as blood vessels and the gastrointestinal tract. Type III fibers are often associated with type I fibers and may occur as often as 9% to 12% in ligaments but are not detectable in tendons. They function in structural maintenance. There are several other types of collagen (IV to XII), but they are less abundant and not as involved with the functioning of the soft tissues that support the musculoskeletal system. In fact there is insufficient data to comment on their exact function.[20]

Collagen forms cross-linkages that hold adjacent collagen molecules together and stabilize its overall structure. The number of cross-linkages increases with trauma, immobilization, advancing age, and in states of degeneration.[21]

TENDON

Tendons form physical links between muscle and bone that serve as transmitters of mechanical energy. Therefore they must be able to withstand large tensile forces and be flexible yet relatively inextensible to minimize loss of energy in transmission. Tendons are strong enough to withstand several times the tension that their attached muscles can generate.[22] The ability to resist stretch is the result of their high composition of collagen fiber, most of which is type I. Collagen allows tendon to perform three important functions. The first function is transmission of tensile forces generated by muscles to bone, making movement across a joint possible. The second function of tendon is storage of strain energy, similar to the way a spring works. The third function of tendon is as a safety mechanism. When tendon is pulled or overstretched, it will produce pain, signalling the body that something is wrong.

LIGAMENT

Ligaments are usually cordlike or bandlike structures made of dense collagenous connective tissue. They are composed mostly of type I collagen, with intervening rows of fibrocytes. Type III collagen also is present, perhaps contributing to the specific structural-functional properties of ligament. Interwoven with the collagen are elastin fibers, allowing ligamentous tissue greater extensibility. The amount of elastin varies from ligament to ligament.[23] The primary function of ligaments is to check excessive motion in joints and guide joint motion. Ligaments have a less parallel arrangement of collagen fibers than tendon, and they have the addition of more elastin. The result is that ligaments have somewhat less tensile strength per unit than tendon but have slightly more yield.

Ligamentous contracture has been identified as a possible mechanism for joint stiffness, although this phenomenon may only occur with long-standing immobilization.[24] Extensibility of connective tissue is caused by the infusion of water between layers of proteoglycan molecules. This presence of sufficient water provides lubrication, allowing for a more parallel configuration of fibers and greater stretch under longitudinal tension. Immobilization leads to dehydration, causing fibers to stick together.

ARTICULAR CARTILAGE

Articular cartilage (AC) covers the joint surfaces of synovial joints. It provides a lining to the joint surface that is made of a special variety of very durable hyaline cartilage. It is lubricated by synovial fluid, is compressible, but is able to withstand large compressive forces. AC is made up of water (75%) and solids (25%) that consist of cells imbedded in a firm matrix. The matrix structure is an intricate network of collagen fibers surrounded by proteoglycans and glycoproteins. AC has no nerve supply or direct blood supply. It must receive nutrients through diffusion from blood vessels in the synovial membrane, the synovial fluid, and blood vessels in the adjacent bone. Fluids can move out of AC when the joint is compressed and back in when the joint is distracted.

MUSCLE

Muscles possess two kinds of elasticity. The first is passive, in the same manner as collagen. When muscular tissue in a passive or relaxed state is subjected to a tensile load, it responds with initial extension, deforming similar to other soft tissues. However, when muscle receives a neurologic stimulus, it contracts in length and exerts a tensile force in an active way. Muscular action is an efficient energy-conversion process. Optimal muscular efficiency occurs when contraction is slow. Gordon[10] writes the following:

> The human is an inadequate structure that would buckle and collapse under its own weight as soon as it tried to stand upright were it not that any tendency to buckling is corrected at once by suitable muscular contraction. If this system of active elasticity is interrupted by alcohol, fainting, or death we fall to the ground in short order. There is much to be said for the active muscular approach to countering inherent muscular instabilities.

BONE

Bone provides the compressive structure to the human frame. Bone begins in the embryo as collagen, and early in the growth and development process, the inorganic calcium compound hydroxyapatite is added to the collagen fibers. Hydroxyapatite is much stiffer than collagen. The resulting material is a short column that is quite strong in compression and fairly strong in tension. Bone does, however, demonstrate variable stiffness properties. Slight bending can occur with low loads; with suddenly applied or high loads, bone will be stiffer.

EFFECTS OF IMMOBILIZATION ON JOINT SYSTEMS

The fact has been well documented in the literature that prolonged immobilization of a joint under compression is detrimental to the joint because it causes degeneration of the articular cartilage.[25-27] Connective tissue elements lose their extensibility when their related joints are immobilized.[28] With immobilization, water is released from the proteoglycan molecule, allowing connective tissue fibers to contact one another and encouraging abnormal cross-linking. This results in a loss of extensibility.[29] The clinical importance is the hypothesis that manual therapy can break the cross-linking and any intraarticular capsular fiber fatty adhesions, thereby providing free motion and allowing water imbibition to occur. Furthermore, manual therapy procedures can stretch segmental muscles, stimulating spindle reflexes that may decrease the state of hypertonicity.[30]

Muscle tightness, or shortness, develops following periods of immobilization. Length changes in muscle are associated with changes in sarcomere number and reorganization of the connective tissue elements within the muscle.[31] Muscle immobilized in a shortened position develops less force and will tear at a shorter length than nonimmobilized muscle with a normal resting length.[32] For this reason, vigorous muscle stretching is recommended for muscle tightness.[33] For the stretch to be effective, however, the underlying joints should be freely mobile. Therefore patients may require manipulation before muscle stretching.

Cantu and Grodin[34] reviewed the literature on the effects of manual therapy on fascia. The effects included circulatory changes, blood flow changes, capillary dilation, cutaneous temperature changes, metabolic changes, and reflexive autonomic changes. Although most of the citations are quite old, the review represents a scholarly look at the potential positive effects of manual therapy on soft tissues.

One of the signs that may demonstrate somatic dysfunction is the presence of muscle hypertonicity. Localized increased paraspinal muscle tone can be detected with palpation and, in some cases, with electromyography. Janda[33] recognizes five types of increased muscle tone: limbic dysfunction, segmental spasm, reflex spasm, trigger points, and muscle tightness. Liebenson[35] discusses treatment of these five types using active muscle contraction and relaxation procedures.

Treadwell and O'Brien[36] have also identified apophyseal joint degeneration over prolonged periods in distraction. They found a high incidence of apophyseal joint degeneration in patients who had received halo-pelvic distraction for the correction of spinal deformity. The immobilization and the effects of compressive loads may be important factors in the degeneration of articular cartilage.

EFFECTS OF TRAUMA ON JOINT SYSTEMS

Reflex muscle spasm, or splinting, follows trauma or injury to any of the pain-sensitive structures of the spine. The pain-sensitive spinal tissues include the zygapophyseal joints, posterior ligaments, paravertebral muscles, dura mater, the anterior and posterior longitudinal ligaments, and the intervertebral discs.[37] Mechanical deformation or chemical irritation of any of these tissues can cause muscle spasm, resulting in restricted motion. Manual treatment directed at the tissue source of pain reduces reflex muscle spasm and increases the range of motion. If the muscle spasm has been present for some time, however, it requires direct treatment, as well.

Traumatic events can produce physiologic changes in muscles, ligaments, fascia, and so on capable of projecting reflex effects into various parts of the body, causing pain and dysfunction. Specific techniques of soft-tissue and reflex manipulation designed to affect and eliminate the irritable lesion have been described.[38]

The effect of specific positional exercises for the treatment of low back disorders is uncertain. Flexion exercises and extension exercises have been advocated as forms of treatment.[39-40] Both have been beneficial in cases of low back pain; however, the specific cause for a therapeutic response is unknown. Schnebel et al[41] examined changes in nerve root-compression forces with spinal flexion and extension motion and traction. The amount of compressive force and tension to the nerve root increased with flexion of the spine and decreased with extension of the spine. Sustained traction on a nerve root increased the compressive forces produced on a root traversing a herniated disc.

The normal function of a motion segment includes two important features: providing for support of the spinal column in the upright posture and absorbing shock. The posterior portion of the motion segment, which is composed of the posterior arch and apophyseal joints, controls patterns of joint movement. Although the primary function of the apophyseal joints is control and stabilization of movement of the motion segment, load-sharing between the apophyseal joints and the intervertebral discs also occurs.[42-43]

The apophyseal joints in the lower lumbar spine are oriented in a semicoronal plane. The apophyseal joints in the thoracic spine are oriented at a 60-degree angle toward the coronal plane and away from the transverse plane. This orientation helps resist transverse shear forces. The apophyseal joints in the cervical spine are oriented midway between the coronal and transverse planes. The orientation of the joints in the cervical spine allows some resistance to shear but a large disc height-to-body height ratio allows more intersegmental joint movement than is found in any other region of the spine. The only areas of the spine where the apophyseal joints exhibit poor resistance to shear forces are the middle and upper lumbar spine, where the orientation of the facets approaches the sagittal plane.

Forces applied in the performance of asymmetric activities affect the spinal functional unit. Higher intradiscal pressure was found at the level of the L3 disc for asymmetric loading positions when compared with symmetric loading positions.[44] Intradiscal pressure and intraabdominal pressure increase when the trunk is loaded in lateral flexion or axial rotation.[45] The measured pressures are higher when the trunk is loaded in rotation than when it is loaded in lateral flexion. Under load therefore, when a disc is wedged, the highest compressive stresses are transmitted through the annular fibers on the closed side of the wedge. The lowest compressive stresses are transmitted through the annular fibers and the open side of the wedge. In the flexed posture, the highest compressive stresses are transmitted through the anterior aspect of the annulus; the lowest stresses are transmitted through the posterior annulus.[46]

Torg et al[47] studied the effects of trauma to the cervical spine sustained in athletic injuries. They report that injuries to the middle cervical spine involving the bony, intervertebral disc and ligamentous structures are rare but, when they occur, are typically the result of an axial loading force sustained during an athletic activity. Perhaps, because the weight of the head does not equal the weight of the torso, this suggests that indeed an important factor in developing disc herniation is an axial load.

CLINICAL RELATIONSHIPS

Traditionally, allopathic physicians identify and treat diseases. This has led to the development of a problem-based health care system. Alternative health care practitioners (chiropractors, homeopaths, acupuncturists) emphasize treatment of the constitutional characteristics of the patient rather than treatment of specific disorders. However, because of the third-party payment system of health care, clinicians must report treatment for specific established disorders. In low back pain, one of the most common causes of suffering and disability, a precise diagnosis of the clinical lesion and the site and level of the lesion are important. Nachemson[48] reports that only 20% of patients with acute low back pain can be given a precise diagnosis.

A major problem in development of diagnostic and treatment protocols for patients with joint pain is fitting the disorder into the classic model of health and disease.[49] All but the most severe degenerative changes in the cervical and lumbar spine can exist in asymptomatic individuals. Profound pain and disability can occur in a spine that appears free of pathology.

Under these circumstances, two models should be developed and appreciated. One model considers the pathology and pathogenesis of joint dysfunction leading to pain or impairment. The other model places more importance on the structural and functional relationships of joint systems.

THE STRUCTURAL MODEL

A *structure* is defined as any assemblage of materials intended to sustain loads. Each life-form is contained in a structure. Even the most primitive unicellular organism must be enclosed and protected by cell membranes that are flexible and strong yet capable of accommodating cell division during reproduction. As life-forms advance and evolve, structure requirements become more sophisticated. Most living tissues carry some kind of mechanical load. Muscles also apply loads, changing shape as they do so. By making use of contractile muscles as tension members and strong bones as compression members, highly developed vertebrates withstand necessary loads and are capable of mobility, growth, and evolution.

The upright posture places different demands on the spine than occur in quadrupeds. Parallels have been drawn between the spine and the mast of a ship (Fig. 2-7). Compressive loads are concentrated in the vertebrae of the spine and the wooden mast of the ship. Tension loads are diffused into tendons, skin, and other soft tissues of the body and into the ropes and sails of the ship to maintain an upright position. A ship mast, however, is immobile, rigidly hinged, vertically oriented, and dependent on gravity. These rigid columns require heavy bases to support the incumbent load. The biologic structure of the spine must be a mobile, flexibly hinged, low–energy-consuming, omnidirectional structure that can function in a gravity-free environment.[50] The rigid upright model does not properly characterize the spine.

The model of a truss system such as is used in bridges has been used to make comparisons between the spine and a bridge. The musculoskeletal system of a large four-legged animal, such as a horse, is capable of bearing a substantial load in addition to its own weight, rests on four slender compression members (leg bones), and is supported by tension members (tendons, muscles, skin) (Fig. 2-8). Trusses have flexible, frictionless hinges with no bending moments about the joint. The support elements are either in tension or compression, so applied loads are distributed about the truss as tension or compression.[50] This model seems plausible but does not offer a complete explanation of the spine. Most trusses are constructed with tension members oriented in one direction. They will function in only one direction and therefore cannot function as the mobile, omnidirectional

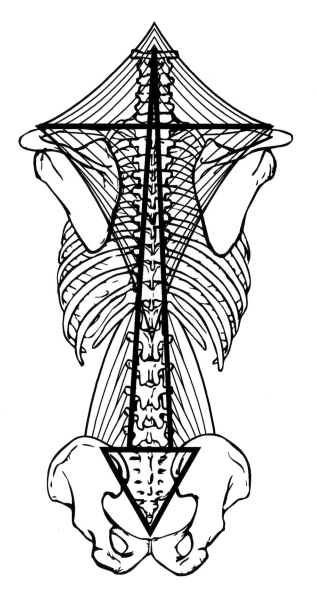

Fig. 2-7 Comparison of a ship's mast with the spine. Both are upright structures supported by a base and stabilized by tensile elements (guy wires, muscles/tendons).

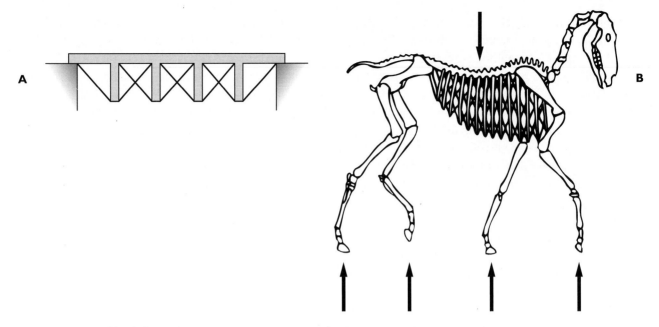

Fig. 2-8 Comparison of **A**, a truss bridge and **B**, the spine of a quadruped (horse) demonstrating that both have compression and tension members that maintain balance and resist applied forces.

structure necessary for describing spinal movements. Moreover, vertebrates have to move, whereas bridges do not. The comparison cannot be directly applied to the human skeleton because it is upright, and forces are applied in the long axis rather than perpendicular to the long axis (Fig. 2-9).

Levin[50] identifies another class of trusses called *tensegrity structures*, which are omnidirectional. The tension elements always function in tension, regardless of the direction of the applied force. A structure that meets the requirements of an integrated tensegrity model has been described as the *tensegrity icosahedron*. In this structure, the outer shell is under tension and the vertices are held apart by internal compression struts that appear to float in the tension network (Fig. 2-10). In architecture, stable form is generated through equilibrium among interdependent structures, each of which is in a state of disequilibrium. Complex architecture cannot be broken into pieces without losing qualities that are inherent to the structural whole. This is extremely important in biologic systems in which each functional unit is more than the sum of its parts.[51]

Many architectural structures depend on compressive forces for structural integrity. Compression-dependent structures are inherently rigid and unsuitable for a rapidly changing environment. Most naturally occurring structures depend on natural forces for integrity.[52] The human body is a tensile structure in which tensional integrity (tensegrity) is maintained by muscles suspended across compression-resistant bones. Fuller[53] describes a universal system of structural organization of the highest efficiency based on a continuum of tensional integrity, or tensegrity. Fuller's theory of tensegrity developed from the discovery of the geodesic dome, the most efficient architectural form, and study of the distribution of stress forces over the dome's structural elements. A tensegrity system is an architectural construction comprised of compression-resistant struts (bones) that do not touch one another but are interconnected by a continuous series of tension elements (muscles, ligaments).[51] Action and reaction are equal and opposite; therefore the tension forces must be compensated for by equal and opposite compressive forces and vice versa.

The most common and successful of structures is the cell, in which the tension membrane encloses a core of fluid that reacts against tension loads by hydrostatic compression. Many other biologic structures (viruses, clethrins, radiolaria, pollen grains, dandelion balls) have an icosahedron tensegrity configuration. The higher, complex animals developed rigid compression members (bones, cartilage) to counteract tension forces. The number of compression elements, however, is kept to a minimum to keep weight down.

Gravitational force is a constant and greatly underesti-

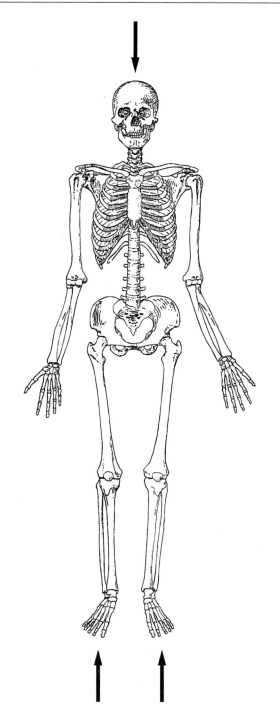

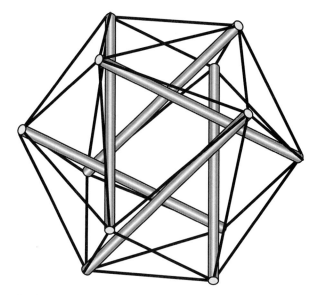

Fig. 2-10 A model of a tensegrity icosahedron showing its rigid compression members and elastic tension members. A series of these with a compression member form a structural model of the spine.

Fig. 2-9 The spine of a biped (human) is not suspended horizontally. Although the spine is composed of tension and compression members, maintaining balance, allowing movement, and resisting applied forces pose a unique biomechanical challenge. *(From* Medical Illustration Library: General Anatomy. *Baltimore: Williams & Wilkins; 1994.)*

mated stressor to the somatic system. The most obvious effect of gravitational stress can be evaluated by careful observation of posture, which is both static and dynamic. The static alignment of body mass with respect to gravity is constantly adjusted by dynamic neuromuscular coor-

dination as the individual changes position. Over time, individual static postural alignment conforms to inherent connective tissue structure and the cumulative functional demands of static and dynamic postural conditions. Musculoligamentous function also is influenced by and responsible for static and dynamic postural alignment.[54]

The musculoskeletal system is a structurally sound and functionally able closed kinetic chain composed of many interconnected tensegrity units. The development of asymmetric functional barriers in the spine has more than one cause. However, a unifying factor is the transfer of forces within the soft tissues, that is, the tensegrity mechanism, which creates altered and asymmetric tension. Manual therapies have the potential to influence the altered and asymmetric tension, thereby restoring homeostatic balance.

THE PATHOLOGIC MODEL

Study of the pathogenesis and pathology of a problem helps the physician better understand the nature of the clinical process, thereby facilitating the formation of a logical plan for treatment. Physicians and patients are most comfortable with a clear-cut relationship between pathology and symptomatology, between health and disease, and between cause and effect. The physician attempts to fit a particular patient's symptoms to a demonstrated pathology supported by various tests.[49]

Kirkaldy-Willis[55] states that the initial cause of lumbar spine dysfunction must be found in pathophysiology but

---

BOX 2-1

FACTORS IMPORTANT IN THE PATHOGENESIS OF JOINT PAIN

1. Aging
2. Acute trauma
3. Mechanical occupational stresses
4. General health
5. Exercise
6. Psychosocial factors

---

follows with the statement that the pathophysiology of low back pain is speculative at present. Haldeman[49] states that the relationship of pathology to symptomatology is extremely complicated and the classic pathology model in its simplistic form cannot explain back pain or disability.

Six important factors in the pathogenesis of joint pain are listed in Box 2-1.[49] The natural effects of aging produce an initial increase in pathology without symptoms, followed by a period of symptom increase. Acute trauma and the effects of inappropriate loads contribute to or produce the classic pathologic changes in joint dysfunction. Mechanical occupational stresses consist of repetitive activities (lifting, postures, vibration, etc.) that would not constitute an acute traumatic event but would result in pathologic changes. The general health of the individual contributes to the incidence and recurrence of joint pain through the negative effects of smoking, obesity, diabetes, cardiovascular disease, fatigue, and illnesses. Lack of exercise produces reduced cardiovascular function, muscle strength, and mobility, which contribute to chronic joint pain and disability. Finally, psychosocial factors (loneliness, coping skills, litigation, financial stability) have been associated with patients with chronic back pain, although the relative importance has yet to be determined.

The pathoanatomy of low back pain has been studied in cadavers. Much of the information, however, can be applied to other spinal regions. Kirkaldy-Willis[55] identifies three phases of the degenerative process affecting the structure and function of the lumbar spine. He suggests that a rotational strain or compressive injury to the lumbar spine begins the process of change within the three-joint complex, resulting in posterior joint and annular strain. This first step, the *dysfunction phase*, is characterized by changes that take place in the facet joints and intervertebral discs. The discs develop small circumferential tears in the annulus fibrosus. Because of small capsular and annular tears, joint subluxation takes place. The posterior joint capsule or synovial membrane may be injured, leading to reactive synovitis or capsulitis and joint hypomobility. The posterior segmental muscles protect the joint by sustained hypertonic contraction. The muscles become ischemic and this causes more pain. Accumulation of metabolites in muscle further aggravates the pain and sustains the hypertonic state of contraction. The posterior joints continue to be splinted, and subluxation is maintained. The changes lead to fibrosis. The three-joint complex is dysfunctional, and the result of these changes in the facet joints and disc is restriction in normal movement of the three-joint complex.

If this process continues, the articular cartilage begins degenerating and the joint capsule attenuates, leading to laxity of the capsule and the potential for hypermobility of the posterior joints. Circumferential tears in the annulus coalesce to form radial tears that allow passage of nuclear material into the defect. This eventually leads to internal disruption of the disc and bulging of the annulus. These changes in the posterior joints and disc lead to increased movement of the three-joint complex and the next stage of the degenerative process, called the *unstable phase* (not to be confused with segmental instability).

If the process continues, further damage occurs to the posterior joints and disc. The body reacts to the excessive movement and the cartilage of the facet joints is destroyed, leading to fibrosis within the joint. Hypertrophy of the facet joints occurs to decrease joint movement. At the same time, loss of hydration takes place in the nucleus, with a loss of height allowing approximation of the vertebral bodies. The vertebral endplates are destroyed, leading to fibrosis within the disc and the production of osteophytes and spondylophytes. The result of these changes in the facets and disc is increased stiffness and restabilization of the three-joint complex. This is called the *stabilization phase*. With hypertrophy of facet joints and the loss of disc height with spondylophyte and osteophyte formation, space is lost, resulting in spinal stenosis. This may occur primarily in the canal (central stenosis) or in the area of the intervertebral foramen (lateral stenosis). In either case, neurologic compromise may affect the spinal cord (cauda equina) or the nerve roots.

The basis for this three-phase degenerative process is an alteration in the biomechanics and the tensegrity structure of the spine. The use of manual therapy has been discussed for treatment of patients undergoing this process.[55] There appears to be the most beneficial effects from thrust techniques applied in the dysfunction phase. Thrust techniques applied in the unstable and stabilization phases seem to have only minimal benefit. However, no other forms of manual therapy were attempted.

Disc disorders have been recognized as pathoanatomic entities since Luschka described them in 1858.[56] In 1934, Mixter and Barr[57] described the association of disc problems with low-back pain and sciatica. Until recently the only explanation for disc involvement in clinical pain syndromes has followed this same model of the association of disc problems to low back pain and sciatica. The association is not strong between the intervertebral disc as an anatomic concept and the clinical syndrome that accompanies it. Removal of a compressive neural lesion is effective in some, but not most, cases of low back and leg pain. Asymptomatic degeneration is well-known, and the finding of disc lesions in asymptomatic patients is also well-documented. Even in cases of sciatica with radiologically documented disc herniations, the clinical presentation is not uniform and suggests that there is more than one biologic source of pain and dysfunction. Lipson[58] hypothesizes, on the basis of experimental disc degeneration, that the herniated disc is newly synthesized proliferative metaplastic fibrocartilage and not herniation of preexisting disc tissue, particularly that of the nucleus pulposus. Using histologic procedures, evidence of proliferative fronts of fibroblastic cells was revealed in herniated discs with hypocellular interiors. Further biochemical assays determined that the age of the material was less than that of material in the in situ annulus fibrosus and the material was not from the nucleus pulposus. Lipson's conclusion is that herniated discs are proliferative metaplastic fibrocartilage, synthesized by annular fibroblasts and not herniation of preexisting disc tissue. Although this work is revolutionary, no repeat studies corroborating these conclusions have been undertaken nor has there been acceptance or promotion of these conclusions by others. Lipson's work, however, represents an interesting hypothesis with some unanswered questions. Furthermore, results from these studies will not influence treatment considerations. The emphasis remains on pathologic findings and diagnostic criteria that support specific established disorders.

CONCLUSION

The understanding and clinical application of the basic principles of biomechanics to the evaluation and treatment of joint pain of mechanical origin is essential and appropriate. However, because no one model can be used to explain every cause of joint dysfunction, pain, and disability, it is necessary to address the larger picture of joint pain and disability in society. The one common characteristic that may have a major effect on the structural relationships and pathologic processes in the musculoskeletal system is the effects of axial loading. Axial loads produce compression at all weight-bearing joints. This concept would support the use of therapeutic procedures that are capable of producing distraction that would unload the joints. This will be the premise used to justify the need for the techniques in the chapters that follow.

REFERENCES

1. White AA, Panjabi MM. *Clinical Biomechanics of the Spine.* Philadelphia: JB Lippincott; 1979.
2. Nordin M, Frankel VH. *Basic Biomechanics of the Musculoskeletal system.* 2nd ed. Philadelphia: Lea & Febiger; 1989.
3. Goal VK, Weinstein JN. *Biomechanics of the Spine: Clinical and Surgical Perspective.* Boca Raton: CRC Press; 1990.
4. Pope MM, Andersson GBJ, Frymoyer JW, Chaffen DB. *Occupational Low Back Pain: Assessment, Treatment, and Prevention.* St Louis: Mosby; 1991.
5. Farfan HF. *Mechanical Disorders of the Low Back.* Philadelphia: Lea & Febiger; 1973.
6. Gracovetsky S. *The Spinal Engine.* New York: Springer-Verlag; 1988.
7. Levin SM. The sacrum in three-dimensional space. In Dorman TA, ed. Prolotherapy in the Lumbar Spine and Pelvis. *Spine.* 1995;9(2):381-388.
8. Bergmann TF, Peterson DH, Lawrence DJ. *Chiropractic Technique.* New York: Churchill Livingstone; 1993.
9. Andersson GBJ. Biomechanics of the lumbar spine. In Kirkaldy-Willis WH, Burton CV. *Managing Low Back Pain.* 3rd ed. New York: Churchill Livingstone; 1992.
10. Gordon JE. *The Science of Structure and Materials.* New York: Scientific American Books, Inc; 1988.
11. Garg A. Occupational biomechanics and low back pain. *Occup Med.* 1992;7(4):609-628.
12. Fiorini GT, McCammond D. Forces on the lumbo-vertebral facets. *J Biomed Eng.* 1976;4:354-363.
13. Farfan HF, Cossette J, Robertson G, et al. Effects of torsion on the intervertebral joint: the roll of torsion in the production of disc degeneration. *J Bone Joint Surg.*1970;52A:468-497.
14. Adams MA, Hutton WC. The relevance of torsion to the mechanical derangement of the lumbar spine. *Spine.* 1981;6:241-248.
15. Schultz AB, Warwick DN, Berkson MH, et al. Mechanical properties of the human lumbar spine motion segments: part 1. Response in flexion, extension, lateral bending, and torsion. *J Biomech Eng.* 1979;101:46-52.
16. Skipor AF, Miller JAA, Spencer DA, et al. Stiffness, properties, and geometry of lumbar spine posterior elements. *J Biomech Eng.* 1985;18:821-830.
17. Broberg KB. On the mechanical behavior of intervertebral discs. *Spine.* 1983;8(2):151-165.
18. Perry O. Fracture of the vertebral endplate in the lumbar spine. *Acta Orthop Scand.* 1957;25(suppl).
19. Adams MA, Hutton WC. Prolapsed intervertebral disc: a hyperflexion injury. *Spine.* 1982;7(3):184-191.
20. Stathopoulos PC, Cramer GD. Microscopic anatomy of the zygopophyseal joints and intervertebral discs. In: Cramer GD, Darby SA, eds. *Basic and Clinical Anatomy of the Spine, Spinal cord, and ANS.* St Louis: Mosby; 1995.
21. Lanz CA. The vertebral subluxation complex. In: Gatterman MI. *Foundations of Chiropractic Subluxation.* St Louis: Mosby; 1995.
22. Davison PF. Tendon. In: Weiss JB, Jayson MIV, eds. *Collagen in Health and Disease.* Edinburgh: Churchill Livingstone; 1982.
23. Injeyan HS, Fraser IH, Peek WD. Pathology of musculoskeletal soft tissues. In: Hammer WI, ed. *Functional Soft Tissue Examination and Treatment by Manual Methods.* Gaithersburg, Md: Aspen; 1991.
24. Woo SL-Y, Matthews JV, Akenson WH, Amiel D, Covery FR. Connective tissue response to immobility: corrective study of biomechanical and biochemical measurements of normal and immobilized rabbit knees. *Arthritis Rheum.* 1975;18:257.
25. Salter RB, Field P. The effects of continuous compression on living articular cartilage: an experimental investigation. *J Bone Joint Surg.* 1960;42A:31-41.
26. Baker WD, Thomas TG, Kirkaldy-Willis WH. Changes in cartilage of the posterior intervertebral joints after fusion. *J Bone Joint Surg.* 1969;51B:736-746.
27. Enneking WF, Horowitz M. The intra-articular effects of immobilization on the human knee. *J Bone Joint Surg.* 1972;54A:973-985.
28. Akeson WH, Amiel D, Woo SLY. Cartilage and ligament: physiology and repair processes. In: Nicholas JA, Hershman EB, eds. *The Lower Extremity and Spine in Sports Medicine.* St Louis: Mosby; 1995.
29. Akeson WH, Amiel D, Mechanic GL, Woo S, Harwood FL, Hamer ML. Collagen cross linking alterations in joint contractures: changes in reducible cross links in periarticular connective tissue collagen after 9 weeks of immobilization. *Connect Tissue Res.* 1977;5:5.
30. Burger AA. Experimental neuromuscular models of spinal manual techniques. *Manual Med.* 1983;1:10.
31. Garrett W, Tidball J. Myotendinous junction: structure, function, and failure. In: Woo SLY, Buckwalter JA, eds. *Injury and Repair of the Musculoskeletal Soft Tissues.* Park Ridge, Ill: American Academy of Orthopaedic Surgeons; 1988.
32. Jones VT, Garrett WE, Seaber AV. Biomechanical changes in muscle after immobilization at different lengths. *Trans Orthop Res Soc.* 1985;10:6.
33. Janda V. Muscle spasm: a proposed procedure for differential diagnosis. *J Manual Med.* 1991;6:136-139.
34. Cantu RI, Grodin AJ. *Myofascial Manipulation: Theory and Clinical Application.* Gaithersburg, Md: Aspen; 1992.
35. Liebenson C. Active muscular relaxation techniques: part 1. Basic principles and methods. *J Manipulative Physiol Ther.* 1989;12(6):446-454.
36. Treadwell SJ, O'Brien JP. Apophyseal joint degeneration in the cervical spine following halo-pelvic distraction. *Spine.* 1980;5(6):497-501.
37. Bogduk N, Twomey LT. *Clinical Anatomy of the Lumbar Spine.* 2nd ed. Melbourne: Churchill Livingstone; 1991.
38. Bergmann TF. Chiropractic reflex techniques. In: Gatterman MI, ed. *Foundations of Chiropractic: Subluxation.* St Louis: Mosby; 1995.
39. Williams PC. Lesions of the lumbosacral spine: part 2. Chronic traumatic postural destruction of the lumbosacral intervertebral disc. *J Bone Joint Surg.* 1937;19:690-703.
40. McKenzie RA. *The Lumbar Spine: Mechanical Diagnosis and Therapy.* Upper Hutt, New Zealand: Wright and Carman, Ltd; 1981.

41. Schnebel BE, Watkins RG, Dillin W. The role of spinal flexion and extension in changing nerve root compression in disc herniations. *Spine*. 1989;14(8):835-837.

42. Andersson GBJ. The biomechanics of the posterior elements of the lumbar spine. *Spine*. 1983;8(3):326.

43. Miller JAA, Haderspeck KA, Schultz AB. Posterior elements in lumbar motion segments. *Spine*. 1983;8(3):331-337.

44. Ortengren R, Andersson GBJ, Nachemson AL. Studies of relationships between lumbar disc pressure, myoelectric back muscle activity, and intra-abdominal (intragastric) pressure. *Spine*. 1981;6:98-103.

45. Andersson GBJ, Ortengren R, Nachemson A. Intradiscal pressure, intra-abdominal pressure and myoelectric back muscle activity related to posture and loading. *Clin Orthop*. 1977;129:156-164.

46. Adams MA, Hutton WC. The effects of posture on the lumbar spine. *J Bone Joint Surg*. 1985;67B:625-629.

47. Torg JS, Sennett B, Vegso JJ, Pavlov H. Axial loading injuries to the middle cervical spine segment: an analysis and classification of 25 cases. *Am J Sports Med*. 1991;19(1):6-20.

48. Nachemson AL. Advances in low back pain. *Clin Orthop*. 1985;200:266-278.

49. Haldeman S. Presidential address, North American Spine Society: Failure of the pathology model to predict back pain. *Spine*. 1990;15(7):718-24.

50. Levin SM. The importance of soft tissue for structural support of the body. In: Dorman TA, ed. Prolotherapy in the lumbar spine and pelvis. *Spine*. 9(2):357-363.

51. Ingber DE, Jamieson JD. Cells as tensegrity structures: architectural regulation of histodifferentiation by physical forces transduced over basement membrane. In: Andersson LC, Gahmberg CG, Ekblom P, eds. *Gene Expression During Normal and Malignant Differentiation*. London: Academic Press; 1985.

52. Thompson DW. *On Growth and Form*. New York: Cambridge University Press; 1977.

53. Fuller BR. *Synergetics*. New York: McMillan; 1975.

54. Kuchera ML. Gravitational stress, musculoligamentous strain, and postural alignment. In: Dorman TA. Prolotherapy in the lumbar spine and pelvis. *Spine*. 1995;9(2)243-490.

55. Kirkaldy-Willis WH, Burton CV. *Managing Low Back Pain*. 3rd ed. New York: Churchill Livingstone; 1992.

56. Luschka H. Die Halbgeleke des menschlichen Korpers. Reimer, Berlin; 1858. Ein monographie.

57. Mixter WJ, Barr JS. Rupture of the intervertebral disc with involvement of the spinal cord. *N Eng J Med* 1934;211:210.

58. Lipson SJ. 1988 Metaplastic proliferative fibrocartilage as an alternative concept to herniated intervertebral disc. *Spine*. 1988;13(9):1055-1060.

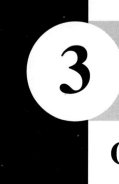

3

Overview of Manual Therapy

Manual therapy has been described clinically since the days of Hippocrates. There is a dearth of information, however, about the scientific foundations of the indications for and the specific effects of all forms of manual therapy.[1] The chiropractic profession is dedicated to the use of manual therapy and, specifically, the adjustment as a form of clinical intervention. Manual therapy has been used for centuries and still occupies a small niche in medical, osteopathic, and physical therapy practices. The chiropractic profession has promoted the use of manual therapy in the treatment of neuromusculoskeletal dysfunction.[2] However, the profession has yet to substantiate experimentally the clinical value of any uniquely chiropractic method of health care.[3] Studies designed to compare the effectiveness of the many forms of chiropractic technique systems have not yet been performed. No technique system or evaluative procedure has been demonstrated to be more or less effective than any other procedure for any condition. Therefore studies comparing the effectiveness and efficiency of different technique systems are long overdue.

Curricula from accredited chiropractic colleges are designed to ensure that certain information is imparted to the student body. The colleges offer a comprehensive program that includes elements of basic science and clinical science while also providing a clinical experience. Although the curriculum is standardized to assure the public that the graduates have been provided a competent education, each college does not necessarily teach its students the same chiropractic techniques. The forms of chiropractic technique have elements in common; however, there are substantial differences in the approaches applied and nomenclature used. Furthermore, many technique procedures are available to the profession in the form of postgraduate seminars, many of which are not under the influence of any regulatory body or accrediting process.

ROLE OF MANUAL THERAPY

Manual therapy has been proposed as a treatment for a variety of conditions but is most commonly associated with disorders that have their origins in pathomechanical or pathophysiologic alterations of the locomotor system and its synovial joints. Identification of the common functional components of the dysfunctional joint lesion is critical to management of conditions affecting the neuromusculoskeletal system. This has, however, contributed to the misconception that all manipulative disorders have the same pathologic basis. The disorders that seem to have the most favorable response to chiropractic manipulative procedures display joint and somatic functional alterations; however, many pathologic processes are capable of inducing dysfunction of the locomotor system. When joint dysfunction is perceived as the sole cause of the disorder being considered for treatment, adjustive therapy may stand alone. However, when dysfunction is secondary to other disorders, therapy directed to treat the source of the problem should be provided or made available to the patient.[4]

Manual therapy, with its emphasis on joint movement, has become increasingly important for the treatment of pain and dysfunction of the musculoskeletal system. The rationale for the apparent success of manual therapy has changed radically in recent years. Current biologic research shows the value of movement in maintaining the health and strength of collagenous, muscular, and bony tissues and emphasizes the need for joint movement and relatively high levels of activity throughout the life cycle. The musculoskeletal system thrives on stress and movement and reacts adversely to prolonged rest or immobilization.[5]

Forms of manual therapy are used to restore optimal joint range of motion. Rahlmann[6] identifies the mechanisms for increasing range of motion as releasing minor adhesions, altering the position of an intraarticular loose body, reducing a displaced articular meniscoid, and reducing discrete muscle spasm by affecting the input through the gamma-loop system. Lamb[7] reports that repetitive, rhythmic movement will perform the following four functions: (1) affect the hydrostatics of the disc and vertebral bodies; (2) activate the type I and II mechanoreceptors in the capsule of the facet joint, influencing the spinal gating mechanism; (3) alter the activity of the neuromuscular spindle in the intrinsic muscles of the segment subsequently affecting bias in the gray matter cells; and (4) assist the pumping effect on the venous plexus of the vertebral segment.

EFFECTS OF MANUAL THERAPY

The goals for the application of manual therapy include a combination of mechanical, soft tissue, neurologic, and psychologic effects. Although these categories seem to be specific and distinct from one another, they actually represent only academic divisions, because it is impossible to produce a singular effect. That is, when a therapeutic procedure is applied to create a desired mechanical effect, it also affects the soft tissues and/or the neurologic elements. These categories are given only for easier understanding of the principles for applying the forms of manual therapy.

MECHANICAL EFFECTS

The mechanical effects of manual therapy include changes in joint alignment, dysfunctional joint motion, and spinal curvature dynamics. Generally, the mechanical effects of an adjustment will be on derangements of the somatic structures that have altered joint function. Causes of altered joint function are acute injury, repetitive use injury, faulty posture or coordination, aging, congenital or developmental defects, and primary disease states.

There are several causes of acute and chronic mechanical joint dysfunction (Box 3-1). Gatterman[8] and Rahlmann[6] conclude that more than one mechanism is probably involved in the development of joint dysfunction, although immobilization as a result of adhesions has the strongest literature support. Therefore, all mechanisms will be considered in this discussion.

Intraarticular meniscoids are leaflike, fibroadipose folds of synovium that are attached to the inner surface of the joint capsule and project into the joint cavity. These meniscoids are present in all posterior joints of the spine. Bogduk and Jull[8] suggest that extrapment of these meniscoids may cause restricted joint motion. On flexion, the inferior articular process of a zygapophyseal joint moves upward, taking the meniscoid with it. On attempted extension, the inferior articular process returns toward its neutral position but, instead of reentering the joint cavity, the meniscoid contacts the edge of the articular cartilage and buckles, representing a space-occupying lesion under the capsule. Pain occurs as a result of capsular tension, and extension motion is restricted. The application of a procedure that will separate the articular surfaces may release the extrapped meniscoid.[9]

Cyriax[10] believes that displaced nuclear material along an incomplete radial fissure is the source of joint fixation. Postmortem dissection studies of degenerated discs have demonstrated radial fissures in the annulus fibrosus. Nuclear migration along these radial fissures has also been demonstrated by CT discography and correlated with the patient's pain.[11] However, questions remain regarding the disc's ability to restrict motion. First, annular fissures apparently are irreversible and do not mend with manipulation, yet manipulation can have an immediate and often lasting effect on joint dysfunction. Moreover, joint dysfunction and fixation can occur at segments where there are no intervertebral discs, such as the atlantooccipital articulation, the atlantoaxial articulation, the sacroiliac articulations, and the extremity joints. Finally, disc pathology can lead to spinal fixation through reflex muscle spasm. A painful and inflamed annular tear or disc herniation causes reflex muscle spasm that restricts motion.

Specific joint derangements are thought to create a mechanical blockage of movement and an unleveling of the motion segment, resulting in tension on the joint capsule and posterolateral annulus. Because the joint capsule and posterior annulus are pain-sensitive structures, tension on these elements may reflexively induce muscle splinting with further joint restriction. Mechanical joint dysfunction is therefore considered to be a major and frequent cause of spinal pain and a potential source of spinal degeneration.

An intriguing but not necessarily clinically important mechanical effect of manipulation is the process of joint cavitation. Studies performed by Roston et al[12] and Unsworth et al[13] demonstrate that as tension is applied, causing a separation of the joint, there is a point at which the joint surfaces jump apart, coinciding with a cracking noise. Once the tension is removed from the joint, the surfaces approximate themselves once again but at a distance slightly more apart. As the elastic barrier is passed, the articular surfaces separate suddenly, the cracking noise is heard, and a radiolucent space appears within the joint space. The explanation of the radiolucent space rests with the fact that there is normally a small negative pressure present in a synovial joint. The purpose of this pressure is to maintain the cartilage surfaces in apposition and help maintain the stability of the joint. Separation of the joint surfaces beyond the elastic barrier creates a drop in the interarticular pressure, and gas is suddenly liberated from the synovial fluid to form a bubble in the joint space. The bubble bursts almost immediately with an audible crack. More than 80% of the gas produced by synovial fluid cavitation is carbon dioxide.[13] The only definitive effect of this cavitation response is a temporary increase in resting joint space. This implies an increase in the range of motion for the joint, but this has not been adequately established nor has the length of time for increased movement or joint space been established. The sound of the crack and feel of the joint release may also have a placebo effect on the patient. There may be other explanations for the sounds heard when applying manual procedures. A tendinous snap can be produced as a tendon is quickly drawn over a bony prominence. Also, capsular adhesions or collagenous cross-linkages may produce a sound as they are broken.

SOFT TISSUE EFFECTS

The soft tissue effects of manipulation include changes in the tone and strength of supporting musculature and influence on the dynamics of supportive capsuloligamentous connective tissue (viscoelastic properties of collagen). With immobilization, connective tissue elements lose their extensibility and water is released from the proteoglycan molecule, which allows connective tissue fibers to contact one another, encouraging abnormal cross-linking and resulting in loss of extensibility.[14,15] Certain manual therapies may break the cross-linking and

---

BOX 3-2

EFFECTS OF IMMOBILIZATION

MICROSCOPIC EFFECTS:
Loss of parallelism of collagen fibers
Distorted cellular alignment
Increased randomness of matrix organization
Increased collagen cross-link formation

PERIARTICULAR EFFECTS:
Thickening of joint capsule
Raised capsular tension
Connective tissue shrinkage
Muscle atrophy
Bone demineralization

INTRAARTICULAR EFFECTS:
Proliferation of fatty tissue
Obliteration of joint space
Pressure necrosis of the articular cartilage
Extension of marrow space into the subchondral plate
Cartilage erosion and ulceration in noncontact areas
Adhesions to articular cartilage
Articular cartilage tears at the site of adhesions

BIOMECHANICAL EFFECTS:
Decreased ligament strength
Decreased lineal stiffness
Decreased energy-absorbing capacity

Modified from Akeson WH, Amel D, Woo SLY. Cartilage and ligament: physiology and repair processes. In: Nicholas JA, Hershman EB, eds. *The Lower Extremity and Spine in Sports Medicine*. St Louis: Mosby; 1986.

---

any intraarticular capsular fibroadipose adhesions, thereby providing free motion and allowing water imbibition to occur. The action of these manual therapies can stretch segmental muscles, causing spindle reflexes that may decrease the state of hypertonicity.[16] The effects of immobilization are summarized in Box 3-2.[17]

Joints become stiff after immobilization. Although some stiffness results from intraarticular adhesions to surfaces that normally glide past one another, ligamentous structures can shorten (contract) and therefore limit joint motion.[18,19] Joint stiffness probably results from a combination of adhesion formation between normally gliding surfaces and active changes in ligament length. Manual therapy applied to restricted joints presumably will tear the collagen cross-links and fibrous adhesions formed during joint immobilization. However, when articular or nonarticular soft tissue contractures are encountered, incorporation of procedures that minimize inflammation and maintain mobility should be considered. Viscoelastic structures are more amenable to elongation and deformation if they are first warmed and then stretched for sustained periods.[20] Therefore the application of moist heat, ultrasound, or other warming therapies might be considered before application of sustained manual traction or home-care stretching exercises.[21]

NEUROLOGIC EFFECTS

The neurologic effects of manipulation include reduction in pain; influence on spinal and peripheral nerve conduction, which alters motor and sensory function; and influence on autonomic nervous system regulation. Wyke[22] reports that manipulative procedures may stimulate the mechanoreceptors associated with synovial joints and thereby affect joint pain. He identifies four types of joint receptors. Types I, II, and III are corpuscular mechanoreceptors that detect static position of the joint, acceleration and deceleration of the joint, direction of movement, and overdisplacement of the joint. The type IV receptor is a network of free nerve endings that have nociceptive capabilities. Type IV receptors are inactive under normal conditions. However, in response to noxious mechanical or chemical stimulation, or if types I, II, and III receptors are not able to function, type IV receptors become active and the sensation of pain is perceived. If manipulative therapy can restore normal function to the joint, allowing types I, II, and III receptors to function, the type IV pain receptors should be inhibited, thereby decreasing the patient's pain. The structures most sensitive to noxious stimulation are the periosteum and joint capsule.

Evidence supports the theory that spinal adjustment increases pain tolerance in the skin and deeper muscle structures, raises β-endorphin levels in the blood plasma, and has an impact on the nerve pathways between the body wall and viscera that regulate general health.[23-28] A major factor in musculoskeletal function is the musculature and its nervous control. Each individual has a "postural personality" that is an expression of the individual's muscular patterns and posture. A frequent cause of joint dysfunction may be faulty neuromotor patterns caused by muscular imbalance and postural strain or an inability on the part of the patient to consciously control musculoskeletal function.[29]

Controversy exists on the application of manual therapy. A major area of discussion is the role of pain in the appropriateness of manual procedures. Mitchell[30] states that treatment of the area where the patient experiences pain usually results in treatment of the wrong part of the body. He quotes Osler, stating "pain is a liar." Mitchell bases this idea on the concept that in the musculoskeletal system, pain almost always develops and persists in the structures that are stressed the most by the adaptation to the dysfunction. The opposite idea is stated by Lewit[29] who suggests that if a manual therapy treatment is successful, it will usually produce immediate relief of pain. He adds that the most frequent cause of pain is disturbed function. This may involve passive joint mobility or active movement patterns. Manual therapy is directed to movement restriction of joints or motion segments of the spinal column. Pain in the locomotor system is therefore seen as a warning sign of harmful functioning that should be corrected before it causes permanent damage. Lewit[29] also emphasizes that undiagnosed impairment of motor function is the most frequent cause of pain without a specific diagnosis, and treatment of the pain itself, without a thorough understanding of the functioning of the locomotor system, is courting failure.

PSYCHOLOGIC EFFECTS

The psychologic effects of the laying on of the hands cannot be denied. Paris[31] states that with the addition of a skilled evaluation involving palpation for soft tissue changes and altered joint mechanics, the patient becomes convinced of the interest, concern, and manual skills of the clinician. If, at the conclusion of the examination, a manual procedure is performed that results in an audible crack, the placebo factor will be undeniably high. Paris[31] states that some patients report total relief within a second or two after such a procedure, a period that he considers far too short for any genuine benefit to be appreciated. The astute clinician accepts and reinforces this phenomenon, recognizing that the patient is in need of all possible assistance. It should be noted, however, that the response rate to manipulative treatment cannot be accounted for totally by the placebo effect.

FORMS OF MANUAL THERAPY

Although manual therapy is a term broadly used to define the therapeutic application of a manual force, chiropractors emphasize the application of specific adjustive techniques. Many methods of manual therapy exist, and the assumption that all forms are equivalent is incorrect.[32] Nearly 100 techniques have been identified with-

BOX 3-3

**FACTORS THAT INFLUENCE
THE SELECTION OF
MANIPULATIVE PROCEDURES**

1. Age of patient
2. Acuteness or chronicity of the problem
3. Patient's size and flexibility
4. General physical condition of the patient
5. Clinician's size and ability
6. Effectiveness of previous and/or present therapy

Modified from Greenman P. *Principles of Manual Medicine*. Baltimore: Williams & Wilkins; 1989.

BOX 3-4

MANUAL THERAPY TERMINOLOGY

MANUAL THERAPY:
Procedures by which the hands directly contact the body to treat the articulations and/or soft tissues.

MOBILIZATION:
Movement applied singularly or repetitively within or at the physiologic range of joint motion without imparting a thrust or impulse, with the goal of restoring joint mobility.

MANIPULATION:
A manual procedure that involves a directed thrust to move a joint past the physiologic range of motion, without exceeding the anatomic limit.

ADJUSTMENT:
Any chiropractic therapeutic procedure that uses controlled force, leverage, direction, amplitude, and velocity that is directed at specific joints or anatomic regions. Chiropractors commonly use such procedures to influence joint and neurophysiologic function.

Data from Gatterman MI, Hansen D. Develoment of chiropractic nomenclature through consensus. *J Manipulative Physiol Ther.* 1994;17:302-309.

in the chiropractic profession.[1] There are, however, factors that should influence the selection of manipulative procedures (see Box 3-3).[33]

The term *technique* should not be confused with the terms *therapy* or *treatment*. Technique describes a specific manual procedure, whereas therapy and treatment include the application of all the primary and ancillary procedures appropriate in the management of a health disorder. These procedures are limited by individual statutory practice acts but may include procedures such as joint mobilization, therapeutic muscle stretching, soft tissue manipulation, sustained and intermittent traction, meridian therapy, physiologic therapeutic modalities, application of heat or cold, dietary and nutritional counseling, therapeutic and rehabilitative exercises, biofeedback, and stress management.[21] Through a consensus process, Gatterman and Hansen[34] defined the terms manual therapy, manipulation, mobilization, and adjustment (see Box 3-4). Controversy exists over some of the definitions. Those outside the chiropractic profession continue to use manipulation as an umbrella term over all forms of manual therapy. Many chiropractors consider manipulation to be a general, nonspecific procedure, whereas an adjustment is a specific high-velocity, low-amplitude thrust applied to a short lever. However, many chiropractic techniques do not use a high-velocity, low-amplitude thrust yet are still called an adjustment when there is no thrust applied. There apparently is still work to be done on terminology and nomenclature.

Manual therapy is applied in many forms, including massage, mobilization, traction, muscle energy techniques, adjustment, and manipulation (Fig. 3-1). The common characteristic of these methods is the application of external forces to affect the flexibility and pain-free

function of the spine and its contiguous tissues.[35] All of these methods act on sensory receptors, usually in the region where the pain is felt or where it originates, to produce a reflex response.[29] Pain warns us mainly against harmful functioning, and disturbance of function is the most common cause of pain originating in the locomotor system. Movement restriction (blockage) at the segmental level and disturbed motor patterns at the central level may serve as examples.[36] The therapy used must be appropriate for the structures on which it is to act. Manual therapy is a valuable treatment for joint or spinal segment movement restriction.[29]

Sandoz[37] defines the chiropractic adjustment as a passive manual maneuver during which the three-joint complex is suddenly carried beyond the normal physiologic range of movement without exceeding the boundaries of anatomic integrity. However, various forms of manual therapy exist that affect different aspects of joint function without the use of a thrust. Regardless of the procedure used, the therapeutic emphasis is not on forcing a particular anatomic movement of a joint but on restoring normal joint mechanics. Most forms of manual therapy result in movement of joint surfaces either actively or passively, restoring normal articular relationships and function, restoring neurologic integrity, and influencing

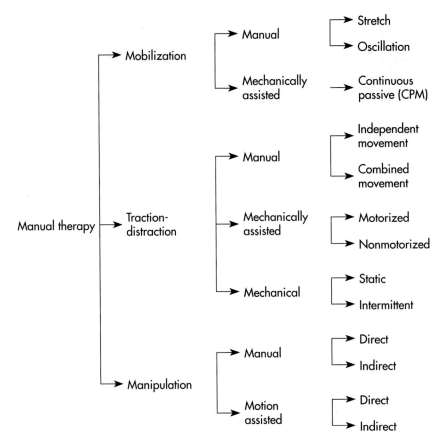

Fig. 3-1 Forms of manual therapy.

physiologic processes. The nature and extent of individual joint motion is determined by the joint structure and, specifically, by the shape and direction of the joint surfaces. No two opposing joint surfaces are perfectly matched or perfectly geometric. Because of the incongruence between joint surfaces, some joint space and "play" must be present to allow free movement and normal functioning of the joint.[19] Leverage is used to influence the direction and amount of joint movement.

The levers used to produce motion at an articulation or group of articulations are simple machines (tools) for reducing work through increased mechanical advantage. The longer the lever, the greater the mechanical advantage and applied force. However, the situation becomes more complex when consideration is given to the vectors of forces and effects of soft tissues on the intervertebral joint. The levers and generated forces are used in such a way that the applied force causes motion between the affected segments and is not dissipated by the elasticity or mobility of other spinal or appendicular structures.[38]

White and Panjabi[20] state that regardless of what the external forces or manipulation may be, the movement of

a vertebra is limited to the combinations possible within the six degrees of freedom. They describe the manual application of forces directly to the spinous process and posterior elements of a given vertebra, loading and displacing it along or around the x, y, or z axis. Sufficient force must be applied to spinous processes or lateral processes (articular, transverse, or mammillary) in the spine to move one segment relative to the other. The implied importance or rationale for the use of a short-lever procedure is increased specificity, which is thought to be important in influencing a specific joint complex for specific joint dysfunction. However, only opinion and reasoned conclusion support this idea.[39]

A widely used form of manual therapy is characterized by a specific high-velocity and low-amplitude thrust. This thrust is achieved by a transmission of force, combining the muscular power and body weight of the practitioner. The force is delivered with controlled speed, depth, and magnitude through a specific contact on a particular structure, such as the transverse or spinous process of a vertebra.[40]

Haldeman[41] states that, although many techniques with

different therapeutic goals are being administered according to different biomechanical or physiologic principles, the most commonly used manipulative technique is the short-lever, high-velocity adjustment. He describes this technique as a quick, small-amplitude, high-velocity thrust that is delivered in a specific direction to one of the small vertebral processes.

Hoag et al[38] state that a major subdivision of osteopathic manipulative therapy involves technique directed mainly to osseous structures and designed to restore normal joint mobility and weight distribution. They describe the procedure used as positioning the patient in such a way that the applied force causes motion between the affected segments that is not dissipated by the elasticity or mobility of other spinal or appendicular structures. After tension is taken up in muscles and ligaments from above and below the site to be manipulated, a force is delivered, usually to the upper of the two segments and in a direction that should restore normal motion or apposition.[38] This procedure implies a specific hand contact on a short lever (spinous process or transverse process) and uses a rapid (high-velocity) and short-distance (low-amplitude) thrusting movement. Greenman[33] writes that the high-velocity, low-amplitude thrust technique is one of the oldest and most frequently and widely used forms of manual medicine. He states further that these procedures are usually applied as precisely as possible to a single joint level and for a specific joint motion loss. He believes the high-velocity, low-amplitude thrust is much more effective in subacute and chronic conditions than in acute somatic dysfunction. However, he offers no support for the statements.

A long-lever technique may use a specific or general primary contact on the body part but the second contact is remote from the segment, forming a broad or long leverage system of forces.[42] All side-posture lumbar- and pelvic-thrust techniques employ a long lever, the bent leg, as a means to apply preadjustive tension or the thrust itself. Long and short lever combinations are frequently used procedures. The long lever provides the necessary leverage for general distraction and articular prestress to the spine; a short-lever contact focuses the force to a smaller section.

Kappler[43] uses velocity and amplitude to describe the nature of the final activating force in a thrust technique, stating that a high-velocity, low-amplitude technique involves a quick thrust carried through a short distance, and a low-velocity, high-amplitude procedure is one in which the rate of motion is slow and the distance is great.

Although he gives no instruction as when to use a certain procedure, he does identify inappropriate applications. It is his opinion that techniques that use a rebound thrust in which the force is directed away from the barrier and not into the barrier would be inappropriate. He also states that the use of a high-velocity, high-amplitude thrust in which the barrier is not engaged (i.e., starting point is the neutral midrange) is also inappropriate. His reasoning is that these procedures produce excessive force that may be harmful.[43]

Manual traction is another form of manual therapy in which joint surfaces are held in sustained separation. Traction may be accomplished solely through contacts made by the clinician or may be applied with the use of a mechanized table or other device, allowing forces to be applied manually, mechanically, or in combination. Traction techniques aid in the application of an adjustment by allowing the area to rest, relieving compressive pressure caused by weight bearing (axial loading); applying an imbibing action to the synovial joints and discs; and opening the intervertebral foramina to allow disruption of reflex neurologic cycles. Many of these procedures are useful for elderly patients when a high-velocity, low-amplitude thrust may not be indicated or is contraindicated. Traction maneuvers produce long axis distraction in the joint to which they are applied. There is a long axis distraction movement of joint play at every synovial joint.[44] Little attention is paid to this important joint movement in the spine as being necessary for normal function of the joint. Perhaps this is because long axis distraction of the spinal joints is difficult to perform manually.

JOINT ASSESSMENT PROCEDURES

A primary health care provider must use findings derived from the case history, physical examination, clinical laboratory tests, and indicated special tests to assess a patient's state of health and determine the nature and extent of any ailments. The steps leading to a decision about treatment are the most important interaction between doctor and patient.[45] The differentiation of the many conditions responsible for joint pain is sometimes based on clinical intuition rather than true objective procedures. This is especially the case, for example, when back pain is not classic for an intervertebral disc lesion or facet (articular) involvement. To make the diagnosis through clinical procedures without the benefit of sophisticated and expensive imaging methods or to administer

---

BOX 3-5

CATEGORIES OF THE EXAMINATION PROCEDURE

1. History
2. Observation
3. Physical evaluation
4. Orthopedic/neurologic evaluation
5. Chiropractic evaluation
6. Diagnostic imaging/laboratory testing

BOX 3-6

INFORMATION FROM THE HISTORY NECESSARY FOR DESCRIPTION OF JOINT PAIN PROBLEMS

1. Past occurrences
2. Location of the pain
3. Onset of the pain
4. Quality of pain
5. Pain rating
6. Aggravating factors

---

anesthetic injections into the joint space requires an understanding of the anatomy of the area and familiarity with the statistical occurrence of the events. Assessment is the process of weighing the significance and priority of the information as it applies to the patient. Box 3-5 lists examination categories. Fig. 3-2, *A* and *B* are charts demonstrating examination procedures for low back and neck pain.

HISTORY

The history provides patients an opportunity to express a subjective description of the symptoms and problems bothering them. The information necessary to begin to determine the nature and extent of the problem and to localize it to a specific level is elicited from the history (Box 3-6).

Past Occurrences. It is important to note any previous experience with similar problems, because this will begin to form a pattern that may be characteristic of a specific problem. Most disc injuries are products of a gradual and progressive process that has a history of previous events consistent with the stages of the degeneration characteristic to the disc. The exceptions are those events that have an associated major trauma that exceeds the resistance of the relatively healthy tissue.

Location and Onset of Pain. The location of the pain and how it was first experienced is an important factor in localizing the site of the lesion. Consideration should also be given to when the particular areas became involved and if any have disappeared since their original occurrence. A pain drawing (Fig. 3-3) should be used to have the patient graphically localize the pain. The site of pain does not always correspond well with the site of lesion.

Quality of Pain. The patient often describes radiating patterns of pain, cutaneous patterns of hyperalgesia or hypalgesia, and tenderness to palpation at sites distant from the site of pathophysiology. Most of these patterns do not correspond to any one muscle or nerve nor do they conform to the well-known and often overused dermatome patterns.

When patients describe the pain as being deep, aching, and difficult to localize, the pain is probably coming from deep somatic lesions following sclerotome patterns.

Pain Rating. A visual analog scale (VAS) and functional status questionnaires (Oswestry, Roland-Morris, Neck Disability Index) are used to rate the intensity of pain and the effects of pain on activities of daily living (Figs. 3-4 and 3-5). These are good monitoring tools to establish whether the pain is improving, staying the same, or worsening.

Aggravating Factors. Identification of the positions or activities that relieve or intensify the discomfort may help differentiate the type of lesion and involved tissues.

EXAMINATION

Much of the examination process is directed at reproducing the patient's signs and symptoms that relate to the chief complaint. The examination must be thorough and accurate and, although the format can vary, it should be systematic to ensure that all tests and procedures are performed. It affords the clinician an opportunity to observe objective signs necessary to confirm, refute, or modify the patient's account of the problem.

The physical evaluation includes assessment of the vital signs (blood pressure, heart rate, respiratory rate, temperature, height, and weight) and any systems assessment deemed necessary (heart, lungs, abdomen, and so on), including clinical laboratory tests (blood, urine). The orthopedic and neurologic evaluations involve tests to identify dysfunctional interactions of the bones, ligaments, tendons, joints, and nerves. Range-of-motion, muscle-stretch reflex, superficial sensation, motor-strength tests, and specific provocative tests are performed. The specific tests are described fully elsewhere.[46,47] Diagnostic imaging procedures include plain film radiographs and advanced imaging to visualize osseous and soft tissue relationships.

For patients having musculoskeletal problems of an

Text continued on p. 47.

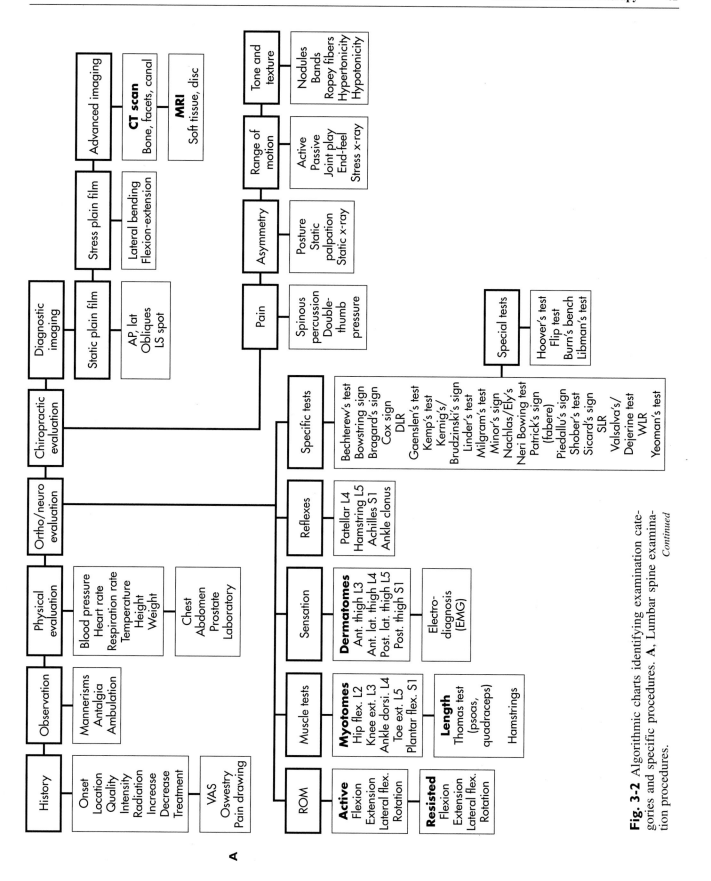

Fig. 3-2 Algorithmic charts identifying examination categories and specific procedures. A, Lumbar spine examination procedures.

Continued

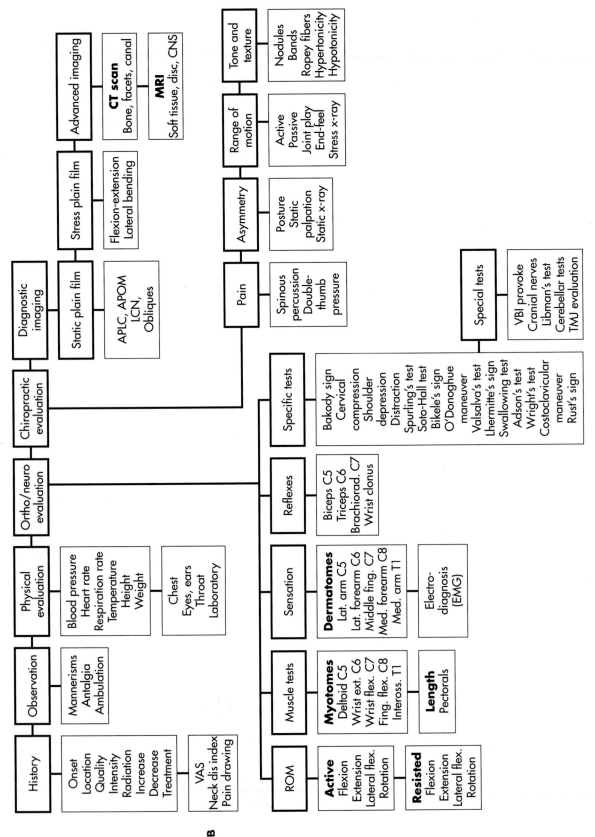

Fig. 3-2, cont'd B, Cervical spine examination procedures.

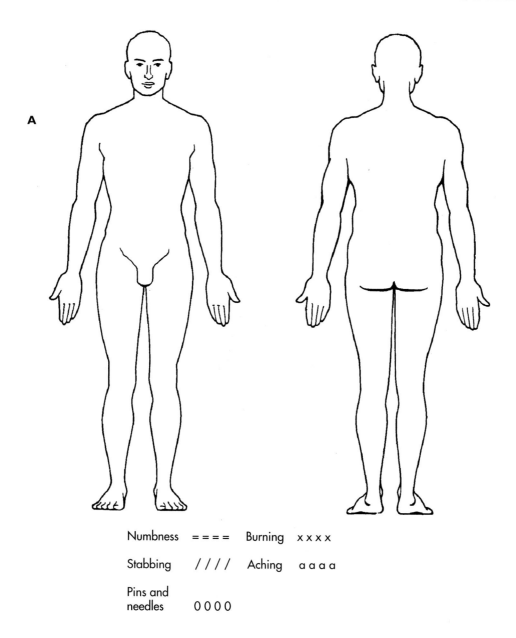

Numbness	= = = =	Burning	x x x x
Stabbing	/ / / /	Aching	a a a a
Pins and needles	0 0 0 0		

Scoring for pain drawing

Writing anywhere	1
Unphysiologic pain pattern	1
Unphysiologic sensory change	1
More than one type of pain	1
Both upper and lower areas of the body involved	1
Markings outside the body	1
Unspecified symbols	1

Score: 1= Normal; 5 or more = Psychologic overlay

Fig. 3-3 Pain drawing. **A,** Patients are asked to localize and describe the character of their pain using the supplied symbols.

Continued

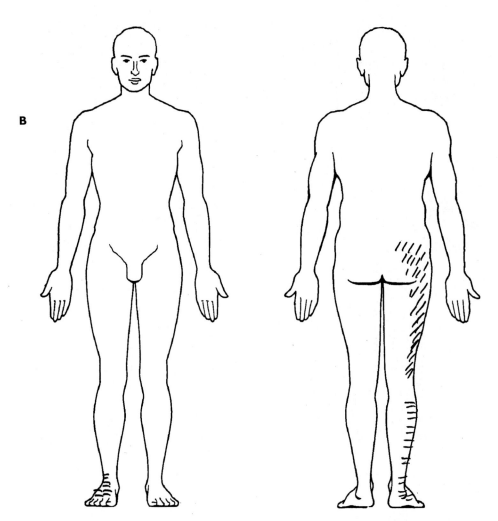

Fig. 3-3, cont'd B, A completed pain drawing characteristic of L5 nerve root compression neuropathy.

INSTRUCTIONS: Please make a mark on the line provided below to correspond to how you presently feel.

NO PAIN ━━━━━━━━━━━━━━━━━━━━━━━━━━━ WORST PAIN EVER

Fig. 3-4 Visual analog pain severity scale (VAS). The patient is asked to mark a dot or an X on the line to rate pain from absence to extreme; the examiner measures the distance from no pain in millimeters (0 to 100 scale). A verbalized, numeric system from 0 to 10 or 0 to 100 can also be used.

Oswestry Low Back Questionnaire

Name_____ Date_____ / _____ / _____ File #_____

Instructions: Please mark the ONE BOX in each section which most closely describes your problem.

Section 1—Pain Intensity
- [ ] 0. The pain comes and goes and is very mild.
- [ ] 1. The pain is mild and does not vary much.
- [ ] 2. The pain comes and goes and is moderate.
- [ ] 3. The pain is moderate and does not vary much.
- [ ] 4. The pain comes and goes and is severe.
- [ ] 5. The pain is severe and does not vary much.

Section 2—Personal Care (Washing, Dressing, etc.)
- [ ] 0. I would not have to change my way of washing or dressing in order to avoid pain.
- [ ] 1. I do not normally change my way of washing or dressing even though it causes some pain.
- [ ] 2. Washing and dressing increase the pain but I manage not to change my way of doing it.
- [ ] 3. Washing and dressing increase the pain and I find it necessary to change my way of doing it.
- [ ] 4. Because of the pain I am unable to do some washing and dressing without help.
- [ ] 5. Because of the pain I am unable to do any washing or dressing without help.

Section 3—Lifting
- [ ] 0. I can lift heavy weights without extra pain.
- [ ] 1. I can lift heavy weights but it gives extra pain.
- [ ] 2. Pain prevents me lifting heavy weights off the floor.
- [ ] 3. Pain prevents me lifting heavy weights off the floor, but I can manage if they are conveniently positioned, e.g., on a table.
- [ ] 4. Pain prevents me from lifting heavy weights but I can manage light to medium weights if they are conveniently positioned.
- [ ] 5. I can only lift very light weights at the most.

Section 4—Walking
- [ ] 0. I have no pain on walking.
- [ ] 1. I have some pain on walking but it does not increase with distance.
- [ ] 2. I cannot walk more than 1 mile without increasing pain.
- [ ] 3. I cannot walk more than 1/2 mile without increasing pain.
- [ ] 4. I cannot walk more than 1/4 mile without increasing pain.
- [ ] 5. I cannot walk at all without increasing pain.

Section 5—Sitting
- [ ] 0. I can sit in any chair as long as I like.
- [ ] 1. I can sit only in my favorite chair as long as I like.
- [ ] 2. Pain prevents me from sitting more than 1 hour.
- [ ] 3. Pain prevents me from sitting more than 1/2 hour.
- [ ] 4. Pain prevents me from sitting for more than 10 minutes.
- [ ] 5. I avoid sitting because it increases pain immediately.

Section 6—Standing
- [ ] 0. I can stand as long as I want without pain.
- [ ] 1. I have some pain on standing but it does not increase with time.
- [ ] 2. I cannot stand for longer than 1 hour without increasing pain.
- [ ] 3. I cannot stand for longer than 1/2 hour without increasing pain.
- [ ] 4. I cannot stand for longer than 10 minutes without increasing pain.
- [ ] 5. I avoid standing because it increases the pain immediately.

Section 7—Sleeping
- [ ] 0. I get no pain in bed.
- [ ] 1. I get pain in bed but it does not prevent me from sleeping well.
- [ ] 2. Because of pain my normal nights sleep is reduced by less than 1/4.
- [ ] 3. Because of pain my normal nights sleep is reduced by less than 1/2.
- [ ] 4. Because of pain my normal nights sleep is reduced by less than 3/4.
- [ ] 5. Pain prevents me from sleeping at all.

Section 8—Social Life
- [ ] 0. My social life is normal and gives me no pain.
- [ ] 1. My social life is normal but increases the degree of pain.
- [ ] 2. Pain has no significant effect on my social life apart from limiting my more energetic interests, e.g., dancing, etc.
- [ ] 3. Pain has restricted my social life and I do not go out very often.
- [ ] 4. Pain has restricted my social life to my home.
- [ ] 5. I have hardly any social life because of the pain.

Section 9—Traveling
- [ ] 0. I get no pain when traveling.
- [ ] 1. I get some pain when traveling but none of my usual forms of travel make it any worse.
- [ ] 2. I get extra pain while traveling but it does not compel me to seek alternative forms of travel.
- [ ] 3. Pain restricts me to short necessary journeys under 30 minutes.
- [ ] 4. Pain restricts all forms of travel.
- [ ] 5. Pain prevents all forms of travel except that done lying down.

Section 10—Changing Degree of Pain
- [ ] 0. My pain is rapidly getting better.
- [ ] 1. My pain fluctuates but overall is definitely getting better.
- [ ] 2. My pain seems to be getting better but improvement is slow.
- [ ] 3. My pain is neither getting better nor worse.
- [ ] 4. My pain is gradually worsening.
- [ ] 5. My pain is rapidly worsening.

A

Fig. 3-5 Pain questionnaires. Patients are asked to answer questions on the way in which the pain or problem is affecting their activities of daily living. Examples shown are **A**, the Oswestry Low Back Pain Disability Questionnaire.   *Continued*

Neck Disability Index

Name_____ Date_____ / _____ / _____ File #_____

Instructions: Please circle the ONE NUMBER in each section which most closely describes your problem.

Section 1—Pain Intensity

0. I have no pain at the moment.
1. The pain is very mild at the moment.
2. The pain is moderate at the moment.
3. The pain is fairly severe at the moment.
4. The pain is very severe at the moment.
5. The pain is the worst imaginable at the moment.

Section 2—Personal Care (Washing, Dressing, etc.)

0. I can look after myself normally without causing extra pain.
1. I can look after myself normally but it causes extra pain.
2. It is painful to look after myself and I am slow and careful.
3. I need some help but manage most of my personal care.
4. I need help every day in most aspects of self care.
5. I do not get dressed, I wash with difficulty and stay in bed.

Section 3—Lifting

0. I can lift heavy weights without extra pain.
1. I can lift heavy weights but it gives extra pain.
2. Pain prevents me from lifting heavy weights off the floor, but I can manage if they are conveniently positioned, for example on a table.
3. Pain prevents me lifting heavy weights, but I can manage light to medium weights if they are conveniently positioned.
4. I can lift very light weights.
5. I cannot lift or carry anything at all.

Section 4—Reading

0. I can read as much as I want with no pain in my neck.
1. I can read as much as I want with slight pain in my neck.
2. I can read as much as I want with moderate pain in my neck.
3. I can't read as much as I want because of moderate pain in my neck.
4. I can hardly read at all because of severe pain in my neck.
5. I cannot read at all.

Section 5—Headaches

0. I have no headaches at all.
1. I have slight headaches which come infrequently.
2. I have moderate headaches which come infrequently.
3. I have moderate headaches which come frequently.
4. I have severe headaches which come frequently.
5. I have headaches almost all the time.

Score [   ]

Section 6—Concentration

0. I can concentrate fully when I want with no difficulty.
1. I can concentrate fully when I want with slight difficulty.
2. I have a fair degree of difficulty in concentrating when I want to.
3. I have a lot of difficulty in concentrating when I want.
4. I have a great deal of difficulty in concentrating when I want.
5. I cannot concentrate at all.

Section 7—Work

0. I can do as much work as I want.
1. I can only do my usual work, but no more.
2. I can do most of my usual work but no more.
3. I cannot do my usual work.
4. I can hardly do any work at all.
5. I can't do any work at all.

Section 8—Driving

0. I can drive my car without any neck pain.
1. I can drive my car as long as I want with slight pain in my neck.
2. I can drive my car as long as I want with moderate pain in my neck.
3. I can't drive my car as long as I want because of moderate pain in my neck.
4. I can hardly drive at all because of severe pain in my neck.
5. I can't drive my car at all.

Section 9—Sleeping

0. I have no trouble sleeping.
1. My sleep is slightly disturbed (less than 1 hr. sleepless).
2. My sleep is mildly disturbed (1-2 hrs. sleepless).
3. My sleep is moderately disturbed (2-3 hrs. sleepless).
4. My sleep is greatly disturbed (3-5 hrs. sleepless).
5. My sleep is completely disturbed (5-7 hrs. sleepless).

Section 10—Recreation

0. I am able to engage in all my recreation activities with no neck pain.
1. I am able to engage in all my recreation activities with some pain in my neck.
2. I am able to engage in most, but not all, of my recreation activities because of pain in my neck.
3. I am able to engage in only a few of my usual recreation activities because of pain in my neck.
4. I can hardly do any recreation activities because of pain in my neck.
5. I can't do any recreation activities at all.

B

Fig. 3-5, cont'd B, Neck Disability Questionnaire. Other pain questionnaires include the Roland-Morris questionnaire and the Sickness Impact Profile. (*A, Modified from Fairbanks JCT, Davies JB, Mboat JC, Eisenstein S, O'Brian JP. The Oswestry low back pain disability questionnaire. Physiotherapy. 1980;66:13; B, From Vernon H. The neck disability index: a study of reliability and validity. J Manipulative Physiol Ther. 1991;14(7):409.*)

apparently mechanical nature the chiropractic examination process emphasizes the assessment of the joint systems and their relationship to the nervous system. This process must employ all reliable evaluative procedures to identify musculoskeletal derangements that may be impairing the normal function of the nervous system.

Although chiropractic and other physicians have shown increased attention in recent years to quantitative evaluation of the reliability of joint examination procedures, this area of investigation is still considered embryonic.[48] The available literature on the reliability of evaluative procedures for manipulative lesions identifies great variation in the evaluative tools used. Reliability studies for spinal segmental changes have included visual observation[49]; static (misalignment) palpation[50,51]; osseous and soft tissue pain[52-54]; motion, movement, and percussive palpation[50,52-62]; instrument measurements[54,63,64]; soft tissue texture changes[52,61]; static and stress radiograph changes[65-69]; and leg-length evaluation.[64,70] Most of the reliability studies have been performed on single evaluative tools, implying that single evaluative tools are employed in clinical practice. However, clinical experience indicates that doctors frequently employ an informal system of combined clinical indicators to decide on those joints in greatest need of intervention.[48] The use of multiple evaluative approaches to spinal assessment has been suggested and is highly recommended.[71]

Because the human body, particularly the neuromusculoskeletal system, is complex, the use of an evaluative system that combines clinical indicators to decide which joints are in greatest need of intervention is appropriate. No single evaluative procedure should be relied on to make clinical decisions. The structural evaluation of the spinal column should be viewed in terms of a multidimensional index of segmental abnormality. Using the acronym PARTS, the five diagnostic criteria for spinal dysfunction (subluxation) are identified as follows[21,72]:

P: Pain and tenderness. The perception of pain and tenderness may be evaluated in terms of location, quality, and intensity. Most primary musculoskeletal disorders manifest initially by a painful response. The patient's description and location of pain are obtained and the location and intensity of tenderness produced by palpation of osseous and soft tissues noted. Pain and tenderness findings are identified by observation, percussion, and palpation (Fig. 3-6, *A, B*). Furthermore, changes in pain intensity can be objectified using Visual Analog Scales (Fig. 3-4), algometers (Fig. 3-6, *C*), pain questionnaires (Fig. 3-5), and so on.

A: Asymmetry. Asymmetric qualities on a sectional or segmental level are noted. The homeostatic processes in the body seek a balance in structure and function. The human body, particularly the frame, is never completely or perfectly symmetric; however, focal changes in symmetry may be clinically significant. Body symmetry is evaluated using postural examination (Figs. 3-7 and 3-8), static palpation (Fig. 3-9), and static radiograph interpretation (Fig. 3-10). This evaluation should include observation of posture and gait, palpation for misalignment of vertebral segments, and evaluation of static plain film radiographs for malposition of vertebral segments.

R: Range-of-motion abnormality. Changes in active, passive, and accessory joint motions are noted. These changes may be identified as an increase or a decrease in mobility. A decrease in motion is a common component of joint dysfunction that should be amenable to manipulation. An increase in segmental motion represents a nonindication to thrusting forms of manipulation. Global range-of-motion changes are measured with goniometers or inclinometers (Fig. 3-11). Segmental range-of-motion abnormalities are identified through motion palpation (Figs. 3-12 to 3-14) and stress radiographs. The mechanical assistance of a moving table section can be used to assess passive joint movement. The advantage of this procedure is adding the assessment of long axis distraction movement in the spinal joints (Fig. 3-15).

T: Tissue tone, texture, temperature abnormality. Changes in the characteristics of contiguous and associated soft tissues, including skin, fascia, muscle, and ligament are noted. These changes are identified through observation, palpation (Fig. 3-6, *D*), instrumentation, and tests for length and strength.

S: Special tests. Those testing procedures that are specific to a technique system can be performed (leg check, arm fossa test, therapy localization, and so on). Additionally, visceral relationships are considered, as well as other testing procedures deemed necessary from previously obtained data.

The findings derived from the PARTS evaluation can be used to determine which areas are in need of an adjustment. The clinical decision as to whether an adjustment will be made, how it should be performed, and where and when it should be applied can be made by determining the area with the most findings from each category. Minimum findings can be established; for example, one from each of the first four categories. This multidimen-

Text continued on p. 65.

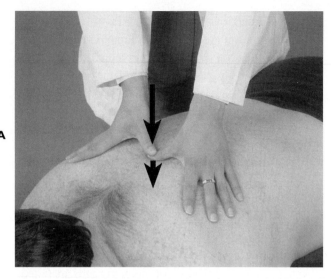

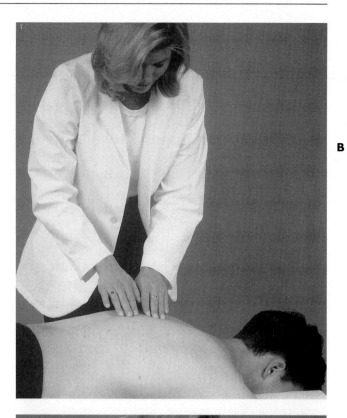

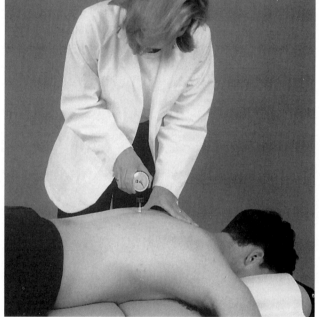

Fig. 3-6 Evaluation for osseous pain and soft tissue change.

A.   Palpatory production of localized pain. Double-thumb percussion of the spinous process applies a posterior to anterior pressure to produce a springing, gliding movement that is normally pain free. With joint dysfunction, pain may be reported and the clinician will feel a different quality of movement. A softer spring may be indicative of an acute, inflammatory problem, whereas a hard quality may indicate a more chronic, fibrotic condition.

B.   Palpatory evaluation for soft tissue tone, texture, and tenderness. Digital palpation of the right thoracic paraspinal muscles (surface temperature can also be evaluated using the dorsum of the hand or a temperature-detection instrument).

C.   Pressure threshold meter (algometer) used for quantitative assessment of osseous and soft tissue tenderness.

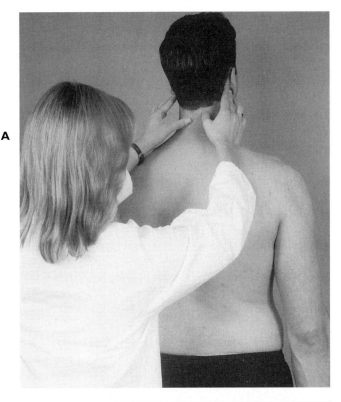

A

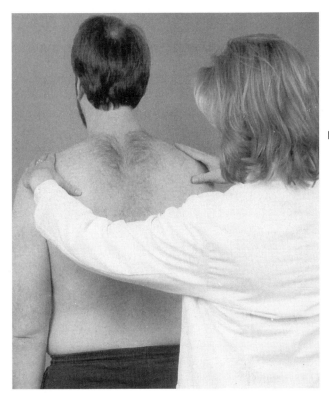

B

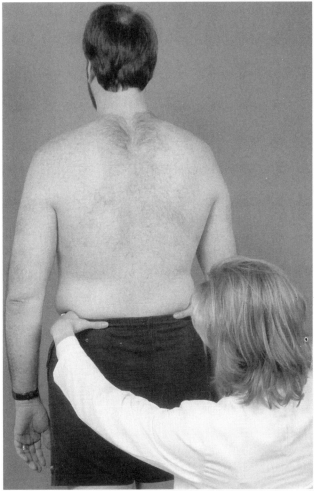

C

Fig. 3-7 Posture examination in the upright, weight-bearing position for sectional or global asymmetry. The clinician observes the patient from the posterior aspect to assess for symmetry.

A. The hands are placed over the mastoid processes to identify head tilt (unleveling) and/or rotation.

B. The hands are placed over the distal aspects of the shoulders to identify upper torso unleveling and/or rotation;

C. The hands are placed over the iliac crests to identify pelvic unleveling and/or rotation.

A

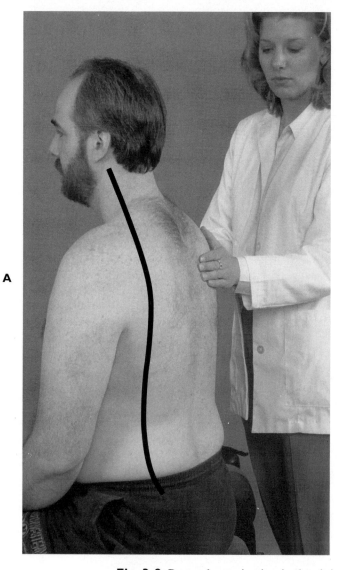 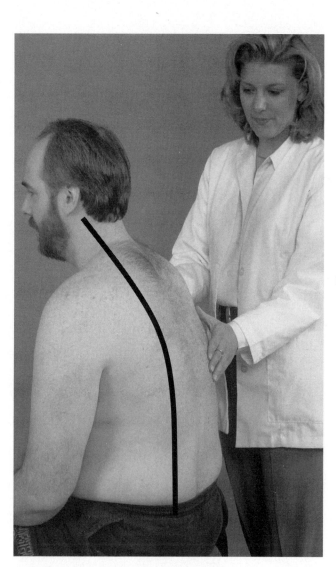

B

Fig. 3-8 Postural examination in the sitting position for sectional or global asymmetry. The clinician observes the patient from the lateral aspect to assess for changes in the anterior-to-posterior curves.

A.   Near-normal curves.

B.   Increased thoracic kyphosis, decreased lumbar lordosis; rounding of shoulders can be visualized.

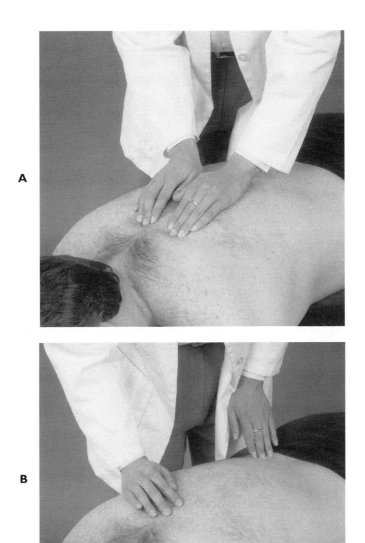

Fig. 3-9 Static palpation for segmental asymmetry; clinician palpates osseous landmarks, comparing one vertebral segment to the ones above and below.

A. Palpation of the transverse processes in the thoracic spine to identify rotation (prominence of one TP posteriorly) and lateral flexion malposition (one TP more superior).

B. Palpation of the interspinous spaces for flexion or extension malpositions.

A 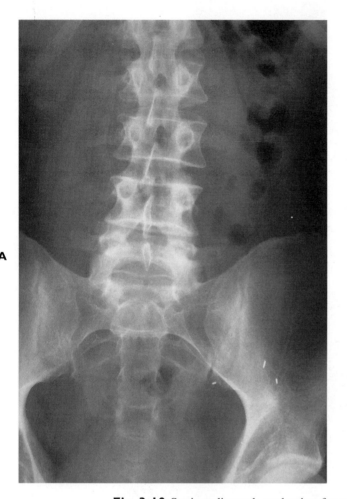 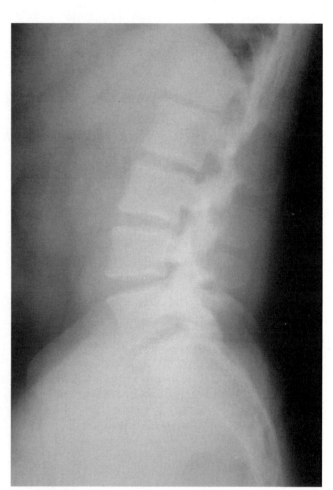 B

Fig. 3-10 Static radiograph evaluation for segmental and sectional asymmetry. A rationale for use of plain film imaging in the chiropractic office is (1) to rule out the presence of pathology that contraindicates manipulative therapy, (2) to identify any anomalies or structural changes that may influence the way an adjustment will be applied, and (3) to obtain static and functional biomechanical relationships that may have clinical relevance to the patient's symptoms or health. Each vertebra is observed for its relationship to the one above and below for rotational and lateral flexion malpositions on the posterior-to-anterior view and for flexion or extension malpositions on the lateral view.

A.   In the anterior-to-posterior view of the lumbar spine a right rotational and right lateral flexion malposition of L4 on L5 can been seen.

B.   In the lateral view of the lumbosacral spine an extension of L4 on L5 can be seen.

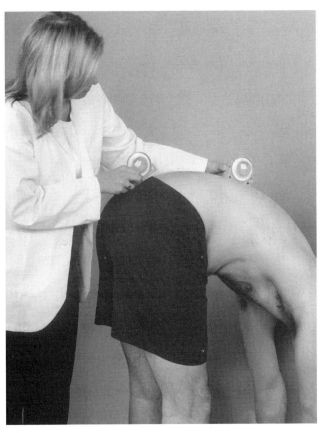

A

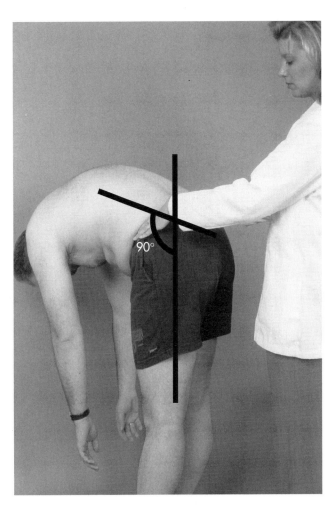

B

Fig. 3-11 Active range of motion. The clinician assesses the patient's ability to move in the rotational degrees of motion, noting the extent of movement and grading any pain that occurs during movement. The feet must be separated sufficiently to serve as a stable base. The amount of movement can be estimated, or duel inclinometers can be used to quantify the movement.

A. Duel inclinometers are used to quantify the amount of lumbar spine flexion.

B. To assess lumbar flexion the clinician asks the patient to bend over to touch the toes without bending the knees. The normal amount of lumbar spine flexion is 90 degrees, though this patient is capable of only 75 to 80 degrees.

Continued

C

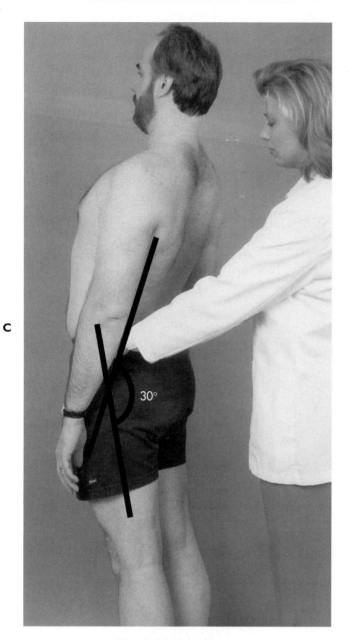

D

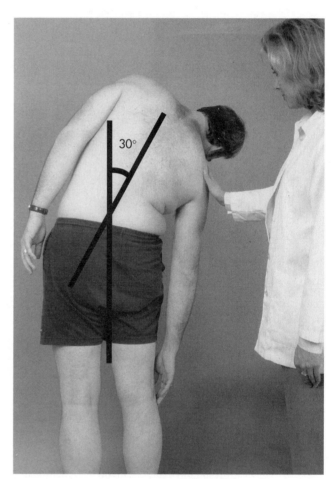

Fig. 3-11, cont'd

C. Lumbar extension is assessed by asking the patient bend backward as far as possible. The clinician stabilizes the pelvis by holding both iliac crests or by placing a hand over the sacrum to serve as a fulcrum. The normal amount of lumbar spine extension is 30 degrees.

D. To assess lumbar lateral flexion the clinician asks the patient to bend to one side as far as possible without lifting the opposite-side foot off the ground. This movement is then repeated to other side. The normal amount of lateral flexion to each side is 30 degrees.

Continued

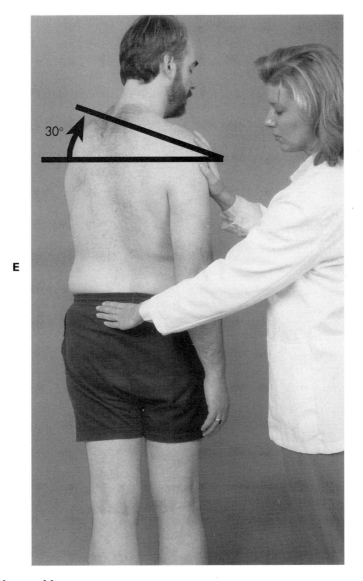

Fig. 3-11, cont'd

E.   To assess lumbar rotation the clinician asks the patient to turn to one side as far as possible. This movement is then repeated to other side. The normal amount of rotation to each side is 30 degrees.

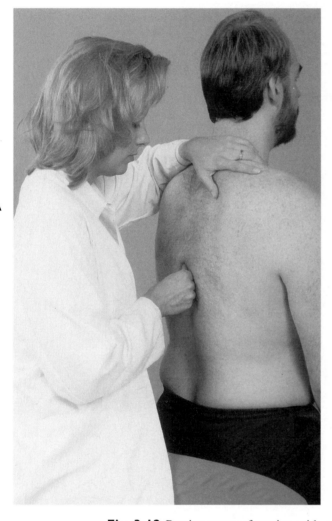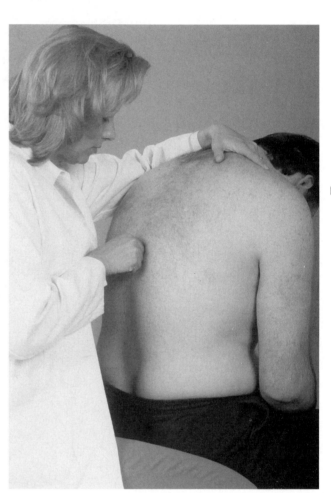

A

B

Fig. 3-12 Passive range of motion with overpressure to determine the presence of the accessory movement of end-play.

A.   Starting position with patient sitting upright, clinician grasping shoulder for directing the movement desired.

B.   The patient is prestressed in flexion; overpressure is applied to the spinous process to assess for springing end-feel in flexion.

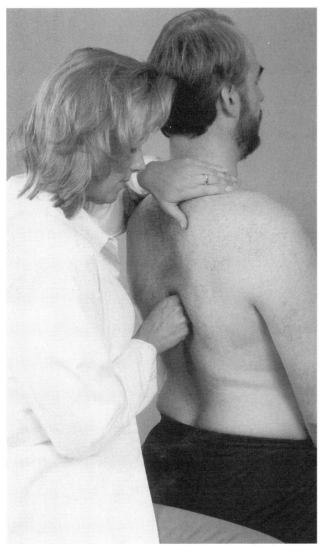

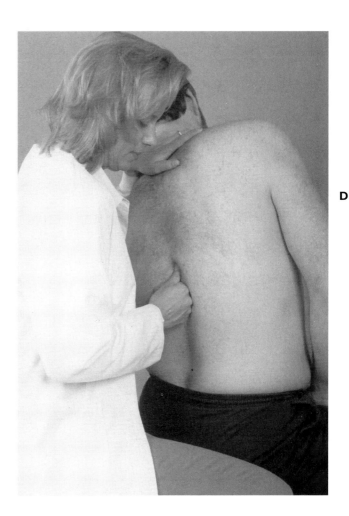

Fig. 3-12, cont'd

C.   The patient is prestressed in extension; overpressure is applied to the spinous process to assess for springing end-feel in extension.

D.   The patient is prestressed in left lateral flexion; overpressure is applied to the spinous process to assess for springing end-feel in left lateral flexion.

Continued

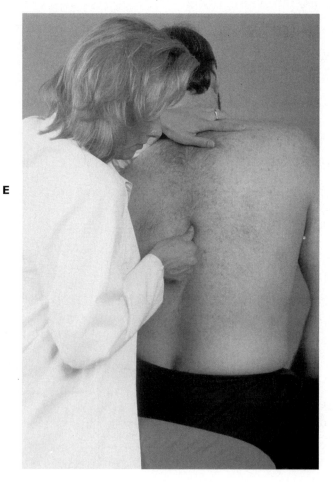

E

Fig. 3-12, cont'd
E.   The patient is prestressed in rotation; overpressure is applied to the spinous process
     to assess for springing end-feel in rotation (an alternative point of contact is the lat-
     eral process—AP, TP, MP).

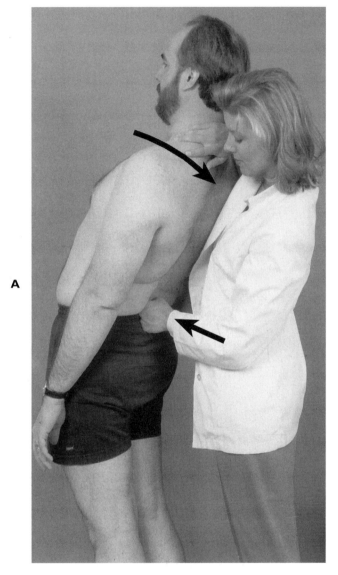

Fig. 3-13 Combined active and passive movements.

A.   The patient is asked to actively extend as the clinician applies overpressure in extension to determine whether pain is produced, taking note if the pain is centralized or peripheralized. Peripheralization of the pain is a nonindication for the use of that position with manual therapy procedures.   *Continued*

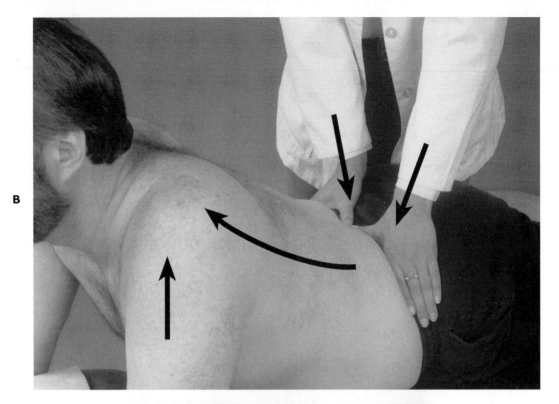

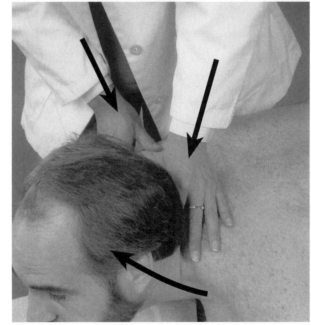

Fig. 3-13, cont'd

B.   In the prone position, the patient is asked to push up into extension while the clinician applies posterior-to-anterior overpressure, keeping the patient's pelvis on the table, to determine whether pain is produced. The clinician notes if pain is centralized or peripheralized. Peripheralization of the pain is a nonindication for the use of that position with manual therapy procedures.

C.   In the prone position, the patient is asked to raise the head up into extension while the clinician applies overpressure to the lower cervical spine, keeping the shoulders on the table, to determine whether pain is produced. The clinician notes if pain is centralized or peripheralized. Peripheralization of the pain is a nonindication for the use of that position with manual therapy procedures.

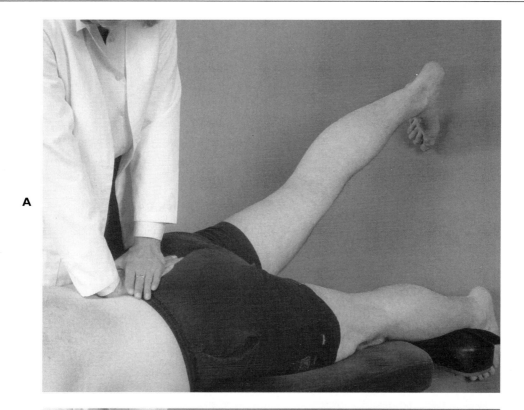

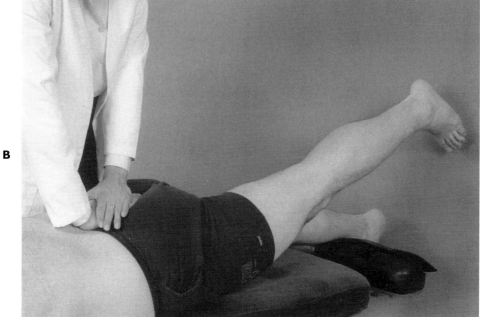

Fig. 3-14 In the prone position, the patient is asked to raise one leg and then the other while the clinician applies posterior-to-anterior pressure against the sacrum to keep the pelvis on the table.

A.   The side that rises higher is the relatively anterior innominate side.

B.   The side that does not rise as high is the relatively posterior innominate side.

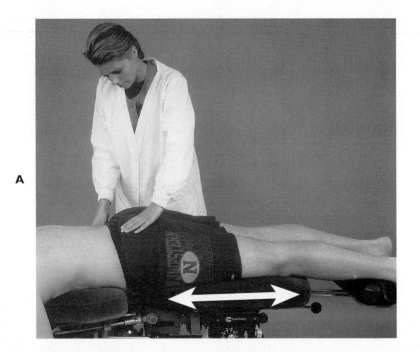

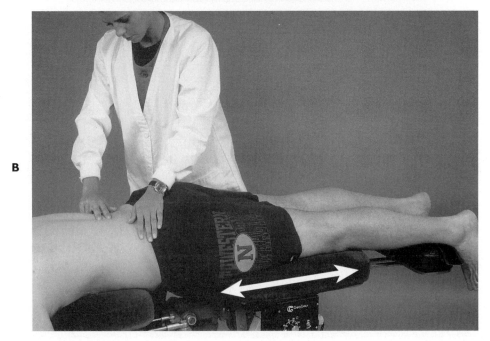

Fig. 3-15 Motion (mechanically) assisted palpation (MAP). A table that produces linear distraction can be used to assess long axis distraction (y-axis translation) in the following areas:

A.   Sacroiliac articulation: The clinician's hands are placed over the sacroiliac articulations, contacting the PSISs and sacral base to identify separation movement as the pelvic section of the table distracts.

B.   Lumbar spine: The clinician's fingers are placed over two spinous processes to identify passive separation movement of the lumbar segments as the pelvic section distracts.

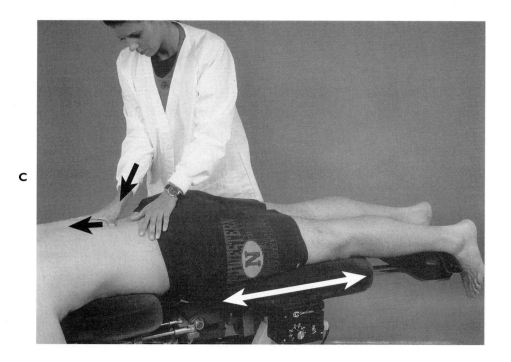

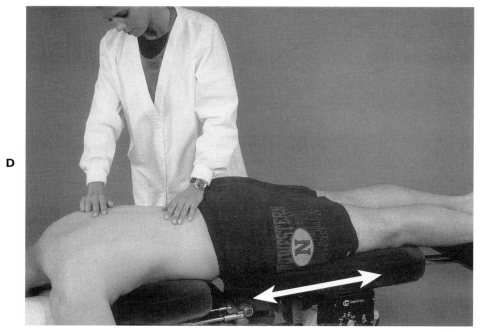

Fig. 3-15, cont'd

C. Long-axis end-play of the lumbar motion segments can also be assessed by placing a thumb at the inferior aspect of the superior vertebra of the motion segment and applying an inferior-to-superior overpressure as the pelvic section of the table moves caudally.

D. Thoracic spine: The clinician's fingers are placed over two spinous processes to identify passive separation movement of the thoracic segments as the pelvic section distracts.

Continued

E

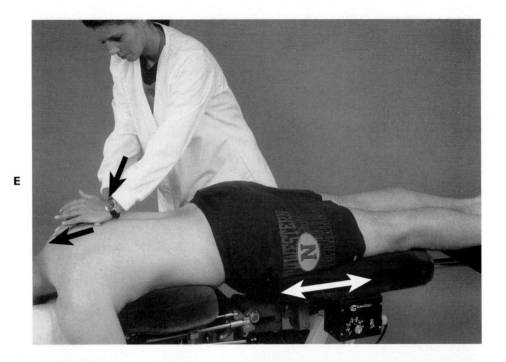

F

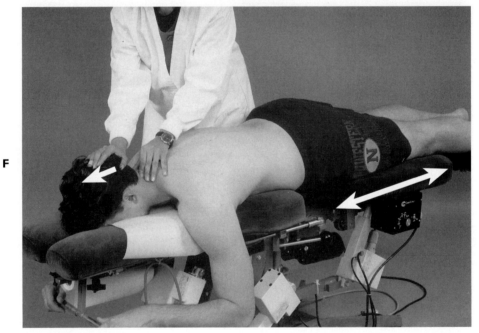

Fig. 3-15, cont'd

E.   Long-axis end-play of the thoracic segments can also be assessed by placing a thumb at the inferior aspect of the superior vertebra of the motion segment and applying an inferior-to-superior overpressure as the pelvic section of the table moves caudally.

F.   Cervical spine: The clinician's cephalad hand stabilizes the occiput while digital contacts of the caudal hand are placed over the posterior aspects of the articular pillars to identify passive separation movement of the cervical segments as the pelvic section distracts.

sional examination procedure can be used with any technique applications. It is used to assess joint function leading to the application of mechanically assisted distraction and motion assisted thrust techniques described in later chapters.

If the examination is inadequate and fails to reveal the source or the extent of the problem, treatment cannot be maximally effective. The use of joint assessment procedures should be part of a critical, continual assessment of the patient to monitor the effects of care. Perceiving when to stop is as important as knowing how to start and recognizing whether to continue. Even if a complete and thorough examination can be completed during the first visit, signs and certainly symptoms must be rechecked during the course of treatment to determine the extent of patient progress. This ongoing evaluation and assessment forms the basis for treatment modification and is a key factor in total patient management. The initial examination, no matter how thorough, cannot be expected to provide all the answers. A treatment trial should be instituted and its effects assessed to determine whether it should be continued or a different plan devised. The examination forms the foundation for treatment, guiding the practitioner in selecting appropriate treatment techniques, frequency, and course. If clinicians were to standardize their evaluations, comparisons of treatment effectiveness and efficiency could be performed.

REFERENCES

1. Bergmann TF. Various forms of chiropractic technique. *Chiropr Tech.* 1993;5(2):53-55.
2. Bergmann TF. Short lever, specific contact articular chiropractic technique. *J Manipulative Physiol Ther.* 1992;15:591-595.
3. Keating JC. Traditional barriers to standards of knowledge production in chiropractic. *Chiropr Tech.* 1990;2(3):78-85.
4. Peterson DH, Bergmann TF. Joint assessment principles and procedures. In: Bergmann TF, Peterson DH, Lawrence DJ, eds. *Chiropractic Technique.* New York: Churchill Livingstone; 1993.
5. Twomey LT. A rationale for the treatment of back pain and joint pain by manual therapy. *Phys Ther.* 1992;72:885-892.
6. Rahlmann JF. Mechanisms of intervertebral joint fixation: a literature review. *J Manipulative Physiol Ther.* 1987;10:177-187.
7. Lamb DW. A review of manual therapy for spinal pain. In: Grieve G, ed. *Modern Manual Therapy.* 2nd ed. Edinburgh: Churchill Livingstone; 1994.
8. Gatterman MI. Indications for spinal manipulation in the treatment of back pain. *ACA J Chiropr.* 1982;19(10):51-66.
9. Bogduk N, Jull G. The theoretical pathology of acute locked back: a basis for manipulative therapy. *J Manual Med.* 1985;1:78-82.
10. Cyriax J. *Textbook of Orthopedic Medicine.* 9th ed. London: Ballier Tindall; 1974; 2.
11. Vanharanta H, Sachs BL, Spivey MA et al. The relationship of pain provocation to lumbar disc deterioration as seen by CT discography. *Spine.* 1987;12:295-298.
12. Roston JB, Wheeler-Haines RW. Cracking in the metacarpophalangeal joint. *J Anat.* 1947;81:165.

13. Unsworth A, Dowson D, Wright V. Cracking joints, a bio-engineering study of cavitation in the metacarpophalangeal joint. *Ann Rheum Dis.* 1971;30:348.

14. Akeson WH, Amiel D, Woo S. Immobility effects of synovial joints: the biomechanics of joint contracture. *Biorheology.* 980;17:95.

15. Akeson WH, Amiel D, Mechanic GL, Woos, Harwood FL, Hamer ML. Collagen cross-linking alterations in joint contractures: changes in reducible cross-links in periarticular connective tissue collagen after nine weeks of immobilization. *Connect Tissue Res.* 1977;5:5.

16. Burger AA. Experimental neuromuscular models of spinal manual techniques. *Manual Med.* 1983;1:10.

17. Akeson WH, Amel D, Woo SLY. Cartilage and ligament: physiology and repair processes. In: Nicholas JA, Hershman EB, eds. *The Lower Extremity and Spine in Sports Medicine.* St Louis: Mosby; 1995.

18. Evans EV, Eggers GWN, Butler JK et al. Experimental immobilization and remobilization of rat knee joints. *J Bone Joint Surg.* 1960;42a:737-758.

19. Dahners LE. Ligament contraction: a correlation with cellularity and actin staining. *Trans Orthop Res Soc.* 1986;11:56.

20. White AA, Panjabi MM. *Clinical Biomechanics of the Spine.* 2nd ed. Philadelphia: JB Lippincott; 1990.

21. Bergmann TF, Peterson DH, Lawrence DJ. *Chiropractic Technique.* New York: Churchill Livingstone; 1993.

22. Wyke BD. Articular neurology and manipulative therapy. In: Glasgow EF, Twomey LT, Schull ER, Kleynhans AM, eds. *Aspects of Manipulative Therapy.* New York: Churchill Livingstone; 1985.

23. Terrett ACJ, Vernon H. Manipulation and pain tolerance. *Am J Phys Med.* 1984;63(5):217-225.

24. Vernon HT, Dhami MSI. Spinal manipulation and beta-endorphin: a controlled study of the effect of a spinal manipulation on plasma beta-endorphin levels in normal males. *J Manipulative Physiol Ther.* 1986;9(2):115-123.

25. Vernon HT. Pressure pain threshold evaluation of the effect of spinal manipulation on chronic neck pain: a single case study. *JCCA.* 1988;32(4):191-194.

26. Tran TA, Kirby JD. The effectiveness of upper cervical adjustment upon the normal physiology of the heart. *ACA J Chiropr.* 1977;11:58-62.

27. Sato A, Swenson RS. Sympathetic nervous system response to mechanical stress of the spinal column in rats. *J Manipulative Physiol Ther.* 1984;7(3):141-147.

28. Briggs L, Boone WR. Effects of a chiropractic adjustment on changes in pupillary diameter: a model for evaluating somatovisceral response. *J Manipulative Physiol Ther.* 1988;11(3):181-189.

29. Lewit K. *Manipulative Therapy in Rehabilitation of the Motor System.* London: Butterworths; 1985.

30. Mitchell FL. Elements of muscle energy technique. In: Basmajian JV, Nyberg R, eds. *Rational Manual Therapies.* Baltimore: Williams & Wilkins; 1993.

31. Paris SV. Spinal manipulative therapy. *Clin Orthop.* 1983;179:55-61.

32. Haldeman S. Spinal manipulative therapy and sports medicine. *Clin Sports Med.* 1986;5(2):277-293.

33. Greenman P. *Principles of Manual Medicine.* Baltimore: Williams & Wilkins; 1989.

34. Gatterman MI, Hansen D. Development of chiropractic nomenclature through consensus. *J Manipulative Physiol Ther.* 1994;17:302-309.

35. Triano JJ. Studies on the biomechanical effect of a spinal adjustment. *J Manipulative Physiol Ther.* 1992;15:71-75.

36. Nachemson A. A critical look at the treatment for low back pain. *Scand J Rehabil Med.* 1979;11:143-147.

37. Sandoz R. Some physical mechanisms and effects of spinal adjustments. *Ann Swiss Chiropr Assoc.* 1976; 6:91.

38. Hoag JM, Cole BW, Bradford SG. *Osteopathic Medicine.* New York: McGraw-Hill Book Co; 1969.

39. Bergmann TF. Short/long lever, nonspecific contact, articular chiropractic technique: a review of the literature. *Chiropr Tech.* 1993;5(3):107-110.

40. Grice AS. Biomechanical approach to cervical and dorsal adjusting. In: Haldman S, ed. *Modern Developments in the Principles and Practice of Chiropractic.* New York: Appleton-Century-Cross; 1980.

41. Haldeman S. Spinal manipulative therapy: a status report. *Clin Orthop.* 1993;179:62-70.

42. Grice A, Vernon H. Basic principles in the performance of chiropractic adjusting. In: Haldeman S, ed. *Principles and Practice of Chiropractic.* 2nd ed. Norwalk, Conn: Appleton & Lange; 1992:443-458.

43. Kappler RE. Direct action techniques. *J Am Osteopath Assoc.* 1981;8(4):239-243.

44. Mennell JM. *The Musculoskeletal System: Differential Diagnosis from Symptoms and Physical Signs.* Gaithersburg, Md: Aspen; 1992;23.

45. Gatterman MI. *Chiropractic Management of Spine-Related Disorders.* Baltimore: Williams & Wilkins; 1990.

46. Evans RC. *Illustrated Essential in Orthopedic Physical Assessment.* St Louis: Mosby; 1994.

47. Ferezy JS. *The Chiropractic Neurological Examination* Gaithersburg, Md: Aspen; 1992.

48. Keating JC, Bergmann TF, Jacobs GE, Finer BA, Larson K. Interexaminer reliability of eight evaluative dimensions of lumbar segmental dysfunction. *J Manipulative Physiol Ther.* 1990;13(8):463.

49. Kappler RE. A comparison of structural examination findings obtained by experienced physician examiners and student examiners on hospital patients. *J Am Osteopath Assoc.* 1980;79:468-471.

50. Aldridge J, Codieux J, Marsh D. *Motion Palpation: Static Palpation—A Comparative Study.* Toronto: Canadian Memorial Chiropractic College; 1975. Thesis.

51. Johnston WL. The role of static and motion palpation in structural diagnosis. *J Am Osteopath Assoc.* 1975;75:421-424.

52. Boline PD, Keating JC, Brist J, Denver G. Interexaminer reliability of palpatory evaluations of the lumbar spine. *Am J Chiropr Med.* 1988;1(1):5-11.

53. DeBoer KF, Harmon R, Tuttle CD, Wallace H. Reliability study of detection of somatic dysfunction in the cervical spine. *J Manipulative Physiol Ther.* 1985;8:9-16.

54. Terrett ACJ, Vernon H. Manipulation and pain tolerance: a controlled study of the effect of spinal manipulation on paraspinal cutaneous pain levels. *Am J Phys Med.* 1984;63:217-225.

55. Dombrowsky N, Dunn G, Millar D. Correlation between the motion palpation of three graduating chiropractic students. Toronto: Canadian Memorial Chiropractic College; 1976. Thesis.

56. LeMoel B, Chadwick G, Goldman C, Spring J, Putnam R. An appraisal of the efficacy of movement palpation. Toronto: Canadian Memorial Chiropractic College; 1976. Thesis.

57. Love RM, Brodeur RR. Inter- and intra-examiner reliability of motion palpation for the thoracolumbar spine. *J Manipulative Physiol Ther.* 1987;10:1-4.

58. Mootz RD, Keating JC, Kuntz HP, Milus TB, Jacobs GE. Inter- and intra-examiner reliability of passive motion palpation of the lumbar spine. *J Manipulative Physiol Ther.* 1989;12(6):440-445.

59. Wiles MR. Reproducibility and interexaminer correlation of motion palpation findings of the sacroiliac joints. *J Can Chiropr Assoc.* 1980;24:59-68.

60. Gonella C, Paris S, Kutner M. Reliability in evaluating passive intervertebral motion. *Phys Ther.* 1982;62:436-444.

61. Johnston WL, Allan BR, Hendra JL et al. Interexaminer study of palpation in detecting location of spinal segmental dysfunction. *J Am Osteopath Assoc.* 1983;82:839-845.

62. Mior SA, King RS, McGregor M, Bernard M. Intra- and inter-examiner reliability of motion palpation of the cervical spine. *J Can Chiropr Assoc.* 1985;19:195-198.

63. Brunarski DJ. Chiropractic biomechanical evaluations; validity in myofascial low back pain. *J Manipulative Physiol Ther.* 1982;7:243-249.

64. Addington ER. Reliability and objectivity of the anatometer, supine leg length test, thermoscribe II, and the derm-therm-o-graph measurements. *Upper Cervical Monographs.* 1983; 3:8-11.

65. Deyo R, McNiesh LM, Cone RO et al. Observer variability in the interpretation of lumbar spine radiography. *Arthritis Rheum.* 1985;28(9):1066-1070.

66. Antos JC, Robinson K, Keating JC, Jacobs GE. Interrater reliability of fluoroscopic detection of fixation in the mid-cervical spine. *Chiropr Tech.* 1990;2(2)53-55.

67. Taylor JAM. Full spine radiology: a review. In: Proceedings 7th Annual Conference on Research and Education; 1992. Palm Springs, Calif. *J Manipulative Physiol Ther.* 1993;16(7):460-474.

68. Mick TJ. The use of functional radiographs in diagnosis: a review of the literature. In: Proceedings 7th Annual Conference on Research and Education; 1992; Palm Springs, Calif. *J Manipulative Physiol Ther.* 1993;16(7):460-474.

69. Phillips R. Plain film radiology in chiropractic. *J Manipulative Physiol Ther.* 1992;15:47-50.

70. Fuhr AW, Osterbauer PJ. Interexaminer reliability of relative leg-length evaluations in the prone, extended position. *Chiropr Tech.* 19891:13-18.

71. Faucret B, Mao W, Nakagawa T, Spurgin D, Tran T. Determination of bony subluxations by clinical, neurological and chiropractic procedures. *J Manipulative Physiol Ther.* 1980;3:165-176.

72. Bergmann TF. The chiropractic spinal examination. In: Ferezy JS, ed. *The Chiropractic Neurological Examination.* Gaithersburg, Md: Aspen; 1992.

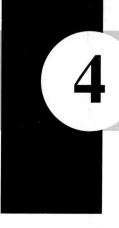

Traction-Distraction Techniques for the Trunk

INTRODUCTION TO MECHANICALLY ASSISTED TECHNIQUES

Presently, there is an interest in the approach of distraction as it is applied to the spine by manual adjusters/manipulators. A specific topic of interest is distraction as applied by chiropractors who use the flexion-distraction method developed by Cox and based on the work of McManis from the early part of this century. This chapter describes the foundation of the techniques developed by allopaths (Cyriax) and osteopaths (McManis) and discusses application of the major flexion-distraction techniques used by chiropractors. The techniques of Cox, Leander, and Hill and the essentials of application as presently understood, are explored in this chapter. Motion-assisted distraction (MAD), a new approach that builds on the earlier work of McManis, Cox, Markey, Leander, Hill, and Jensen, is presented. Motion-assisted thrust technique (MATT) is discussed in Chapter 6.

THE CONCEPT

The practice of manipulation continues to evolve, primarily through the work of chiropractors. Several approaches to manipulation are presently being developed. These approaches are departures from the more traditional short-lever, high-velocity, low-amplitude maneuvers and require the use of special equipment. Manipulation using assistive devices has been performed since the time of Hippocrates, who used the "traction machine" and the spinal lever assist. The flexion-distraction tables and Cox's technique are a refinement of the Hippocrates table and technique (as far as we can derive from history). Other devices that assist in the delivery of the thrust or manipulation include the mechanical assists (drop piece mechanism) of Thompson (Fig. 4-1, A) and a mechanical device, the Activator Adjusting Instrument, developed by Lee and

Fuhr (Fig. 4-1, B). All of these devices are designed to help in the delivery of adjustive treatment.

THE EFFECTS OF TRACTION

The term *traction* refers to the process of pulling one body in relationship to another, which results in separation of two bodies.[1] Traction is passive translational movement of a joint, which occurs at right angles to the plane of the joint between two bones, resulting in separation of the joint surfaces. Kaltenborn[1] grades traction by the three effects it produces. With the first there is no appreciable joint separation, because only enough traction force is applied to nullify the compressive forces acting on the joint. The compressive forces are the result of muscle tension, cohesive forces between articular surfaces, and atmospheric pressure. The second effect produces a tightening in the tissue surrounding the joint that is described as "taking up the slack." The third grade of traction requires more tractive force to produce a stretching effect into the tissues crossing the joint. The principal aim of treatment is restoration of normal, painless range of motion. Grieve[2] identifies a series of treatment goals, adding that the importance of each will vary among clinicians (Box 4-1).

Traction produces measurable separation of vertebral bodies and centripetal forces exerted by the tension applied to surrounding soft tissues.[3] However, traction has other effects as well. Grieve[2] identifies some other effects that are the result of both sustained and rhythmic traction (Box 4-2).

Although traction is mainly used on the lumbar and cervical spine regions, there are descriptions for the application of rhythmic traction to all regions of the spine and extremities. Furthermore, the indications for traction include changes that are common to most synovial joints (Box 4-3).

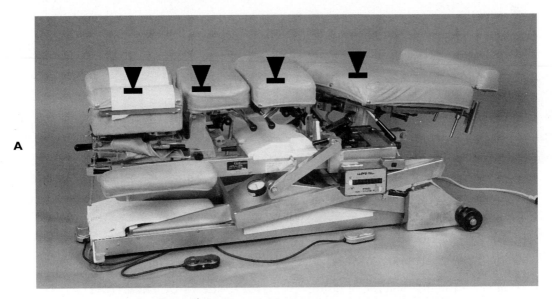

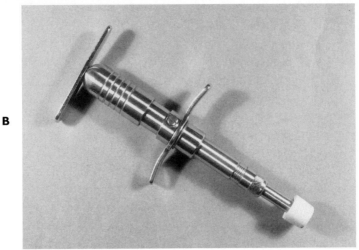

Fig. 4-1 **A,** Table with drop mechanism. **B,** Activator Adjusting Instrument.

Traction is not a unique and separate form of treatment but is simply one form of passive mobilization.[4] Traction can be varied in many ways; almost any form of passive handling may be used with some form of oscillation or as a static hold. Therefore a longitudinal movement may be performed as an oscillatory mobilization, as a slow rhythmic stretch, or as a static traction. Traction may be manual or mechanical, static or rhythmic, or fast or slow; the force applied may be strong or gentle, and it may be applied symmetrically or asymmetrically. These variations must be explored to determine which combination is most appropriate for the patient's needs and the clinician's abilities. The effects of traction are not necessarily localized but may be made more specific by careful positioning.

Maximization of the effect at any degenerative levels will occur, regardless of whether these areas contribute to the patient's current problem. Traction can be a very powerful tool when used with precision. To achieve maximum success in the minimum amount of time, the patient must be positioned accurately, the minimum effective force must be used, and each patient's treatment must be based on the signs and symptoms rather than the diagnosis.

THE MAJOR TECHNIQUES

Mechanically assisted distraction (MEAD) is the nonmotorized form of distraction manipulation represented by techniques such as McManis and Cox (flexion-distraction). Motion-assisted distraction (MAD) techniques were developed by Leander (continuous passive motion [CPM]), Thomas Hill (gravity-assisted intermittent traction [GAIT]), and Jensen (circumductive CPM). Additionally, there are techniques commonly associated with the allopaths. Each of the techniques described uses a piece of equipment in the manipulation process. For example, the Cox flexion-distraction technique is best performed on what Cox calls an "instrument," the Zenith-Cox table (Box 4-4).

EQUIPMENT USED IN DISTRACTION TECHNIQUES

Several tables can be used to provide distraction; many of these are used with the techniques described in this chapter. Other equipment also is used in providing the positioning and forces necessary to effect a correction in the appropriate part of the body. Some equipment is manual and requires the force to be provided by the practitioner; other equipment provides power assists. The practitioner must consider the amount of force to be used in treatment. This affects both the practitioner and the patient and dictates the type of equipment used in manipulation.

Some of the equipment used for chiropractic treatment may be used with several techniques, such as the Thompson table (a table with drop pieces) and the Cox table (a table with flexion-distraction capabilities). Clinician preference in the instance of distraction may be based on the action of the springs used in the compression of the lower section, which creates the distractive force. Some practitioners prefer a coil spring, whereas others like the action of a leaf spring or a pneumatic device. A clinician can create traction for a short time over a fulcrum, tractioning the lower trunk with a stabilizing force to the lumbar spine and a tractioning force to the lower leg while striving to avoid undue hyperextension of the knee.

Selected examples of the major tables used in the distraction process are diagrammatically represented in Fig. 4-2. Figs. 4-3 through 4-13 identify the tables' capabilities and characteristics. The problem faced by practitioners when selecting a table is that it is difficult to identify the characteristics of each table and to compare capabilities. Table 4-1 illustrates the characteristics of the manipulation tables that perform distraction, noting manual and power assists that are available. The tables are organized by the developer of the technique or the manufacturer of the table. No single piece of equipment used by allopaths for traction is as outstanding as the McManis table used by osteopaths. The only equipment that is similar is the Lind Autotraction device (Fig. 4-14), which depends entirely on the action of the table and the ability of the patient to apply and control the amount of traction. The operator of this device is only indirectly involved in its operation, unlike the chiropractor or osteopath, who is an integral part of the treatment and the function of the table. Another noteworthy approach was developed by Burton.[5] It uses a gravity traction frame that is adjustable in angle and provides a varying amount of traction that is applied through a body harness (Fig. 4-15). This device is being replaced by the LTX 3000 (Fig. 4-16), also used by Burton in treatment and rehabilitation of low back injuries.[5] This device is discussed in Chapter 7. Some manual tables have been designed and redesigned to require much less effort to operate and allow practitioners and patients of most sizes to use them comfortably. However, powered tables with MAD provide the greatest range of low-force (on the part of the clinician) devices available. One advantage of MAD equipment is that the clinician can use both hands to treat the patient, instead of having to use one hand for powering the flexion action of the table. This increases the amount of control possible in the treatment, a plus for the patient, and control of the required power, a plus for the clinician.

■ TABLE 4-1 Characteristics of the Manipulation Tables That Perform Distraction

Table and Manufacturer	MAD	Head Section (α_1)	Thoracic Section (α_2)	Lumbar Section (β_1)	Ankle Support (β_2)	Full Table Tilt (Δ)	Elevation (EL)	Drop Pieces (DP)
		α		β				
McManis (Fig. 4-3)	No	(+/-)	(0)	(+/- lat flx, circum)	No	No	Yes	No
Zenith-Cox: Williams Healthcare Systems (Fig. 4-4)	No	(+/-, lat flx, and rot)	(0)	(+/- lat flx, circum, rot)	Yes	No	Yes	Yes
Leander: Leander Health Tech. Corp. (Fig. 4-5)	Yes (CPM)	(+/-, lat flx)	(-, lat flx)	(+/- rot) (CPM)	Yes	No	Yes	No
Hill Intertrac: Thomas Hill (Fig. 4-6)	Yes	(0)	(0)	(+/-, lat flx)	Yes	Yes	Yes	No
Chattanooga Spinalator (Fig. 4-7)	No	(+/-)	(-)	(+/-, lat flx, rot, circum)	Yes	No	Yes	Yes
Back Specialist: Health Care Mfg. (Fig. 4-8)	No	(+/-)	(-)	(+/-, lat flx, rot, circum)	Yes	No	Yes	No
Hill Air Flex: Hill Laboratories (Fig. 4-9)	No	(+/-)	(-)	(+/-, lat flx, rot, circum)	Yes	No	Yes	Yes
Titan: Titan Tech Int. (Fig. 4-10)	No	(+/-)	(-, lat flx, rot, circum)	(+/-)	Yes	No	Yes	No
Galaxy McManis: Lloyd Table Co. (Fig. 4-11)	No	(+/-)	(-)	(+/-, lat flx, rot, circum)	Yes	No	Yes	Yes
Jensen: Annova (Fig. 4-12)	Yes	(0)	(0) (lat flx)	(circum)	Yes	Yes	No	No
Spinalight: Spinalight Inc. (Fig. 4-13)	Yes	(+/-)	(-)	(+/-, lat flx, rot, circum)	Yes	No	Yes	Yes

Text continued on p. 86

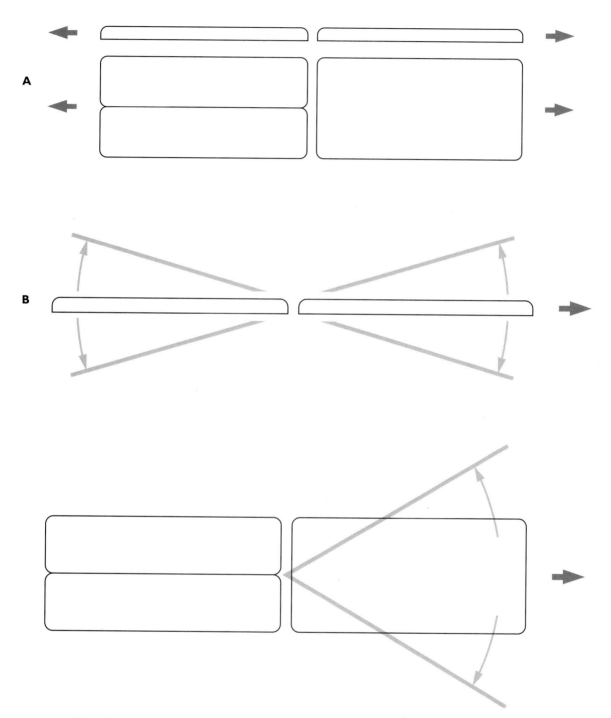

Fig. 4-2 Diagrammatic representation of the major tables. **A,** Allopathic table. **B,** Osteopathic table.

Continued

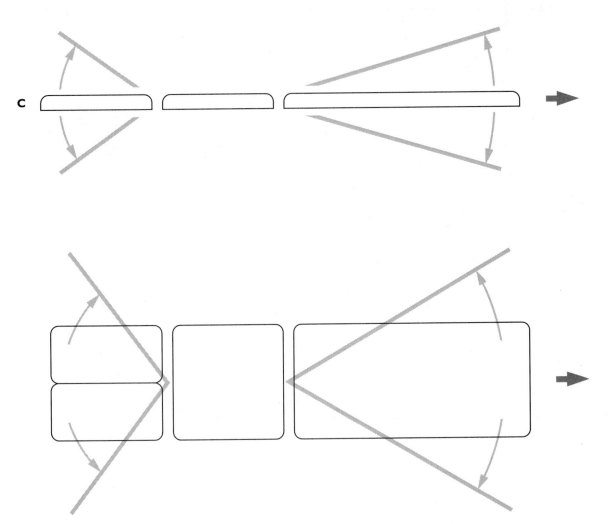

Fig. 4-2, cont'd   C, Cox table.

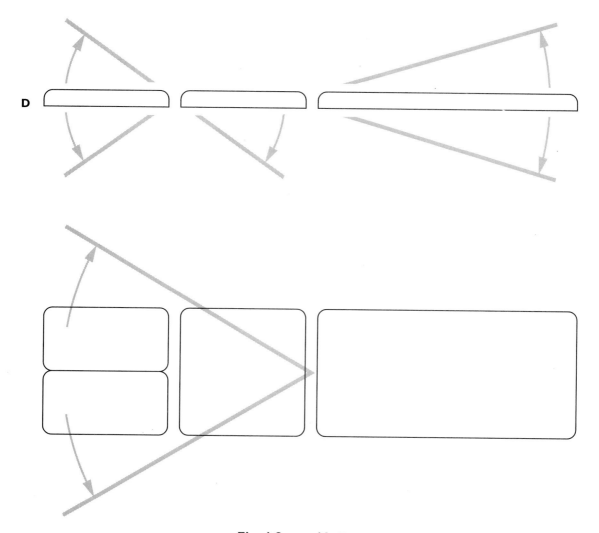

Fig. 4-2, cont'd   **D,** Leander table.

Continued

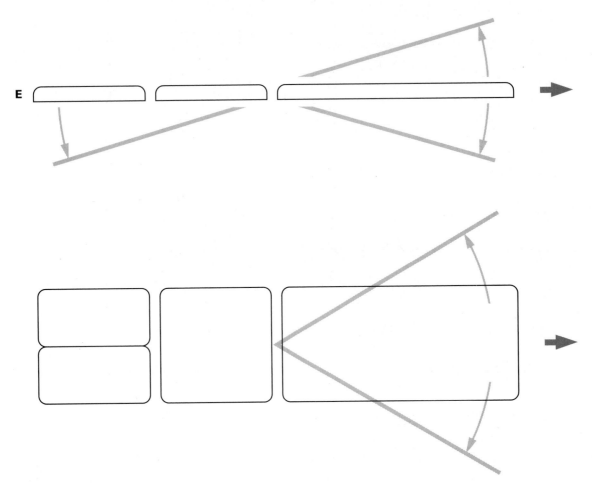

Fig. 4-2, cont'd   **E,** Hill table.

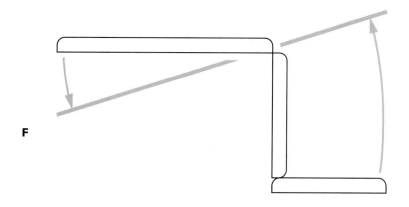

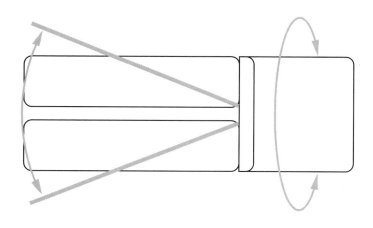

Fig. 4-2, cont'd   **F,** Jensen table.

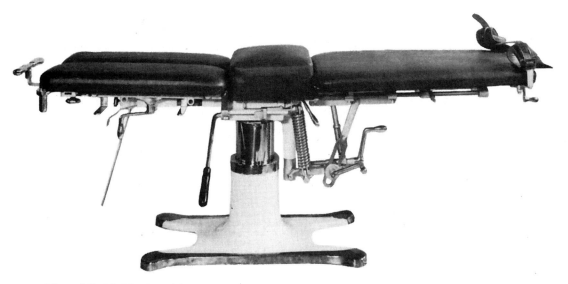

Fig. 4-3 McManis table. *(From McManis JV. McManis Table Technic: Technic Instructions and General Information. Hannibal, Mo: Standard Printing Co; 1938.)*

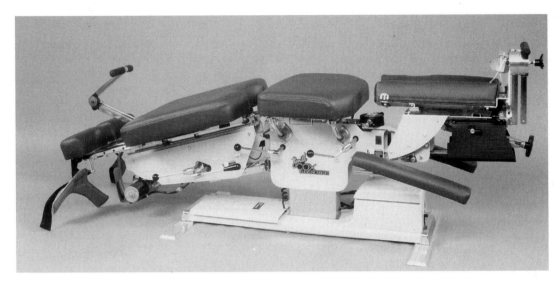

Fig. 4-4 Zenith-Cox table. *(Table by Williams Healthcare Systems, Elgin, Ill.)*

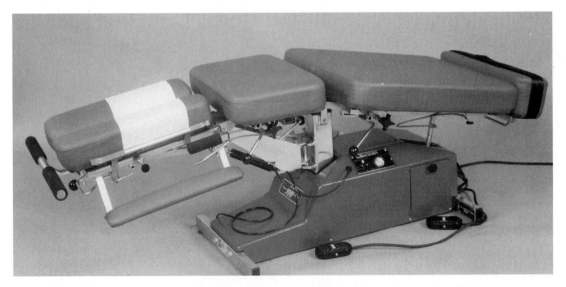

Fig. 4-5 Leander table. *(Table by Leander Health Technologies Corp., Port Orchard, Wash.)*

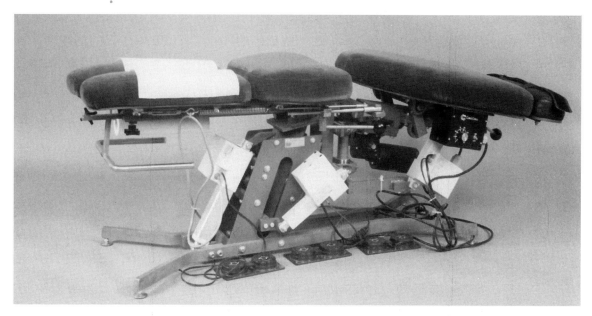

Fig. 4-6 Hill Intertrac table. *(Table by Thomas Hill Tables, Lakefield, Ont.)*

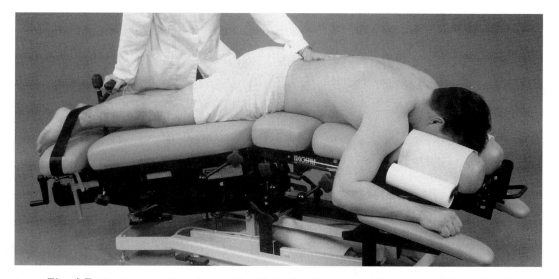

Fig. 4-7 Chattanooga Spinalator table. *(Table by Chattanooga Group, Inc., Hixon, Tenn.)*

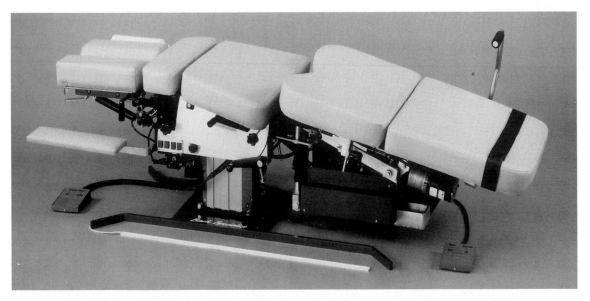

Fig. 4-8 Back Specialist table. *(Table by Health Care Manufacturing, Springfield, Mo.)*

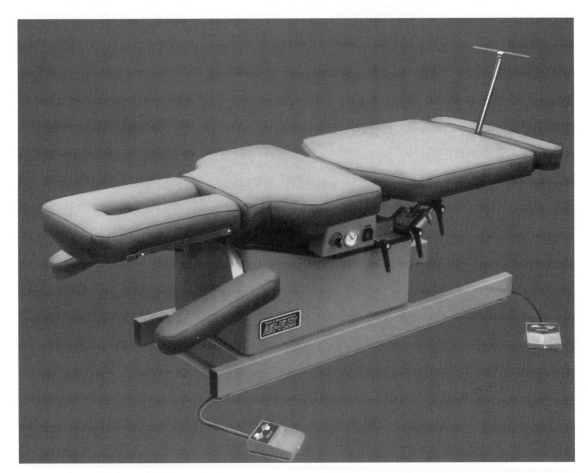

Fig. 4-9 Hill Air Flex table. *(Table by Hill Laboratories Co., Malvern, Pa.)*

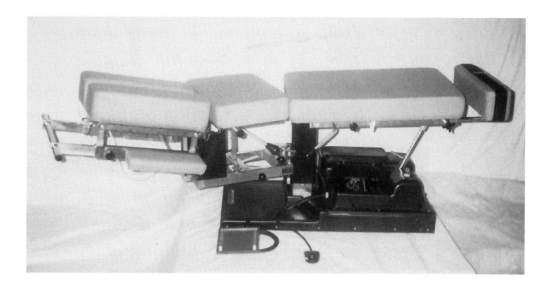

Fig. 4-10 Titan table. *(Table by Titan Technology International, Ellisville, Mo.)*

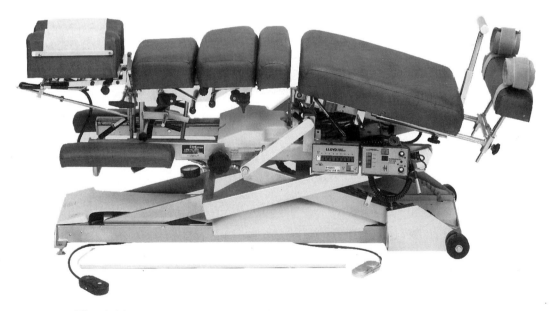

Fig. 4-11 Galaxy McManis table. *(Table by Lloyd Table Co., Lisbon, Iowa.)*

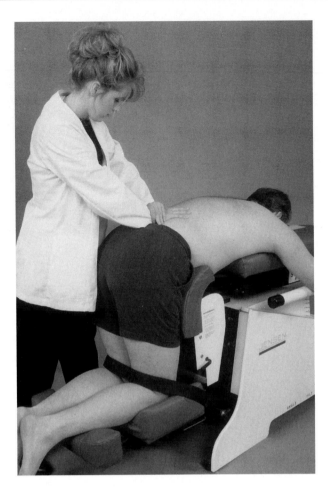

Fig. 4-12 Jensen table. *(Table by Annova, Alexandria, Minn.)*

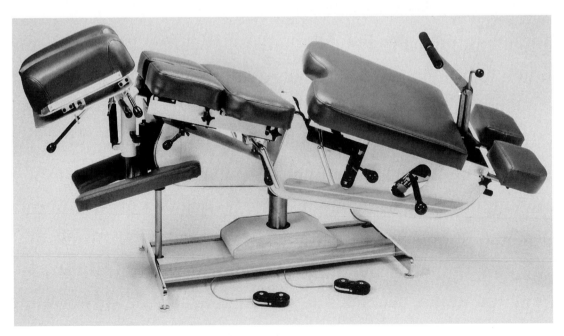

Fig. 4-13 Spinalight table. *(Table by Spinalight, Inc., Woodstock, Ga.)*

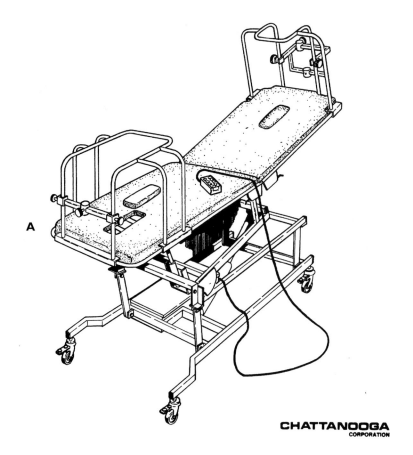

CHATTANOOGA
CORPORATION

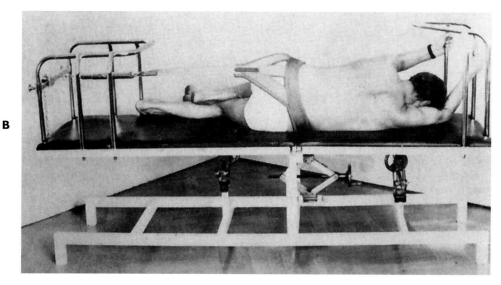

Fig. 4-14 Lind Autotraction table. **A,** Diagram of structure. **B,** Patient performing traction with rotation. (*A, courtesy Chattanooga Group, Inc., Hixon, Tenn.*)

Continued

C

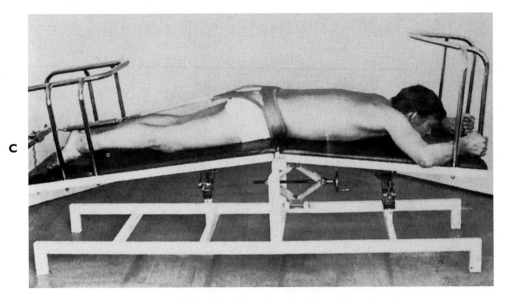

Fig. 4-14, cont'd C, Patient performing distraction with flexion.

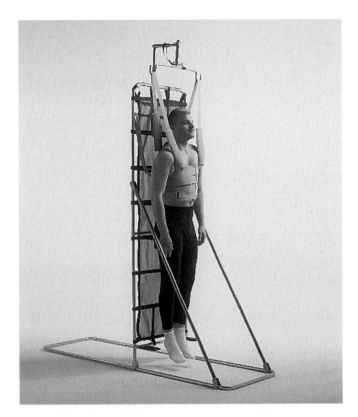

Fig. 4-15 Gravity Lumbar Traction Frame. *(Courtesy Sammons Preston, Bolingbrook, Ill.)*

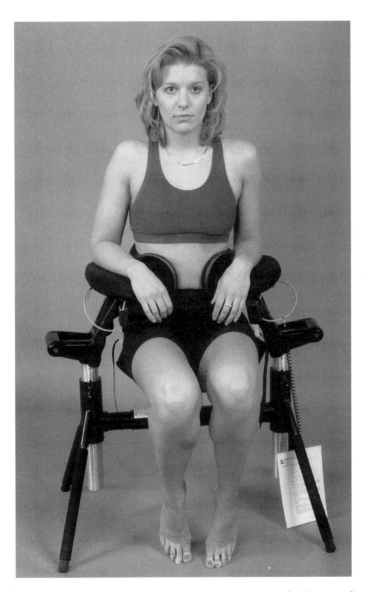

Fig. 4-16 LTX 3000. *(Table by Spinal Designs International, Minneapolis, Minn.)*

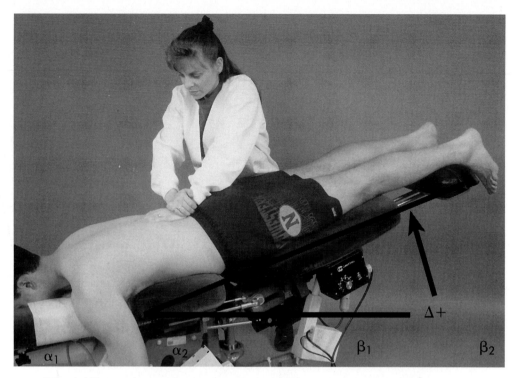

Fig. 4-17 The Hill Intertrac table. *(Table by Thomas Hill Tables, Lakefield, Ont.)*

Multiple positions are possible with distraction equipment, and a common terminology is needed to provide the basis for operating the tables and correctly positioning the patient to obtain the desired treatment. The multiple positions possible are defined by the x, y, and z axes of the body. The treatment table may provide enhancement to the body in any one or more of these axes, with possible positive or negative motion around and/or along the axis.

Certain terminology has been adopted to describe the position of the table and its various sections or components. The section under the head and thorax is identified as the *alpha,* or α, end of the table; this may be subdivided into the α_1 (headpiece) and the α_2 (thoracic) sections of the table. The section of the table that supports the pelvis and lower extremities is called the *beta,* or β section; this may be subdivided into β_1 (pelvis and legs) and β_2 (feet and ankles) sections of the table. The alpha and beta sections together comprise the *delta,* or Δ, section of the table. When these sections are in full horizontal position, they are in a zero (0)-degree position.

The movement of the tables described in this section will be identified by motion along the applicable axis

and by the section of the table that provides the treatment. An example is the Hill Intertrac table, which provides linear distraction along the y axis but also provides additional movement of the β section in the upward (positive [+]) or downward (negative [-]) directions, as well as left and right lateral flexion. If the whole table is tilted, the description includes Δ section positive (+) (Fig. 4-17).

The use of descriptive positioning terms ensures that the position of the patient is clearly defined and that, if appropriate records are kept, the approach to treatment can be duplicated on subsequent visits. This ensures consistency in the treatment and that the method can be clearly described to others, such as insurance carriers and managed care organizations.

INDICATIONS AND CONTRAINDICATIONS FOR APPLICATION OF THERAPY

Much of what is considered in chiropractic focuses on the pathologic model, or the model of disease. The injured disc is the body part that has received the most consideration. Although the disc is indeed a critical component of the musculoskeletal system because it forms a

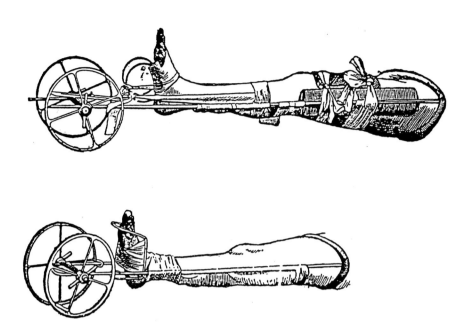

Fig. 4-18 Traction splint for repair of fracture. *(From Peltier LF. A brief history of traction.* J Bone Joint Surg Am. *1968;50:1603-1617.)*

major part of the spinal motion segments, a pathologic model is not necessary to generate concern for its biomechanical function. The structure of the body can have abnormalities without experiencing an illness or a frank injury. A structural joint misalignment or an abnormally moving joint is not necessarily indicative of a pathology; however, it may benefit from a motion-restoring manipulation. Thus the pathologic model of disc injury is not the only model that is applicable to the body. Consideration must be given to a structural model that is demonstrated by an initial simple misalignment or loss of movement of bony joints that progresses to the possible pathology of a disc herniation.

The indications for traction are relatively clear and agreed upon by most adherents of manipulation or manual medicine. The primary effects that traction has on the articulations of the spine or other articulations of the body are mechanical in nature. These effects are summarized by Hinterbuchner[6] as the following: (1) distraction of the vertebral bodies, with enlargement of the intervertebral space producing a suction effect; (2) stretching of muscles and ligaments, with the tautening of the posterior longitudinal ligament exerting a centripetal force on

the adjacent annulus fibrosus; (3) separation of the apophyseal joints; and (4) enlargement of the foramina.

According to Cyriax,[7] contraindications include displacement of a fragment of an annulus, lumbago with twinges, respiratory embarrassment, root pain with loss of conduction, long-standing root pain, elderly patients, and sciatica with deformity. Hinterbuchner[6] describes contraindications as including malignancy, cord compression, infectious diseases of the spine, osteoporosis, hypertension or cardiovascular disease, rheumatoid arthritis, old age, and pregnancy. Through the use of standard examination procedures, including the taking of a health history, these conditions can be identified and the condition that emerges handled appropriately.

The sections that follow present and compare techniques and provide the reader with an understanding of the way each has developed. Some techniques are more defined and refined than others, and more experience is demonstrated in the literature in the use of certain techniques. An objective presentation is given of each technique, including information available on the approaches, even in cases in which there is little documented experience with the technique. Perhaps this presentation will

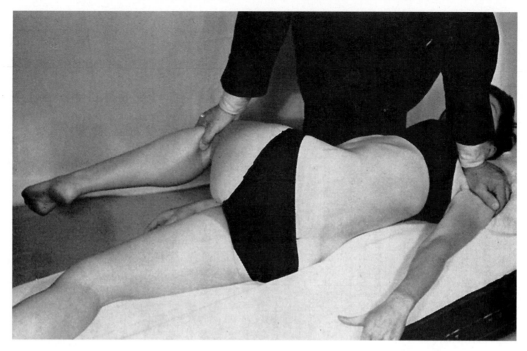

Fig. 4-19 Cyriax positioning for a low back manipulation. *(From Cyriax J.* Textbook of Orthopaedic Medicine. *10th ed. London: Bailliere Tindall; 1980;2.)*

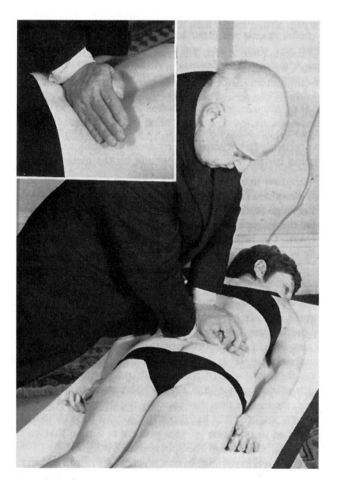

Fig. 4-20 Cyriax treating the low back. *(From Cyriax J. Textbook of Orthopaedic Medicine. 10th ed. London: Bailliere Tindall; 1980;2.)*

spark further discussion and generate additional investigations on these techniques and testing approaches.

THE ALLOPATHIC MANUAL MEDICINE CONTRIBUTION

Allopathic manipulation of the spine is not new; much historical evidence supports its use by allopaths (and other practitioners of manual medical treatment) over several centuries. However, the use of allopathic manipulation in mainstream medicine declined during the Middle Ages with the onset of destructive diseases to the bone (or so it is surmised), and it became a "folk" practice.[8] Even with the emergence of osteopathy and chiropractic, allopathic medicine has been reluctant to incorporate manipulation into mainstream practice. Until recently, allopaths have been reluctant to acknowledge the validity of chiropractic manipulation as a beneficial treatment for any disorders, even those obviously related to mechanical problems of the spine.

Historically, mechanical traction of the spine and other parts of the body has been used by allopaths, primarily for fracture reduction. Various traction splints have been used since as early as the midnineteenth century to improve the potential for normal positioning of bone during the healing process after a fracture (Fig. 4-18).[9]

One of the major proponents of allopathic manual

manipulation of the spine was James Cyriax, an English physician, who wrote extensively on the subject during the midtwentieth century. Although he was not a supporter of chiropractic and some of his writings opposed chiropractic manipulation, referring to its practitioners as "lay manipulators" (this related in part to the position of chiropractors having come from bone-setters in England and the political position of chiropractors at the time of his writing), Cyriax used methods that were similar to adjusting techniques used by chiropractors. Those familiar with Cyriax's writings may recall photos of him applying manipulative force with strong distractive prestress that was sometimes provided with the assistance of one or two other people pulling on the patient's arms and/or legs. He advocated that physical therapists use manipulation in their practices and be recognized for it (Figs. 4-19 and 4-20).[7]

Other allopaths who shared enthusiasm for a manipulative approach to treatment of the human body include Basmajian, Dvorak, Greenman, Mennell, and Janda among the medical establishment (although Greenman is an osteopath). Some of the more prominent practitioners who have written on manipulation (or *manual medicine* as it is referred to in many areas outside the United States, especially in Europe) include Maitland (physiotherapist), Cantu (physical therapist), Nwuga (physical therapist), and Evjenth (manual therapist). Each of these developers of technique has presented forms of manipulative therapy that are used for the treatment of musculoskeletal problems in the human frame. Some of these techniques are related to the bony structure of the skeleton and its joints; others are related to the soft tissues supporting the joints and the myofascial components.

Basmajian[10] identifies three major sections that exemplify his approach and that of the allopaths toward manual therapy as manipulation/mobilization, stretching, and traction/massage. The book detailing his technique was published in 1960. Much of the book is devoted to the spine, and, in the section on traction, Hinterbuchner makes statements regarding traction but notes that she finds it to be unsubstantiated in the literature and thus somewhat irrelevant. In the section on motorized intermittent traction, Rogoff describes methods that involve the use of mechanical traction devices for the spine, from the cervical through the lumbar sections. The traction units rely on both manual and mechanical methods, with variations in the forces applied to areas of the spine. Rogoff notes that the cervical spine is an area in which the results are more clearly identified, but the effects are less clear in the lumbar spine.[10]

This mechanical process appears to provide both a linear and a centripetal effect on the spine and its joints. Traction has a mechanical effect on the disc, pulling the nucleus back within the walls of the annulus fibrosus, enhancing imbibition with the negative pressure created, causing the disc to take on fluids from the surrounding area. With time, this helps rehydrate the disc and, in the process, brings in nutrients for adjacent tissues and flushes waste products from the area.

Colachis and Strohm[11] report a major increase in total mean vertebral separation with 22.7 kilograms of traction, with the greatest increase in posterior separation at the L4-5 level. This separation was measured with lateral radiographs taken during and after traction. Cyriax[7] believes the following:

> If something is to be moved, distraction of the joint surfaces facilitates any maneuver. As the facets are wedge-shaped, the further they are pulled apart the greater the range of movement at the joint. Manipulation during traction has the virtue not only of separating the facet joint surfaces but of abolishing pain (so that the patient relaxes spontaneously), giving room for the loose fragment to move, and applying suction (so that any shift that does occur is towards the center of the joint).

Cyriax[7] cites several instances in which this traction method is applicable, such as nuclear protrusion, cases in which manipulation has failed, primary posterolateral root pain, recurrence after laminectomy, upper lumbar disc lesions, bilateral long-standing limitation of straight leg raising, lower thoracic disc lesions, and bone on bone, as in marked kyphosis.

Another proponent of traction on the human spine is Charles Burton, M.D., who developed gravity traction at Sister Kinney Institute (the hospital of polio treatment fame). His approach is to use a traction frame that is angled to accommodate a patient in a harness, to create an increasing degree of traction in the low back. There are other components to the treatment, such as a regimen of rehabilitating exercises, but this device provides the major effect for the patient (see Fig. 4-15). This frame has largely been replaced by the LTX 3000, which provides the traction with the patient seated, again with the assistance of gravity applied to the lower torso (see Fig. 4-16).[5] The LTX 3000 is discussed in Chapter 7.

APPLICATION OF THERAPY

Cyriax used a traction "couch" of his own design that allowed prone or supine positioning of the patient. It was

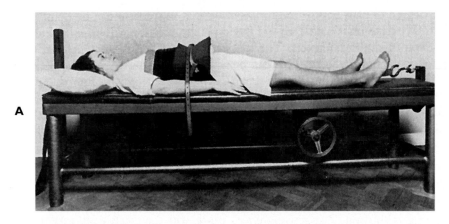

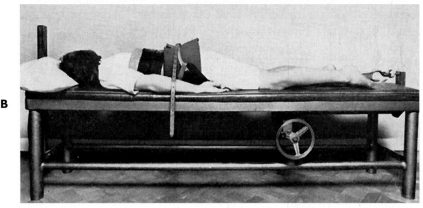

Fig. 4-21 Cyriax traction couch with harness: **A,** supine; **B,** prone. *(From Cyriax J. Textbook of Orthopaedic Medicine. 10th ed. London: Bailliere Tindall; 1980;2.)*

fully manual, with harness attachments for the upper and the lower body and a strapping mechanism attached to either end of the table (couch). A manual crank was located on the side of the table. A strain gauge attached to one end of the table measured the amount of tractive force being applied to the patient in a given traction session. The protocol used by Cyriax applied traction for a brief period (1 or 2 minutes), followed by a period of rest. He contended that this was the best method for reducing a lumbar disc protrusion and, because of the characteristics of traction applied manually, this method would "suck" the nucleus back into the center of the disc, restoring its normal position. Cyriax[7] believes that this device, producing only linear traction with no flexion or extension, places the patient in the best position for restoring the nucleus to its proper location within the disc. No study exists, however, to support Cyriax's contention.

Cyriax's table can best be described as having a section with no deviation toward flexion or extension, keeping a neutral (0-degree) position in the y axis of the body.

The treatment is executed in this manner and, unlike the chiropractic techniques described in the following section, does not allow multiple-plane positioning. The table only operates in the single plane of the y axis and is manual, with no power assists (Fig. 4-21).

ADJUNCTIVE THERAPY

Other allopathic approaches to traction treatment of the spine include that of physical therapists, whose armamentarium has included traction for many years. Studies of physical therapy approaches to traction have included various forms, from constant traction devices to those that are intermittent and incorporate various forces in loading of the spine. In Sweden, Lidstrom[12] (1970) demonstrated that intermittent pelvic traction combined with isometric exercises for the abdominal muscles greatly improved the condition of the injured spine when compared with what was termed *conventional treatment,* including hot packs and massage in combination with mobilizing and strengthening exercises for the spine.

Others who practice joint manipulation techniques use myofascial procedures, which involve pressure, deep massage, and stretching maneuvers over various soft tissues of the body. Some of these procedures incorporate traction but on a limited basis. However, most applications are performed by hand on a table or other equipment consisting of a platform only, with some use of adjustable surfaces on the platform.[13-16]

PROTOCOL/REGIMEN

The Cyriax traction process employs the table shown in Fig. 4-21, which has upper and lower harnesses for attaching to the patient. With a pull or force and the assistance of the table, the harnesses draw the upper and lower halves of the patient in opposite directions. The harnesses strap around the patient and can be used with the patient in either a prone or supine position. The harnesses should be placed adjacent to the patient, with a layer of foam rubber between to pad the surface of the skin. With proper placement of the harness, pull is exerted on the upper body (the thorax) and the lower body (the lumbar area). A spring tensioning device attached to the lower end of the table regulates the amount of traction applied to the patient. The maximum traction possible using this device is 100 kilograms. The spring tension device measures the amount of traction that is applied to the patient and regulates the traction applied so that it is even and consistent.

For the application of traction, the patient is attached to the ends of the table. Cyriax[7] contends that only continuous traction provides the force necessary to effect a correction of the patient's condition. He believes that the traction must be sustained because it only becomes effective after approximately 2 minutes in the tractive state. He notes that in mechanical pull, which is intermittent, the stretch reflex comes into play and the traction is ineffective. He emphasizes that the force must be sustained for a time. He recommends daily treatment for 2 weeks or more, until symptomatic relief is effected and the protrusion of the disc is reduced.

THE OSTEOPATHS (AS EXEMPLIFIED BY McMANIS)

The work of osteopath J.V. McManis has had an osteopathic influence on the manipulative procedures of chiropractors. Much of chiropractor James Cox's initial work in developing his technique of flexion-distraction was based on McManis' work. Moreover, the design of the early Cox table, especially that embodied in the Barnes table, was a direct emulation of the McManis table of the early 1900s.[17-19]

Hilton Taylor, D.C.,[18] a chiropractor from South Africa who used the McManis table in his practice during the 1970s, described his approach to the use of the McManis table. He noted that the patent for the McManis 20th Century table was issued in May of 1909. This manual table, which allowed a multiple-plane approach to manipulation, including flexion-extension and lateral flexion, was a boon to both the patient and the clinician.

Taylor identified the effects of traction on the spine as stretching of the muscles and ligaments, improving glide of the dural root sleeves, freeing fixation of articular facets, reducing hydrostatic pressure in the discs, repositioning nuclear fragments, and improving the blood supply to the spine and its surrounding structures. It should be noted that McManis' approach was more encompassing than Taylor's approach. McManis' use of the table was multifaceted because he placed the patient on it to examine as well as treat. Furthermore, the conditions that he treated were not always of a pathologic nature; in some cases they were related more to the body's structure.[18]

PATIENT POSITIONING

The McManis table incorporated many of the features that appear on contemporary tables, including split headpieces, multiple sections adjustable for patient comfort, and positioning for various adjustive maneuvers. The table also had a lift mechanism, apparently based on that of the barber chair, with either a hand or foot pump for operating the hydraulic lift. This allowed positioning of the patient at a height convenient to the clinician.

The use of the table by the osteopaths was perhaps somewhat different from that of the chiropractors.[19] McManis saw the table being used for gynecologic and proctologic examinations and as a chair for evaluation of patients with eye, ear, nose, and throat problems. Other positions more useful to the chiropractor were also possible, including the prone position, useful, as McManis[20] termed it, "especially for work with the patient on the face, as in adjusting a posterior innominate."

McManis[20] notes that the table was a radical departure from previous models in that its surface was divided into three sections, "capable of various adjustments and the bringing into play of mechanical apparatus to facilitate and reinforce the technique of the clinician." This table, with its manual hydraulic pump to raise and lower the surface, changing the working height for the clinician, was indeed an innovation for the time.

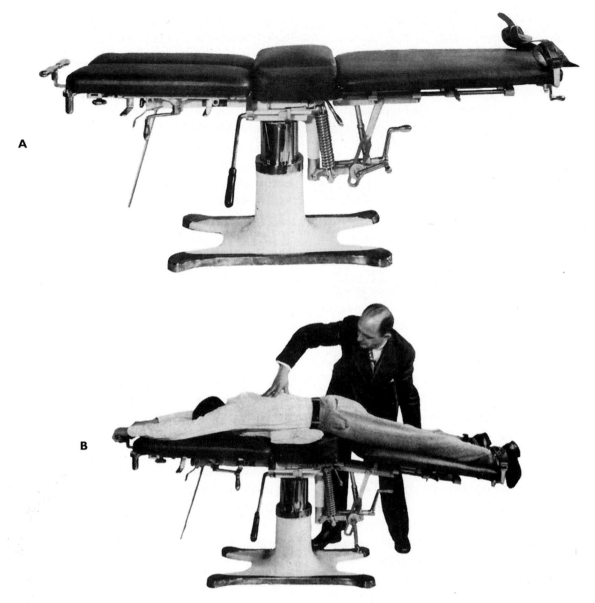

Fig. 4-22 The McManis table: **A,** α, β, and Δ neutral (0) position; **B,** with flexion (β negative [-]); *(From McManis JV. McManis Table Technic: Technic Instructions and General Information. Hannibal, Mo: Standard Printing Co; 1938.)*

The patient typically was placed in a prone or supine position on the table, but also could be placed in the sidelying position. The split headpiece could be positioned from horizontal to a full 90 degrees or any angle between. The middle section, or abdominal pad, could be moved more than an inch toward the foot and could be inclined on either end or raised by 2 inches. Springs attached to the midsection provided a springing action when a thrust was made, enhancing the action. The lower, or foot, section was described as a "swinging" leaf that could be adjusted 4 inches toward the head or foot (linear distraction). This section provided the platform for creating traction of the lower back in a flexion position from the pelvis to the ankles. The lateral flexion position in combination with flexion-extension of the caudal section of the table was also possible.

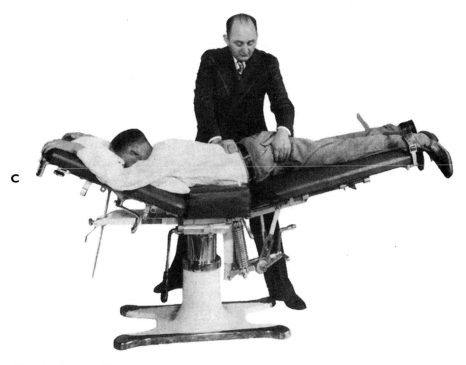

Fig. 4-22, cont'd C, The McManis table with extension (α positive [+] β positive [+]).

APPLICATION OF THERAPY

Although the McManis table was developed by an osteopath, much of its use over the years has been by chiropractors. These practitioners of the manipulative arts found its multiple-positioning capability useful in achieving the high-velocity, low-force adjustments of common use and in the application of a more subtle and gentle therapy that affords a mechanical advantage (through positioning and leverage) to the practitioner.

The McManis table has the potential for multiple positions on both ends of the table, α and β. It is capable of α_1 neutral (0), α_1 tilted upward (+), β tilted downward (-) and upward (+), β rotation (θ z + or -), and β (y + or -) section manual axial distraction. All of the table's functions are manual and require the application of force by an operator (Fig. 4-22).

The use of the McManis table, as described by Taylor,[18] is as follows:

1. The patient is positioned with the assistance of the clinician into a prone position on the table.
2. The feet are fastened into the padded cuffs.
3. The breast harness is fastened into the desired position or the patient is instructed to hold onto the bar at the head of the table.

4. The patient pulls himself or herself forward to take slack from the cuffs.
5. The straps of the breast harness are pulled tight.
6. The table is elevated to the desired height by the hydraulic foot lever.
7. The extension crank at the distal end of the swinging leaf is activated, and the leaf is drawn away from the middle section. This initiates spinal traction in a horizontal plane.
8. The friction clutch, or vertical lock, is released, and the swinging leaf is allowed to move up and down, creating flexion-extension moments of the spine.
9. The lateral lock is released to allow the leaf to swing side to side, creating lateral flexion movement.
10. The torsional lock is released for those cases requiring a tilting of the leaf from one side to the other, permitting an axial rotational movement of the spine and sacroiliac joints.

When the patient is under the desired amount of "stretch," the following movements or combinations of movements can be applied:

1. A straight caudal-axial stretch, which can be achieved in a position either above or below horizontal (β [+] or [-] for - θ x) can be applied. The upward bent, or β (+),

can be sustained in any of the desired angled positions by locking the friction clutch. With the table in this stationary position, the leaf can be extended (drawn out) or repositioned cephalad (drawn in) by turning the crank.

2. Vertical movement with laterality, or β (+) in lateral flexion right and left, is possible.
3. Lateral movement (β lateral right and left in a horizontal plane), β neutral (0) (for - x), or any inclination above or below this level is possible.
4. The swinging leaf, or β, section can be tilted or canted in right and left lateral flexion to a maximum of 35 degrees on the left and right sides. For example, the swinging leaf can be swung in a horizontal plane, in right and left (+ or - θ z) lateral flexion to 20 or 30 degrees, and then tilted down (β [-]), to a maximum of 35 degrees.
5. Circumduction is possible in a 360-degree circular motion around the axis of the pelvis (β circumduct).

The clinician stands adjacent to the table in a lunge position, or fencer's stance, with the cephalad hand contacting the appropriate vertebrae. The hand contact is established over the vertebra above the level of disc involvement, providing a stable resistance for the vertebra. The clinician's caudal hand contacts the distal aspect of the lower leaf of the table (β section), providing the force to flex or extend the leaf and providing the desired force of flexion-extension distraction. The clinician must provide the pumping force for the manipulation.

SPECIAL TREATMENT

McManis used the table for examination and treatment for the eye, ear, nose, and throat and in the evaluation and treatment of various proctologic and gynecologic conditions. Because the table could assume various configurations, the patient could be positioned appropriately for the evaluation and treatment required (Fig. 4-23).

ADJUNCTIVE THERAPY

No particular use by McManis of any adjunctive therapy or equipment has been documented in the articles cited. In his 1938 catalog, McManis shows the use of vibration and massage applied through a device incorporated into the table and operated electrically. He referred to this unit, which was an integral part of the table, as the *Physician's Massage Unit*. It was promoted to provide a "lymphatic drainage" for the patient (Fig. 4-24).

PROTOCOL/REGIMEN

Three basic lines, or directions, of traction are used with the McManis table in treating the patient with low back

pain. Patients are classified in one of these treatment groups, according to the type of low back problem. These groups reflect the capabilities of the table in its flexed, extended, and laterally flexed positions. These groups are as follows:

Group A: Horizontal line of traction. This position allows the swinging leaf to be distracted caudally (axially) parallel to the floor until sufficient stretch is reached. This is the line of traction along the y axis around which treatment motions are administered. (Fig. 4-25, *A*)

Group B: Above horizontal line. The range for this motion is 5 to 25 degrees above horizontal (β [+]), and the swinging leaf reflects this angle above parallel to the ground. The leaf is distracted axially in this angle until the desired stretch is reached. This angle is maintained as the treatment motions are administered. (Fig. 4-25, *B*)

Group C: Below the horizontal line. The range for this motion is 5 to 35 degrees below horizontal (β [-]), and the swinging leaf reflects this angle below parallel to the ground. The leaf is distracted axially in this angle until the desired stretch is reached. The angle is maintained as the treatment motions are administered. (Fig. 4-25, *C*)

Radiographs are made of patients in the upright position. The clinician views the lateral film in the horizontal position in the view box, with the orientation of the body (in the film) in the same plane as the treatment table. According to Taylor, this facilitates the clinician's visualization of the planes and angles within the spine and its segments. The AP film is viewed in the usual upright position in the view box.

For patients in group A, the treatment protocol includes initially positioning the patient on the table with the chest harness and the ankle cuffs attached. The caudal section is distracted axially until a stretch is felt by the patient. Motion palpation is performed by moving the caudal section laterally, seeking abnormal joint movement. Vertical movement is then initiated using the caudal section, slowly and rhythmically, with the clinician palpating the movement of the spine, sensing soft clicks (resulting from the break down of "cobweb" adhesions). Taylor[18] notes that the range of flexion (β [-]) and extension (β [+]) of the spine is about 10 degrees above and below horizontal. The treatment time is about 4 minutes, and Taylor recommends that it be applied twice per week for 2 to 4 weeks.

This series of movements reduces the lumbar curve, opens the IVF, positions the nucleus pulposus normally, and mildly stretches the apophyseal joints. Taylor[18] indicates further that this movement stretches, squeezes, opens, and closes joints and forces movement into the

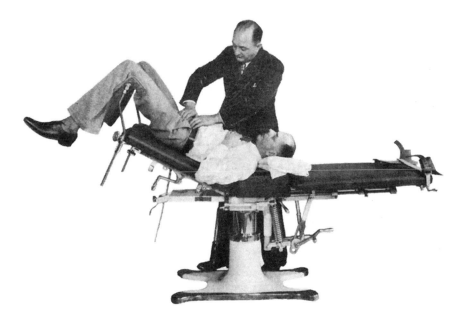

Fig. 4-23 The McManis table in position for special treatment. *(From McManis JV. McManis Table Technic: Technic Instructions and General Information. Hannibal, Mo: Standard Printing Co; 1938.)*

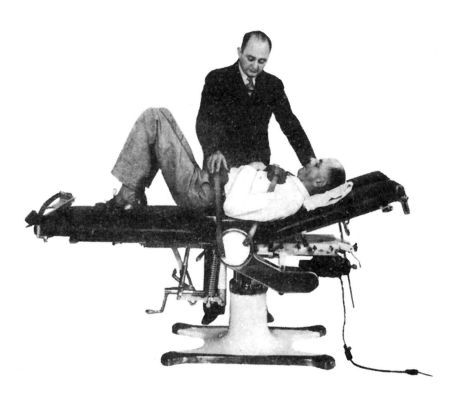

Fig. 4-24 The McManis table with vibration-massage. *(From McManis JV. McManis Table Technic: Technic Instructions and General Information. Hannibal, Mo: Standard Printing Co; 1938.)*

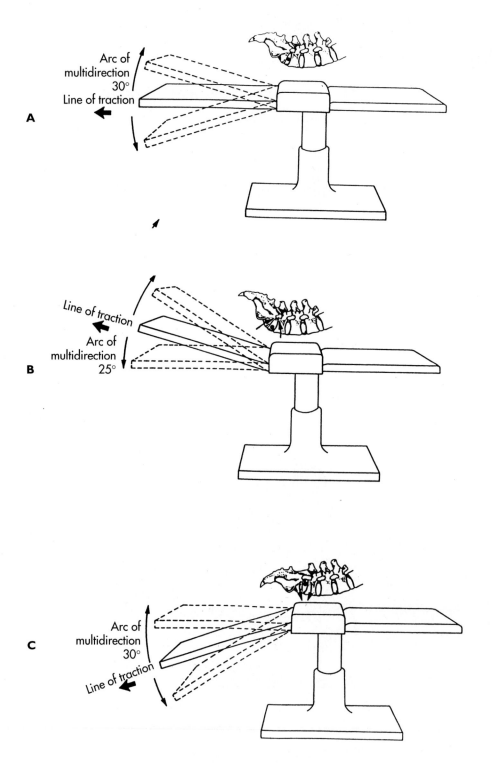

Fig. 4-25 Positioning for patients in **A**, horizontal line of traction, **B**, traction above horizontal line; **C**, traction below horizontal line. *(From Taylor H. The McManis table: professional papers. ACA J Chiropr. 1978;12:100.)*

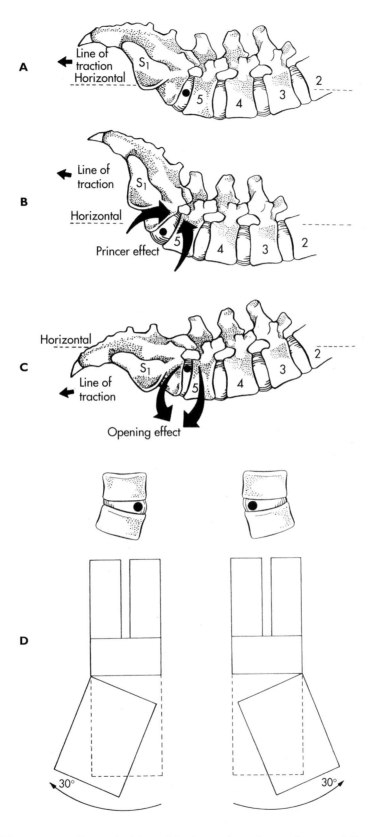

Fig. 4-26 Proposed effects of table positioning and traction on facets and disc **A**, in horizontal line of traction, **B**, above horizontal line of traction, **C**, below horizontal lines of traction, **D**, lateral flexion movement. *(From Taylor H. The McManis table: professional papers. ACA J Chiropr. 1978;12:87-100.)*

nerve roots, where there are dural root adhesions. This category of treatment is potentially applicable for elderly patients with or without arthrosis, because it increases the motion in the involved segments. (Fig. 4-26, *A*)

For patients in group B the same process applies for placing patients on the table and readying them for treatment. The caudal section is adjusted to an angle of 5 to 25 degrees above horizontal (β [+]), and the tensioning springs are adjusted to maintain this position. The caudal section is distracted axially until stretch is felt by the patient. Pain is the guide, and the patient is manipulated in a pain-free state. Slow, rhythmic stretching is desired, and the time of this treatment is between 2 and 4 minutes. The clinician decreases the stretch slowly on completion of the traction. The patient is required to lie prone for a short time after treatment. The average treatment period in this configuration is four to six sessions.

This treatment is thought to increase the lumbar curve, closing the IVF with a pincer effect, increase pressure on the nucleus pulposus toward the anterior of the disc and away from the IVF, and move the apophyseal joints in a slight "overriding position." Taylor[18] notes that a slow, rhythmic movement that creates a stretch is his recommended approach (Fig. 4-26, *B*).

Patients in group C are treated in the flexion (β [-]) mode to "open up" the articulating facets. Attention is given to the nucleus, which is oriented toward the anterior of the disc. The patient is secured in the harness while prone on the table, and the ankle cuffs are fastened. The caudal section is distracted axially 5 to 35 degrees below horizontal (β [-]) until a stretch is felt by the patient. All movements are maintained below the horizontal (β [-]), with emphasis on opening the facets. Four to six treatments are given once or twice per week.

The effect of treatment in patients in group C is that the lumbar curve is decreased, the IVF is opened, the nucleus is forced toward the IVF, and the apophyseal joints are separated. The clinician must keep the lower, or β, section relatively depressed (-) to effect the lumbar stretch and open the facet joints (Fig. 4-26, *C*).

Taylor[18] notes that providing this distractive treatment is not considered a replacement for chiropractic management of spinal problems but rather adjunctive or supplemental by "restoring the functional equilibrium of the vertebral column." He also refers to the early writings of James Cox, D.C., whose technique is discussed in the next section.

COX FLEXION-DISTRACTION (USING TABLES OF WILLIAMS ZENITH-COX, CHATTANOOGA, AND LLOYD AND AS MODIFIED BY MARKEY)

The Cox technique is based on the technique and table developed by McManis. Cox[17] notes that his approach to mechanically assisted manipulation is a blend of osteopathic and chiropractic principles into one technique and one "instrument" (as Cox describes the table). He refers to the technique as "Cox closed reduction of disc protrusion," although he indicates a broader application of the technique for conditions other than lumbar disc protrusions. He identifies appropriate conditions for use of the technique as lumbar disc protrusion, spondylolisthesis, facet syndrome, subluxation, and scoliotic curves of a nonsurgical nature.

Most of Cox's approach to the spine is related to a pathologic model. This model is based on the idea that spine treatment is related to a pathologic problem that involves some disease process or is the result of a traumatic incident. Cox[17] notes several benefits of this form of spinal manipulation, including increasing intervertebral disc height; removal of pressure on the disc; centering of the nucleus of the disc, thus relieving disc pressure; restoration of normal motion to the spine; and improvement of posture. Cox uses a process of analysis that involves a combination of orthopedic and neurologic testing and imaging to establish the presence of a disc lesion, facet syndrome, or other condition of a pathologic or traumatic nature.

Cox[17] states that myelography has consistently shown that flexion of the lumbar spine causes disappearance of the bulge of the posterior annulus and longitudinal ligament as the anterior margins of the vertebral bodies approach each other and the posterior margins separate. The myelographic column becomes flat, and the dural sac closely approximates the back of the posterior longitudinal ligament and annulus. Even though flexion increases the force propelling the nucleus posteriorly, it also tightens the posterior annulus and posterior longitudinal ligament and improves the barrier, with the net effect of reduction of the posterior protrusion.

Paul Markey, who was closely associated with Cox for several years, describes subtle differences in the application of the technique and evaluation. Markey has

Text continued on p. 118

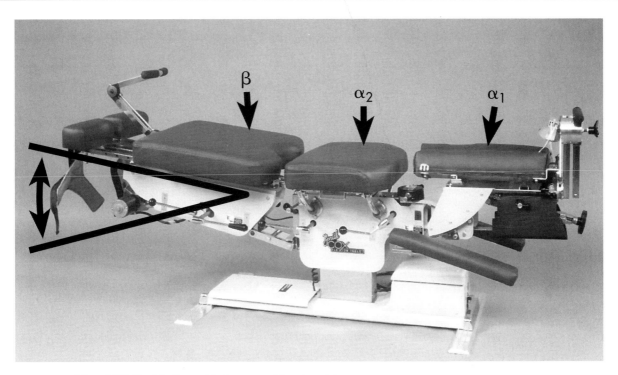

Fig. 4-27 Zenith-Cox table in upward-bent position.
- Table is positioned in neutral. The elevation is at lowest level.
- The α, α_1, β, β_1, and Δ sections are in neutral position, or 0.
- All controls for positioning and control for positive and negative movement of the β section and lateral flexion positions are located on the side of the table.
- The handle for providing distraction is shown in the upright and locked position, ready for use.
- The handle must be repositioned before patient is placed on the table. The handle folds flat into the table. *(Table by Williams Healthcare Systems, Elgin, Ill.)*

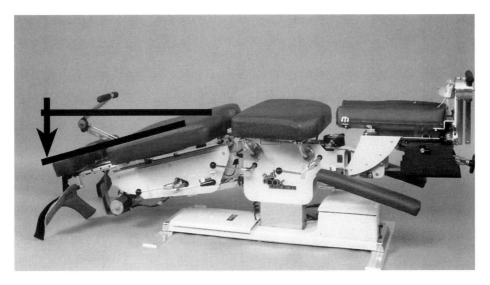

Fig. 4-28 Zenith-Cox table in downward locked position.
- Table is positioned with the β, or pelvic, section moved downward (β [-]). *(Table by Williams Healthcare Systems, Elgin, Ill.)*

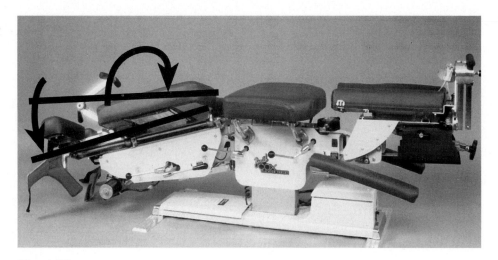

Fig. 4-29
Zenith-Cox table in downward locked position with rotation.
• Table is positioned with the β section locked downward (β [-]) and rotated (- θ y).
(Table by Williams Healthcare Systems, Elgin, Ill.)

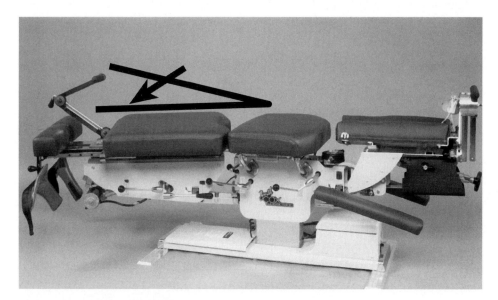

Fig. 4-30 Zenith-Cox table with lateral flexion.
• Table is positioned with the β section 0, or neutral, with lateral flexion (+ θ z). *(Table by Williams Healthcare Systems, Elgin, Ill.)*

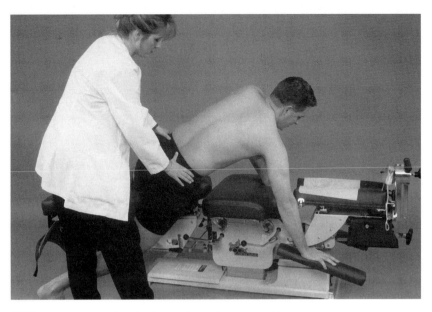

Fig. 4-31 Zenith-Cox table: Patient being placed on table.
- Table is positioned in neutral, with all sections locked. This is an important safety consideration for the patient mounting the table.
- Clinician stands adjacent and carefully monitors the patient's attempt to mount the table. The patient follows instructions from the clinician on the appropriate approach, taking care to maintain balance and rely on the table for support. *(Table by Williams Healthcare Systems, Elgin, Ill.)*

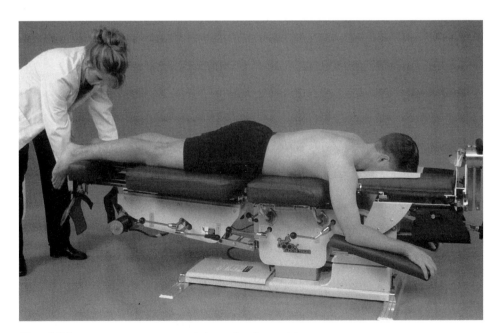

Fig. 4-32 Zenith-Cox table: Clinician adjusting ankle support.
- Clinician adjusting ankle support for length of patient.
- Table is in 0, or neutral, in all sections.
- In this position the clinician can manually adjust the length of caudal section with a crank, thus creating a degree of linear distraction. With a motorized model, the clinician presses a button for the same effect to be created. *(Table by Williams Healthcare Systems, Elgin, Ill.)*

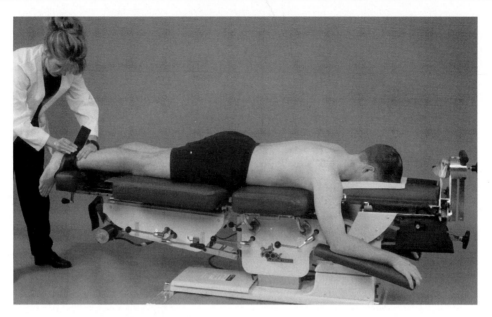

Fig. 4-33 The Zenith-Cox table: Clinician setting hand lever.
- Table is set in 0, or neutral.
- The handle is set to fit the clinician and the patient.
- The handle provides the power for the distraction manipulation or adjustment. *(Table by Williams Healthcare Systems, Elgin, Ill.)*

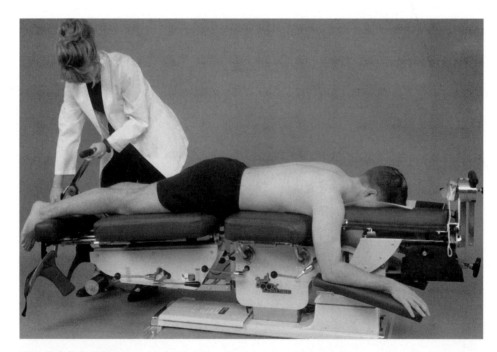

Fig. 4-34 Zenith-Cox table: Clinician attaching the ankle straps.
- Clinician attaches the ankle straps to increase the tractive force of the table.
- The ankle straps are optional, and their use is at the discretion of the clinician. Patient comfort is considered in application of the straps. In acute cases, use of ankle straps should be delayed until the level of pain subsides moderately. The ankle straps will increase the amount of traction to the patient.
- The lower section of the table remains in neutral, or β 0. *(Table by Williams Healthcare Systems, Elgin, Ill.)*

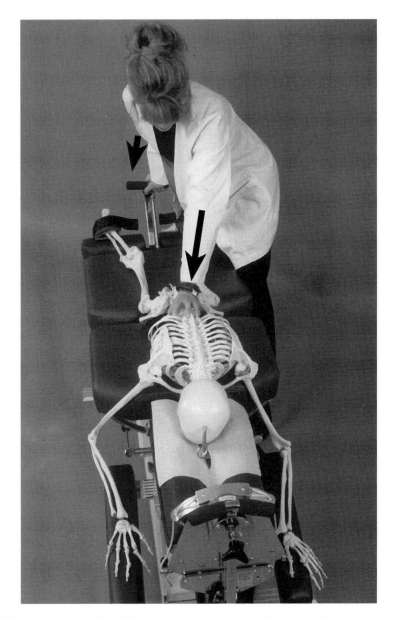

Fig. 4-35 Zenith-Cox table: Clinician showing hand position on skeleton.
- Skeleton is located on table, which is in neutral, 0, position; clinician hand position is shown on spine.
- Clinician body stance is a lunge, or fencer, stance at the side of the table.
- The caudal hand grasps the handle on the lower, or β, section, near the patient's feet.
- The cephalad hand contacts the superior segment over the area of treatment, to effect distraction. *(Table by Williams Healthcare Systems, Elgin, Ill.)*

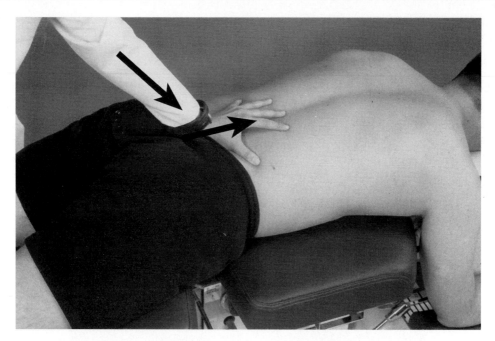

Fig. 4-36 Zenith-Cox table: Close-up of clinician hand position.
- Close-up of clinician hand position, with carpal tunnel indentation over spinous processes and fingers extended (i.e., left hand contacting L5 spinous to distract L5-S1 motion segment). *(Table by Williams Healthcare Systems, Elgin, Ill.)*

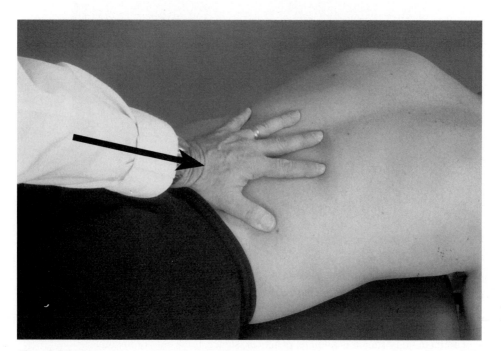

Fig. 4-37 Zenith-Cox table: Close-up of hand position.
- Close-up of hand position on back of patient. *(Table by Williams Healthcare Systems, Elgin, Ill.)*

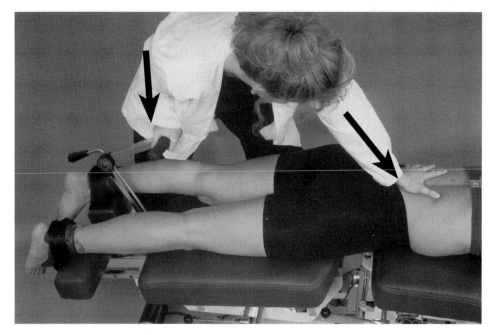

Fig. 4-38 Zenith-Cox table: Clinician using Markey hand position on patient.
- Clinician using Markey hand position, with spinous process located between thumb and second digit (on the web), and leaning over the patient while contacting handle on β section. *(Table by Williams Healthcare Systems, Elgin, Ill.)*

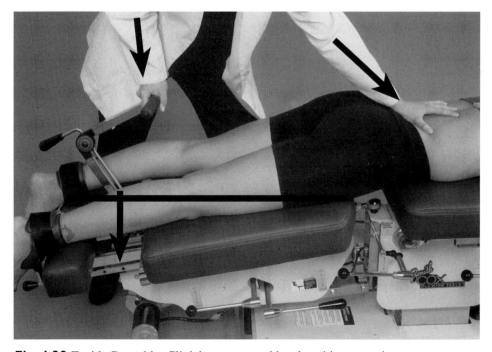

Fig. 4-39 Zenith-Cox table: Clinician stance and hand position on patient.
- Clinician stance, hand position, and contact with handle on β section.
- Table is positioned in β (-), flexing patient and distracting the contacted motion segment. *(Table by Williams Healthcare Systems, Elgin, Ill.)*

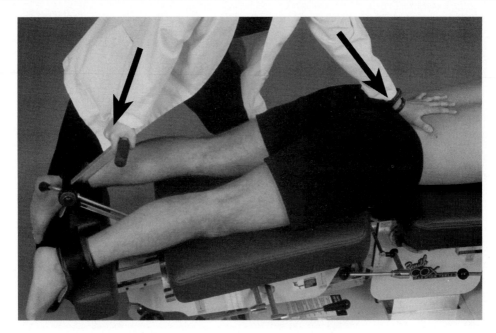

Fig. 4-40 Zenith-Cox table: Stance of clinician, with cephalad lean.
- Clinician stance is forward, with lean toward cephalad end of table.
- The β section of table is (-) negative, flexing patient. *(Table by Williams Healthcare Systems, Elgin, Ill.)*

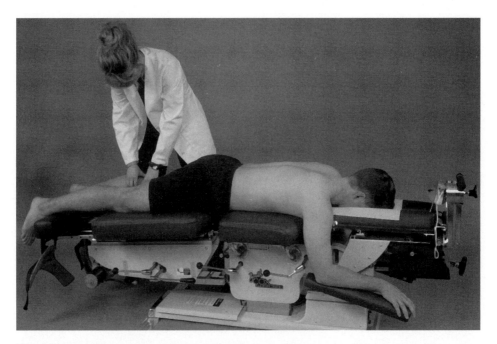

Fig. 4-41 Zenith-Cox table: Clinician goading leg adductors.
- Clinician is seen goading the adductors on the patient's leg.
- Table is in β (0) neutral.
- The ankle straps are not attached.
- This procedure is in preparation for distraction, to assist in relaxation of the muscles. *(Table by Williams Healthcare Systems, Elgin, Ill.)*

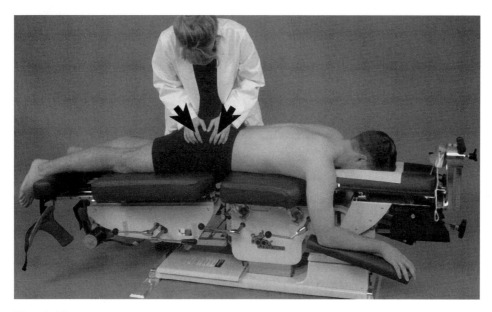

Fig. 4-42 Zenith-Cox table: Clinician goading gluteal muscles.
- Clinician is shown goading the patient's gluteal muscles to achieve muscle relaxation before distraction.
- Table is β (0), or neutral, and ankles are not strapped. *(Table by Williams Healthcare Systems, Elgin, Ill.)*

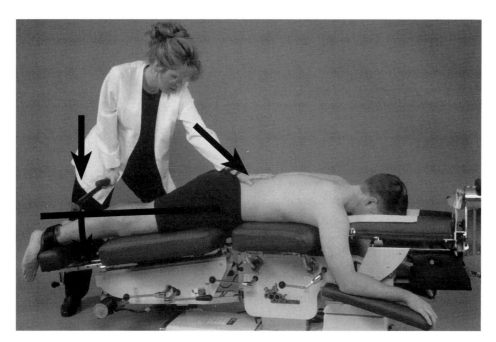

Fig. 4-43 Zenith-Cox table: Clinician demonstrating flexion-distraction of the L5-S1 motion segment.
- Patient is prone in β (-) negative position, with ankles strapped.
- Clinician is standing adjacent, in a lunge position, with treating hand over the L5 spinous process and other hand on handle on β section.
- Clinician depresses β section in pumping action 4 to 5 times while maintaining cephalad pressure on the spine, then repeats the 4 to 5 pumps for 1 or 2 additional cycles, with a 30-second rest between.
- Clinician monitors patient response to pain at all times. *(Table by Williams Healthcare Systems, Elgin, Ill.)*

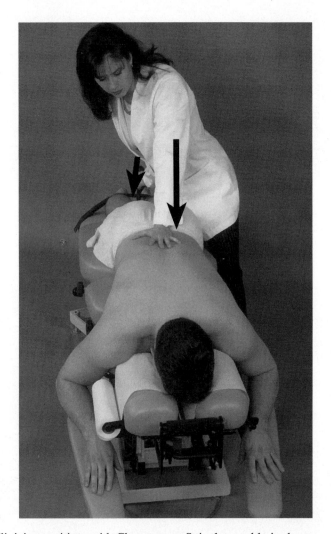

Fig. 4-44 Clinician position, with Chattanooga Spinalator table in downward bend.
- Patient is in β (-) negative position, with ankles strapped.
- Clinician is standing adjacent, with treating hand over lumbar spine and other hand on handle on β section.
- Clinician depresses β section in pumping action 4 to 5 times, then repeats the 4 to 5 pumps 1 or 2 additional cycles, with a 30-second rest between. *(Table by Chattanooga Group, Inc., Hixon, Tenn.)*

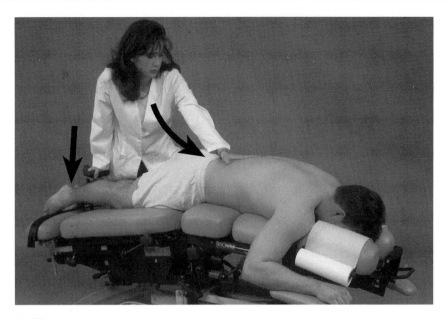

Fig. 4-45 Chattanooga Spinalator table: Clinician position.
- Note the clinician's body position, stance, and hand position.
- The ankles may or may not be strapped, and the table is β (-); the clinician provides movement downward and allows the table to spring back into 0, or neutral, position.
- The ankles are not strapped in this illustration. *(Table by Chattanooga Group, Inc., Hixon, Tenn.)*

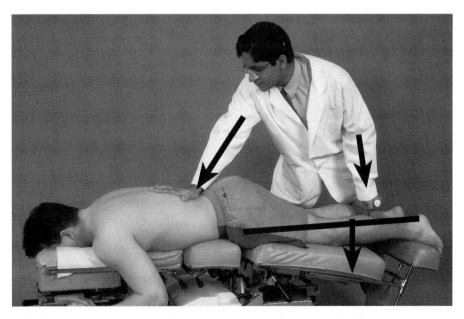

Fig. 4-46 Lloyd Galaxy table: Clinician position, with flexion of table.
- The α_3 section is 0, or neutral, and locked.
- Patient is in β (-) negative position.
- Clinician is standing adjacent, with treating hand over lumbar spine and opposite hand on handle on β section to provide power for down and up motion.
- Clinician depresses β section in pumping action 4 to 5 times, then repeats the 4 to 5 pumps 1 or 2 additional cycles, with a 20- to 30-second rest between. *(Table by Lloyd Table Co., Lisbon, Iowa.)*

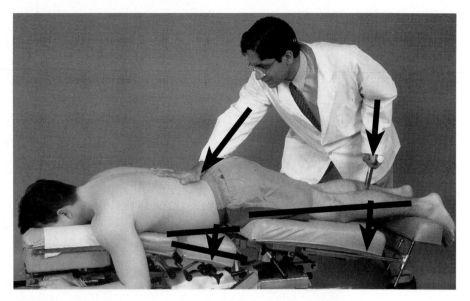

Fig. 4-47 Lloyd Galaxy table: Clinician position.
- Note the clinician position, stance, and hand position.
- Table is β (-) negative, and the clinician provides movement downward and allows the table to spring back into 0, or neutral, position.
- The α_3 section is (-) negative and allowed to spring with the patient's abdomen and maintain the lumbar lordosis. *(Table by Lloyd Table Co., Lisbon, Iowa.)*

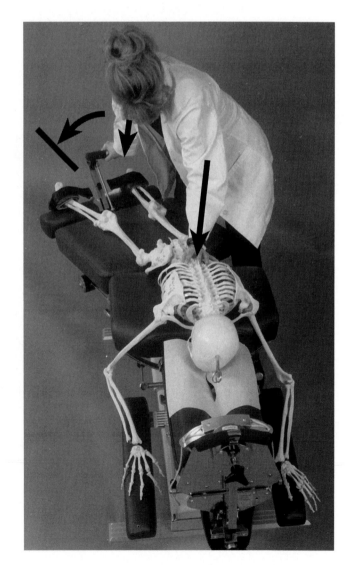

Fig. 4-48 Zenith-Cox table: Clinician performing flexion (β [-]) and lateral flexion on skeleton.
- Clinician stance is alongside the table, and the patient (skeleton) is in a prone position.
- Clinician's hands are placed as shown, with the treating hand on the spine in the prescribed manner. The operating hand is on the handle for flexion force with downward pressure. *(Table by Williams Healthcare Systems, Elgin, Ill.)*

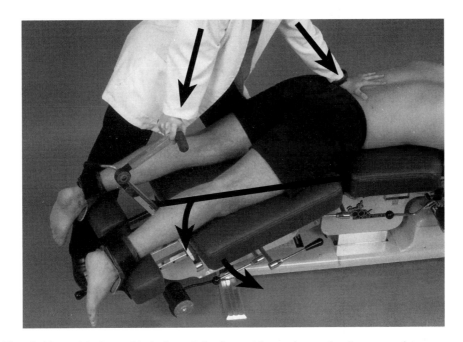

Fig. 4-49 Zenith-Cox table in lateral flexion, with traction on lumbar musculature.
- Clinician is in fencer stance, with hands in contact with left quadratus lumborum musculature and flexion-extension handle.
- The hand contact with the musculature is with the thenar and the hypothenar, the fingers extended fully and separated.
- Table is β (-), flexing and right laterally flexing the patient.
- Clinician laterally flexes the table, and places it in β (-) position, maintaining pressure over the lumbar paraspinal muscles.
- When depressing the β section ([-] negative), the clinician stretches the muscles for a cycle of 4 to 5 times, repeating the cycle 1 additional time. The procedure relaxes the muscles of the low back. *(Table by Williams Healthcare Systems, Elgin, Ill.)*

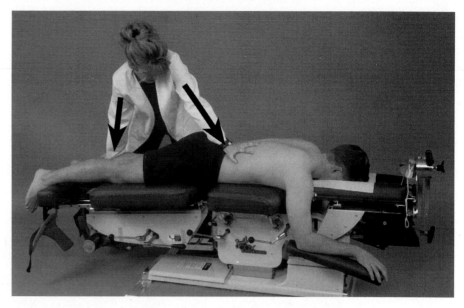

Fig. 4-50 Zenith-Cox table: Clinician stretching quadratus lumborum.
- Patient is positioned prone; ankles may or may not be strapped into the β_2 section, which is adjusted for patient height.
- Clinician laterally flexes the table to right side of patient, followed by a slight β (-) position, maintaining pressure of patient's right paraspinal muscles.
- A pumping motion is maintained through a cycle of 4 to 5 times, then a brief rest and another pumping of the structure 4 to 5 times. (*Table by Williams Healthcare Systems, Elgin, Ill.*)

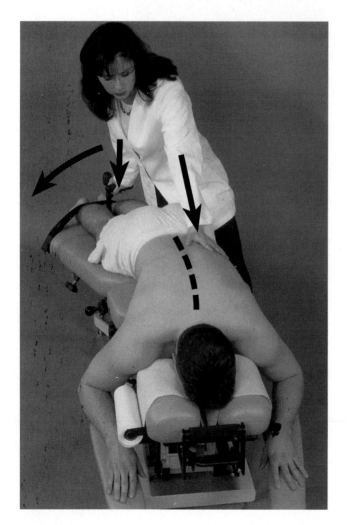

Fig. 4-51 Chattanooga Spinalator table: Clinician laterally flexing patient to right.
- Patient is positioned prone, with the ankles strapped into the β_2 section, which is adjusted for patient height.
- Clinician laterally flexes table to right side of patient, with slight β (-) position, maintaining pressure of patient's left quadratus lumborum muscle.
- A pumping motion is maintained through a cycle of 4 to 5 times, followed by a brief rest and another pumping of the structure 4 to 5 times.
- With a contact over the spine or adjacent to the spine, segmental lateral flexion of a spinal motion segment is performed. (*Table by Chattanooga Group, Inc., Hixon, Tenn.*)

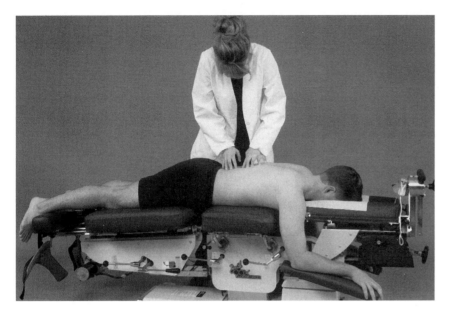

Fig. 4-52 Zenith-Cox table: Clinician using massage over lumbar paraspinal muscles.

- Clinician uses a finger-tip massage over the lumbar paraspinal musculature to assist relaxation.
- Table is in 0, neutral, or in slight β (-) negative.
- The ankle straps are not attached. *(Table by Williams Healthcare Systems, Elgin, Ill.)*

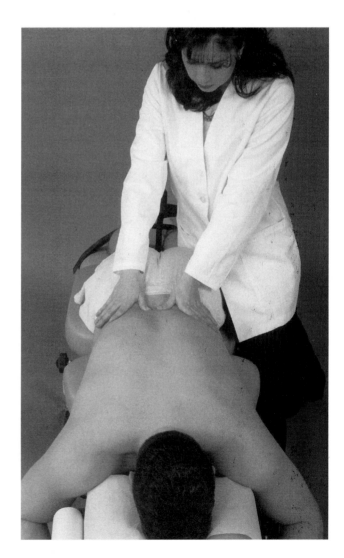

Fig. 4-53 Chattanooga Spinalator table: Clinician applying massage to patient's lumbar musculature.

- Patient is lying prone on the table, which is β (0) neutral or slightly β (-).
- Clinician stands adjacent to the patient and applies muscle massage to the lumbar paraspinal musculature. *(Table by Chattanooga Group, Inc., Hixon, Tenn.)*

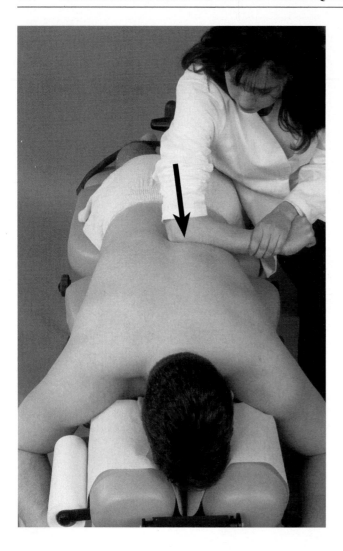

Fig. 4-54 Chattanooga Spinalator table: Clinician applying deep massage to patient's lumbar musculature.

- Patient is lying prone on the table, which is β (0) or slightly β (-).
- Clinician applies deep muscle massage with elbow over the lumbar musculature.
- The β section can also be laterally flexed to provide stretch during the application of deep muscle therapy or other massage of the lumbar musculature. *(Table by Chattanooga Group, Inc., Hixon, Tenn.)*

Fig. 4-55 Zenith-Cox table: Clinician using T-bar.

- Clinician is using a T-bar to apply pressure in goading the lumbar musculature.
- Table is β (0) or slightly β (-), and the ankles are not strapped. *(Table by Williams Healthcare Systems, Elgin, Ill.)*

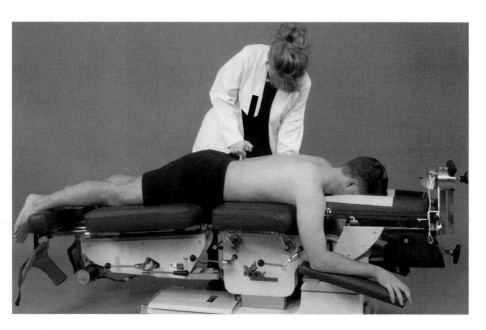

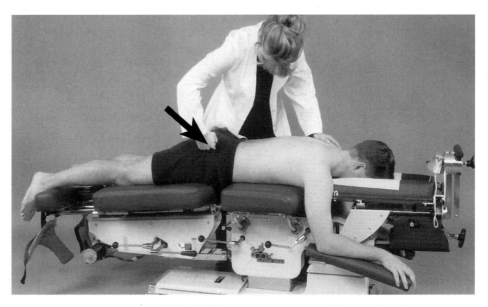

Fig. 4-56 Zenith-Cox table: Clinician using T-bar, alternative position.

- Clinician is using T-bar in alternative position in gluteal muscles.
- Table is β (0) or slightly β (-), and the ankles may or may not be strapped. *(Table by Williams Healthcare Systems, Elgin, Ill.)*

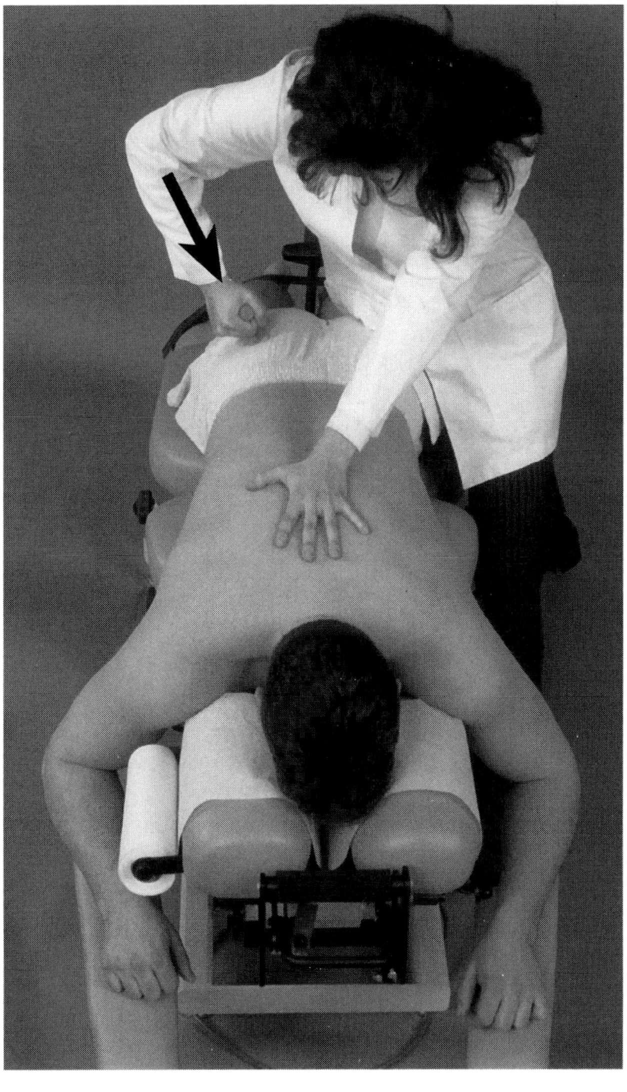

Fig. 4-57 Chattanooga Spinalator table: Clinician using T-bar.

- Clinician is using a T-bar to apply pressure in goading the gluteal musculature.
- Table is β (0) or slightly β (-), and the ankles may or may not be strapped. *(Table by Chattanooga Group Inc., Hixon, Tenn.)*

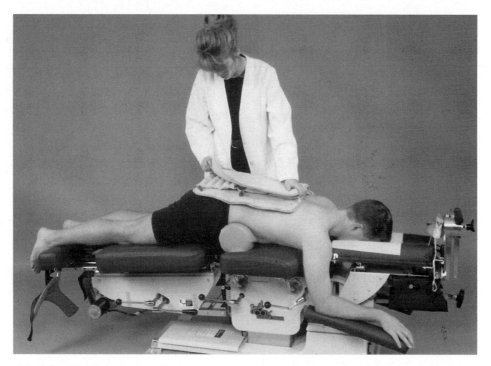

Fig. 4-58 Zenith-Cox table: Clinician applying hot pack to patient.
- Clinician is applying a hot pack to the patient.
- Patient is lying prone, with a lumbopelvic roll under the lower abdomen at the lower part of the β_2 section.
- Table is β (0) or slightly β (-), and the ankles are not strapped. *(Table by Williams Healthcare Systems, Elgin, Ill.)*

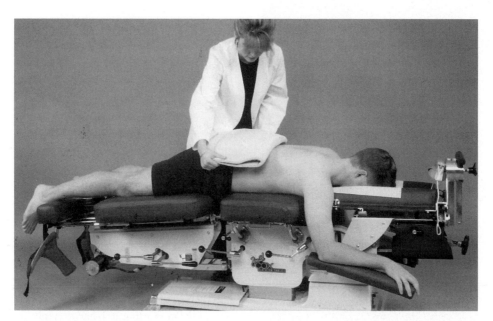

Fig. 4-59 Zenith-Cox table: Clinician applying hot pack to lower back.
- Clinician is applying the hot pack to the patient's lower back.
- Table is β (0) or slightly β (-), and the ankles are not strapped. *(Table by Williams Healthcare Systems, Elgin, Ill.)*

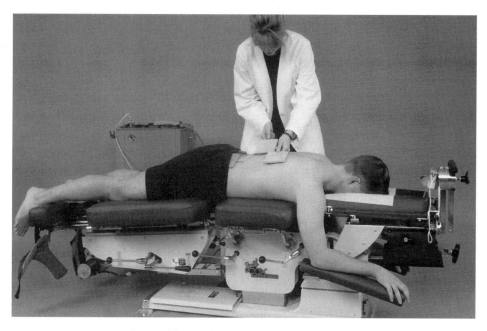

Fig. 4-60 Zenith-Cox table: Clinician applying high-volt therapy to the lumbar spine.
- Clinician is applying high-volt galvanism to the patient's lumbar spine.
- Table is β (0) or slightly β (-), and the ankles are not strapped. *(Table by Williams Healthcare Systems, Elgin, Ill.)*

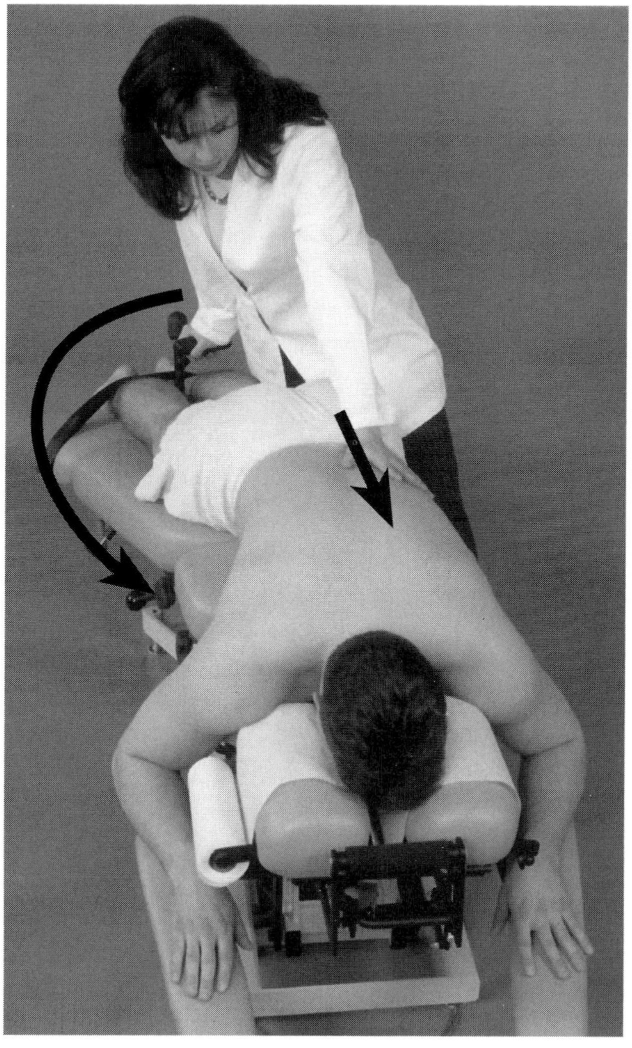

Fig. 4-61 Chattanooga Spinalator table: Clinician performing circumduction in lumbar spine.
- Clinician assumes the usual stance adjacent to the table and applies the treating hand in the manner prescribed.
- Patient is laterally flexed on the table from the right lateral position, with the β section in β (-) position. An arc is then described for circumduction of the area.
- A full revolution is described in one direction then reversed for another revolution.
- The arc described can be repeated several times to achieve increased motion in the lumbar spine at each segmental level. *(Table by Chattanooga Group, Inc., Hixon, Tx.)*

organized areas of evaluation and treatment in a more cogent and understandable form. The work of both men is based almost totally on the pathologic model, but Markey presents his approach through algorithms of evaluation and treatment. (Markey, unpublished data.)

PATIENT POSITIONING

For application of the Cox technique, the preferred table is the Zenith-Cox. However, this technique can be used with many tables, including the Barnes, Spinalight, Titan, Chattanooga, Lloyd, Back Specialist, and others. Markey became an advocate of the Lloyd table, and for several years was on the speaking circuit, demonstrating his approach to the technique of flexion-distraction. All of these tables can be moved to flexion, extension, rotation, and lateral flexion positions (Figs. 4-27 through 4-61).

The patient is positioned prone on the table, with the feet placed over the ankle bar, which is adjustable for length (height) (Fig. 4-32). The placement of the patient on the table is important in the process of applying the therapy. Extreme care should be taken with this table, as with treatment tables of any type, so that the patient is carefully monitored and protected when mounting the table. Anxiety regarding treatment can produce possible confusion and instability in the patient, and this should be carefully observed by the clinician. The patient must be instructed in the proper procedure for getting on and off the table and should be assisted in case of sudden weakness. The clinician should stand adjacent to the patient and provide support to facilitate and monitor placement on the table (Fig. 4-31).

Once appropriately placed, the patient is checked for proper positioning and correct alignment. The arms should be on the arm rests and the hands initially not holding the traction bar at the upper end of the table (Figs. 4-32, 4-33, and 4-34). In some cases, the initial treatment uses a modality of therapy to relieve pain or to relax the musculature in preparation for the distraction (Figs. 4-49 through 4-57). If the musculature is tight and resistant to treatment, therapy such as heat, cold, galvanism, or a combination of these can be applied to provide the desired therapeutic effect (Figs. 4-58, 4-59, and 4-60). Additional lift of the abdomen is sometimes desirable and can be achieved with an abdominal roll approximately 6 to 8 inches in diameter placed under the patient while the table is in the neutral position (Fig. 4-58).

Initially, (with the table distracted in the y axis) the patient is lying prone, and the ankles are not strapped into the ankle restraints. The clinician applies a slight downward positioning of the caudal section of the table (β [-]), creating a slight bending moment over the fulcrum created by the pelvic section and slight flexion to the patient's back (+ θ x) (Fig. 4-44). If the patient can tolerate this 2- to 3-inch deflection of the caudal section, then the table is deflected 1 or 2 inches further. If the flexion (β [-]) is not tolerated by the patient and/or the pain is peripheralized, the process should not continue with further traction but should concentrate on relieving the pain before the therapeutic distraction begins in earnest. Any intolerance is a "red flag" and, although this does not become a clear contraindication for the treatment, it certainly is cautionary and should be treated with respect and restraint. In this instance, more is not better but in fact may make the patient worse.[17]

Once tolerance is determined, the patient can undergo the additional therapy of flexion-distraction to the degree necessary to achieve the desired reduction of pain and a return of normal function.

APPLICATION OF THERAPY

This section discusses Cox's approach to treatment of disc injury. Treatment of areas other than the low back is discussed in Chapter 5. Cox[17] recommends the application of therapy with three 20-second flexion (β [-]) sessions. Once the patient is properly positioned on the table and the tolerance of the patient to flexion is determined, the sessions can begin. The caudal section is used primarily in treating disc injury, facet syndrome, spondylolisthesis, sciatica, and structural problems that are not of pathologic origin. The hand is placed over the spinous process of the superior vertebra of the motion segment to be distracted (e.g., to distract the L5-S1 segment, contact is on the L5 spinous process) (Fig. 4-62). The contact hand is slightly cupped, creating an indentation between the thenar and hypothenar eminence, to receive the protrusion (of the spinous) without placing undue pressure and causing subsequent discomfort to the patient. The patient is encouraged to relax, and the clinician depresses the handle at the foot of the table. If there is no handle, the clinician depresses the foot of the table by hand. The handle is an improvement over placing the hand on the caudal section of the table, improving both the leverage and stance-position of the clinician. Hand position and placement for treatment are demonstrated in Figs. 4-35 and 4-36.

The table is then depressed (β [-]) until the clinician's hand detects that the musculature has reached a point of tautness and all tissue and joint play has been removed from the area under treatment. This point is maintained,

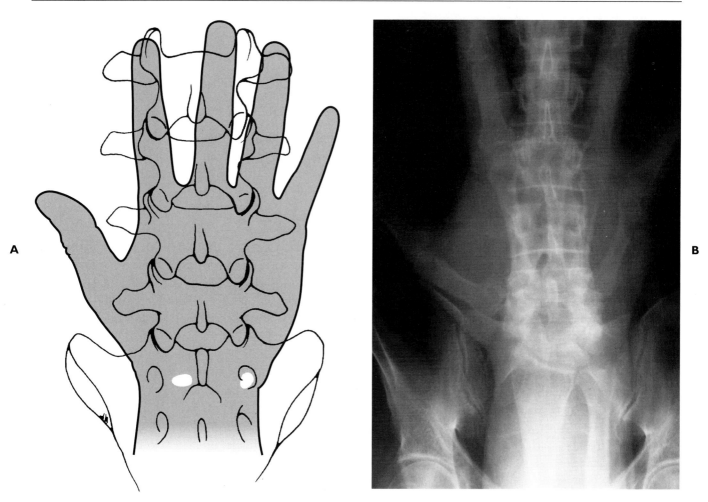

Fig. 4-62 Hand position for contacting the L5 spinous process to distract the L5-S1 segment. (Cox, Leander, Hill, Jensen). **A,** Drawing of hand superimposed on spine. **B,** Radiograph of hand on spine.

and an additional 2 to 3 inches of depression of the table is achieved manually. The caudal section is then allowed to return to the initial taut position or slight flexion (a few degrees β [-]), followed by another downward movement (β [-]) to the previous point over a 20-second period. This process creates the "pumping action" of Cox's distraction technique. This action is repeated 3 times, with a break of a few seconds between each 20-second session. Cox[17] notes that a patient with a protruding disc senses a mild pain on traction; a prolapsed disc will not produce such a sensation. He also warns the clinician not to apply too much traction (β [-]) during the session because this may produce problems in the patient. It may be better to undertreat the patient than to over treat. In the case of disc involvement, the patient is probably sensitive and sore at the point of the injury, and caution is encouraged in the application of the technique.[17]

Markey uses a hand position different than that used by Cox in the execution of the treatment. Markey positions the hands so the spinous process lies between the thumb and the index finger, immediately below the web of the thumb (Fig. 4-38). He believes that this position ensures that the spinous process being treated is not given uncomfortable pressure by the hand. To achieve this position, the practitioner must lean further over the table and maintain that position while providing the treatment. The Markey position contrasts with the position recommended by Cox, in which the hand is cupped slightly, with the spinous process lying below the central crease of the hand, between the thenar and the pisiform, and minimal pressure exerted on overlying tissue. (Markey, unpublished data.)

The following are the essentials of the Cox[17] flexion-distraction treatment:

1. The patient is assisted into a prone position, with the anterior superior spine of the ilium (ASIS) positioned at the base of the thoracic section. The low back is then tested for tolerance to manual distraction. When tolerance has been tested and distraction is found to be tolerable to the patient, the ankle straps can be applied, increasing the tractive force in the area of the proposed treatment.

2. Depression of the caudal section of the table is performed until tautness of the spinal musculature is felt by the clinician.

3. Contact is made and maintained on the spinous process of the vertebra immediately above the disc involvement.

4. Contact on the spinous process of the vertebra is to be maintained with one hand while the other contacts the handle or the foot of the table.

5. Traction is maintained by pressing on the caudal section of the table; patient comfort should be maintained. The subsequent pumping of the caudal section creates a milking action of the disc and, according to Cox, speeds the recovery process.

6. The process outlined above should be repeated to the patient's tolerance. The clinician may palpate a release at the noted vertebral level.

7. One more distraction session (the third) should be performed to patient tolerance for approximately 20 seconds.

8. Following treatment, the caudal section of the table is returned to the neutral position and secured and the ankle straps are released.

9. Musculature in the lower half of the body can be treated manually or with some form of muscle therapy, acupressure, or acupuncture.

10. Modalities of physical therapy can be applied as appropriate.

11. A belt is applied to the patient to provide additional support to the injured area.

12. Home care instructions are provided for the patient.

Cox[17] recommends several accompanying therapies for his disc patients. Home care instructions on activities of daily living (ADL) include suggestions such as avoiding the sitting position; use of alternating hot and cold packs over the back; avoiding constipation to minimize strain on the low back; using a supplement that contains manganese sulfate and other trace minerals, as well as vitamins A, B, and C; eating fruits and vegetables that are high in fiber; and consuming large quantities of fluids. He also advises the patient to use analgesic liniment, avoid certain potentially straining movements, and sleep on a firm mattress. Work can be continued if it does not produce leg pain and, when sitting is possible (later in the treatment), a chair that provides good support should be used. Finally, the patient must perform prescribed exercises as part of the rehabilitation.

SPECIAL TREATMENT

Special treatment on this type of table relates to other forms of illness and injury involving the low back, including scoliosis, spondylolisthesis, facet syndrome, and other problems.

The procedure for treatment of scoliosis differs from that of low back pain, because the lateral curvature is the major focus. Cox[17] identifies this condition as adult scoliosis of an idiopathic origin. He indicates that pain increases with age and degree of scoliotic curvature. Furthermore, he notes that pain usually presents as muscular pain and results from degenerative facets increasingly under structural stress and that radicular pain resulting from foraminal stenosis is possible.[17, 21]

The table used for this treatment is the same as for the other treatment forms (distraction) but also allows tilting of the thoracic and lower sections of the table (α_2 and β rotation). Some tables tilt on a central axis in one or both of these areas; however, in the Zenith-Cox table, both the abdominal and lower sections of the table are on a sliding rocker that allows tilting with a smoother action (less abrupt) than other tables. Both sections tilt (α_2 and β rotation) around a central axis (Figs. 4-63 and 4-64).

The approach to treating scoliosis involves the usual examination, including the taking of a patient history and imaging as necessary to define the problem. Special radiographs may be required to clearly visualize the condition; in some cases these are taken periodically to monitor changes. The table can be positioned in various configurations to accommodate the derotation of the scoliosis, and traction manipulation can be applied manually using the various tables available. Cox[17] indicates that treatment of the patient can be performed with the patient in a side-lying position, should an abdominal position prove uncomfortable. Most of the tables allow many positions to provide the manual manipulative control and thrust necessary (Fig. 4-65).

ADJUNCTIVE THERAPY

Adjunctive therapy includes some of the forms of additional treatment mentioned previously, such as home care, nutritional supplementation, exercise, and application of physical therapy (Figs. 4-58, 4-59, and 4-60). The physical therapy can be applied on the first treat-

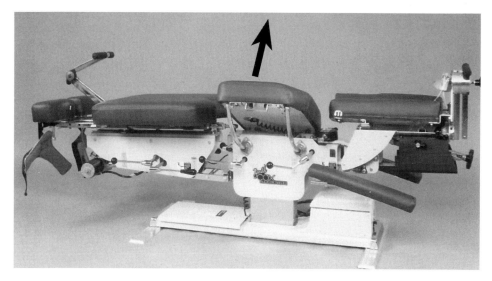

Fig. 4-63 Zenith-Cox table in neutral, with rotation of α_2 section for treatment of scoliosis.
- Patient is positioned prone.
- Table is positioned with the full table in neutral from the α through the β sections.
- The α_2 section is rotated to derotate the curvature of a thoracic scoliosis.
- Additional positioning of the table is possible, with downward bending of the β section and lateral flexing of the β section as required. *(Table by Williams Healthcare Systems, Elgin, Ill.)*

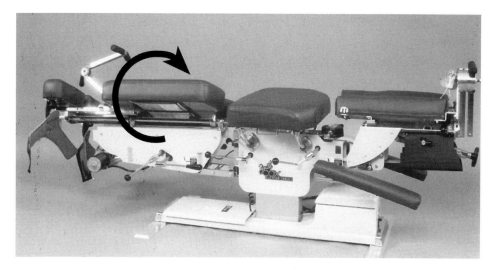

Fig. 4-64 Zenith-Cox table in neutral, with rotation of β section for treatment of scoliosis.
- Table is positioned with the full table in neutral from the α through the β sections.
- The β section is rotated to derotate the curvature of a thoracic and/or lumbar scoliosis.
- Additional positioning of the table is possible, with downward bending of the β section and/or lateral flexing of the β section as required.
- The treatment is run through a cycle of derotation with patient flexing. This is repeated 2 to 3 times, then the patient is allowed rest for a few seconds and the cycle is repeated.
- The objective is derotation of the patient and stretching of the musculature in a manner to reinforce the straightening of the curvature.
- In this manner, extensive leverage is possible with the use of minimum force. *(Table by Williams Healthcare Systems, Elgin, Ill.)*

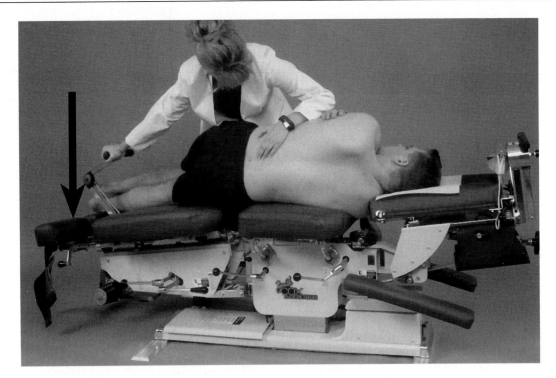

Fig. 4-65 Zenith-Cox table used with patient in side-lying position.
- The side-posture position, used as a stretch for the treatment of scoliosis, may be more readily attained in this position and may be more comfortable to the patient.
- Patient is positioned with the convexity down (e.g., on the right side for a right convex scoliosis).
- Clinician contacts the center of the curve with the cephalad hand and depresses the β section with the caudal hand.
- Cephalad hand applies pressure against the lateral aspect of the spinous processes.
- The number of depressions is 3 to 5, and the number of cycles for a treatment of scoliosis is 2 to 3. *(Table by Williams Healthcare Systems, Elgin, Ill.)*

ment and thereafter for some portion of the treatment period, and the other forms of therapy, such as exercise and patient education, can be applied at different times during the treatment, as appropriate.

PROTOCOL/REGIMEN

The protocol for the Cox technique for treatment of a disc lesion includes an initial intensive treatment that may require the patient to stay in the office for the full day, depending on the severity of the patient's symptoms. Cox advises the patient not to sit but to remain primarily recumbent. A major concern is that when the patient goes home, the movement of entering the car, driving, and stepping out of the car can be detrimental to the patient's condition.

One of the first steps after treatment is to fit the patient with a lumbar support that is to be worn 24 hours a day until the leg pain eases. With improvement of the leg pain, the support is gradually removed. Cox[17] notes that all patients with acute disc lesions are treated for 3 months. Initially, treatment is daily, but as the pain eases the frequency is reduced and the length of time between treatments is increased.

Cox[17] issues a strong caveat to his patients that they are allowed a 3-week period of trial therapy. If leg pain does not decrease by 50% during this period, a neurosurgical consult will be scheduled. He notes that this establishes some parameters for both the clinician and the patient, and, if the expected results are not obtained, the patient is referred.

In the case of conditions such as sprain or strain, the treatment protocol is similar, but emphasis is placed on muscle work. For a scoliosis, the treatment concentrates on derotation and flexing to the side opposite the scoliosis. The objective is to provide movement to which the body is unaccustomed and perhaps incapable of performing or finds difficult to perform. For a spondylolisthesis, the objective is to avoid contacting the affected segment in a manner that could worsen the condition, such as manipulating the segment to the anterior, which is an inappropriate direction for the segment. The best approach is to contact the segment above and to support the involved segment.

For most treatment on this table or a similar model, the caudal section is depressed to the point at which the clinician feels tension in the patient's back. A series of 3 to 5 depressions is made, followed by a 10- to 15-second rest and another set of depressions, for a total of 2 to 3 cycles. This procedure may be repeated 2 to 3 times, depending on the severity of the problem and the tolerance of the patient. The patient may not feel the full effect of the treatment at the time it is given, and therefore the clinician must be careful to not overtreat the patient, because considerable leverage is applied.

LEANDER (FLEXION-DISTRACTION CPM)

RATIONALE: THE CONCEPT OF THE LEANDER TABLE

The Leander table is an example of motion-assisted distraction (MAD) that provides motorized distraction capability. This means that the distraction provided manually and mechanically in the Zenith-Cox table is executed with the assistance of a motor. The clinician contacts the patient directly over the spine, as with the Cox technique, using the same type of hand contacts. The difference is that both hands are free for use on the spine as the motor moves the pelvic piece. The duration of flexion and extension of the spine is usually controlled by a timer. Several tables have incorporated a motion-assist with a motor that provides assisted flexion capability. The Leander table is the only one that currently has this motorized flexion-extension capability. Manufacturers of other tables are experimenting with an air-powered function for flexion-extension. The Hill Intertrac table, which is discussed later, incorporates a motion-assist in the linear axis.

The Leander technique, for which the Leander table was developed, was created by Leander Eckard and is based on the concept of producing continuous passive motion (CPM) during spinal correction. The technique, an example of MAD, was designed to provide continuous motion for the spine and to allow the lumbar spine to assume its normal lordosis while in a prone position. This position allows gravity to pull the abdomen downward and create the lordosis that is deemed essential to the technique. Patient position on the Leander table is drawn from the surgical table, on which the chest and head are supported prone and the knees are drawn up under the abdomen, supposedly creating the lumbar lordosis. This concept of the surgical model appears to be erroneous; the Leander table does not allow such a lordosis because the support of the thighs under the abdomen preclude forming the lordosis to the extent of the surgical position. Eckard[22] asserts that this position enhances biomechanical levers and allows a reduction in venous pressure in the vicinity of the involved nerve root (Figs. 4-66 through 4-74).

CPM is used in the Leander technique in evaluation of the spine to identify fixations, to treat the spine where fixations are found, and to determine if the treatment was successful. The contact established over the spine is similar to that of the Cox technique, using the base of the palm with the spinous process in the indentation corresponding to the carpal tunnel of the contact hand. The other hand is placed over the contact hand (see Fig. 4-72), with the fingers and thumb partially wrapped around the contact wrist.

PATIENT POSITIONING

The three major differences between the techniques of Leander and Cox are as follows: (1) the thoracic section of the Leander table is released, causing it to depress when released (α_2 [-]), and allowing lumbar lordosis to form while the patient is in the prone position; (2) lateral flexion is accomplished with the cephalad section of the table (α_1, α_2); and (3) the flexion-distraction is accomplished by a motorized function of the table. When Cox's technique is applied, the lumbar lordosis is flattened, the thoracic section (α_2) is neutral (0), and the caudal section of the table (β) is capable of lateral flexion. The major difference between the two techniques, however, is that the Leander technique is applied with a motorized table, allowing the application of motion-assisted manipulation or adjusting, whereas Cox's technique is totally manual or mechanically assisted manipulation/adjusting.

Text continued on p. 129

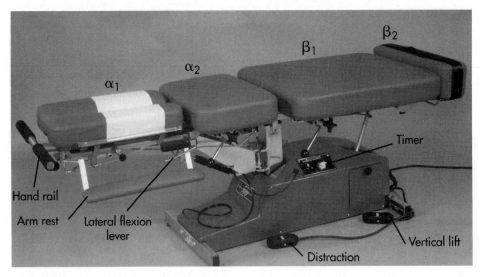

Fig. 4-66 Leander table in neutral position.
- Leander table is positioned in neutral, with all sections at 0.
- Vertical positioning is located at the lowest point.
- Note the foot switches for activating the β section and vertical lift.
- Note the position of the hand rail at the upper end of the table, adjacent to the α_1 section and the arm rests on either side of the α_1 section.
- The switches for the timer and speed control for the Leander table are located on the lower housing, near the vertical shaft.
- A hand control for lateral bending of the α and α_1 sections is located adjacent to the headpiece, or α_1 section.
- A strap for the feet is located on the extensible foot rest at the extreme caudal end of the β section. *(Table by Leander Health Technologies Corp., Port Orchard, Wash.)*

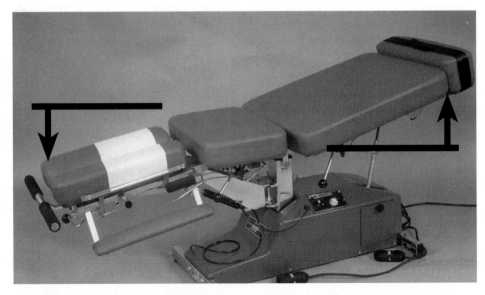

Fig. 4-67 Leander table with facepiece α_1 (-), abdominal α_2 (0), and lower section β (+).
- The Leander table is positioned with α_1 (-), α_2 (0), and β (+).
- Table is at minimum elevation. *(Table by Leander Health Technologies Corp., Port Orchard, Wash.)*

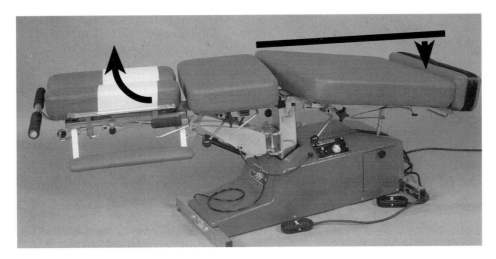

Fig. 4-68 Leander table with facepiece α_1 and abdominal α_2 (0) and right-laterally flexed lower section β (-).
- The Leander table is α_1 and α_2 (0), with β (-).
- Note that α_1 and α_2 are laterally bent to the right, and the elevation of the table is minimal. *(Table by Leander Health Technologies Corp., Port Orchard, Wash.)*

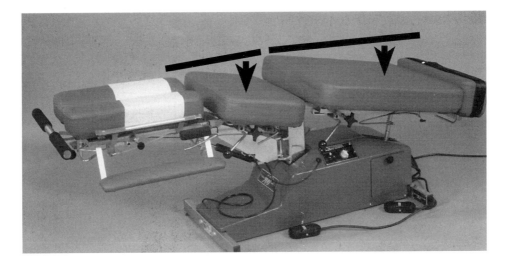

Fig. 4-69 Leander table with facepiece α_1 (0), abdominal α_2 (-), and lower section β (-).
- The Leander table is shown with the α_1 section neutral, α_2 negative, and β negative.
- No lateral bending is shown, and the table is at minimal elevation. *(Table by Leander Health Technologies Corp., Port Orchard, Wash.)*

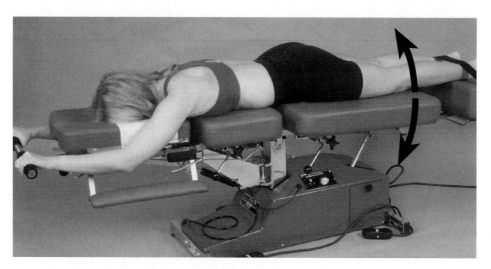

Fig. 4-70 Leander table: Patient positioned with all table sections in neutral.

- Patient is positioned on the Leander table with all the table sections in neutral, the ankles strapped on the extension of the β section, and the hands holding onto the head bar for maximum traction.
- It may not be appropriate for each patient to be strapped at the ankles nor for the hands to hold the bar for the first treatment session because this configuration may produce excessive traction for the patient.
- Traction-distraction should be tested on the patient to determine tolerance before attempting the maximum possible.
- The height of the table may be adjusted to fit the size of the clinician.
- Clinician must give the patient clear directions for mounting the table and assuming the correct position.
- The clinician should stand close by the patient to observe the patient's movements and render assistance as required.
- This assistance is especially important with a patient experiencing severe pain or in the case of the frail elderly. *(Table by Leander Health Technologies Corp., Port Orchard, Wash.)*

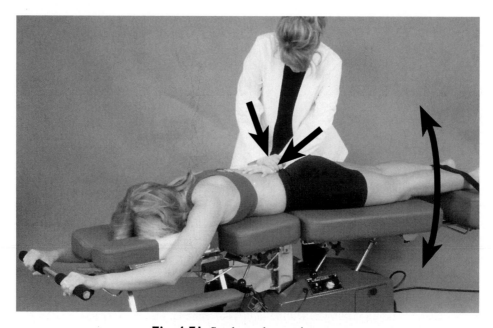

Fig. 4-71 See legend opposite page.

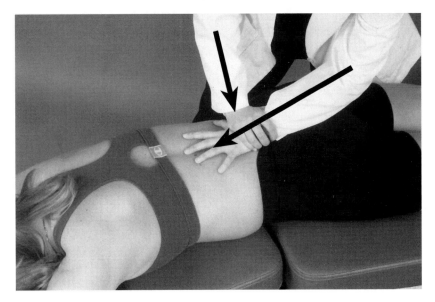

Fig. 4-72 Leander table: Close-up of hand position as used on the Leander table.
- Patient is positioned in the neutral position on the Leander table, and the clinician's hands are placed over the lower lumbar spine in preparation for delivering distraction manipulation to the patient.
- Clinician's position is most advantageous when standing with legs approximately 2 feet apart, with a contact hand resting over the spinous process and the opposite hand used over the contact hand to deliver the stabilizing force.
- The contact hand delivers the force in an inferior-to-superior (I-to-S) direction while the stabilizing hand provides force in the posterior-to-anterior (P-to-A) direction. *(Table by Leander Health Technologies Corp., Port Orchard, Wash.)*

Fig. 4-71 Leander table: Clinician standing adjacent.
- Clinician stands adjacent to the table, with the patient lying prone and the table in the neutral position.
- Table is adjustable for the clinician's height. When the patient is securely, correctly, and comfortably positioned on the table, the clinician can then start the table in β (-) direction at a preset speed and arc by pressing on the foot pedal.
- As the table starts the cycle, the clinician places the hands for appropriate manipulation.
- The ankle strap and hand bar may or may not be used, as deemed appropriate by the clinician. *(Table by Leander Health Technologies Corp., Port Orchard, Wash.)*

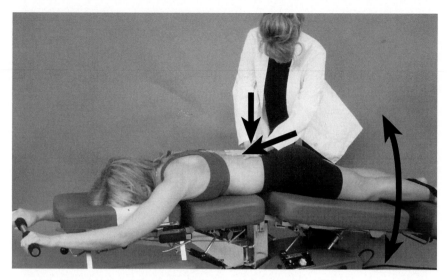

Fig. 4-73 Leander table: Start of cycle.
- Patient is positioned on the Leander table as appropriate for the individual's condition. The β section moves into a negative angle while the clinician resists the resultant flexion of the patient, creating traction on the lumbar spine.
- Note that in this illustration the α_2 section remains in neutral. *(Table by Leander Health Technologies Corp., Port Orchard, Wash.)*

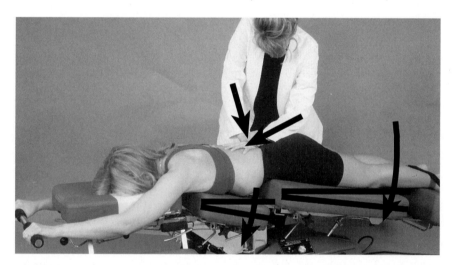

Fig. 4-74 Flexion-distraction on the Leander table, with the abdominal (α_2) section negative.
- Patient is positioned on the Leander table, with the α_2 section negative while the β section is moving from neutral (0) into full negative position.
- Clinician is providing resistance in the lumbar spine as the arc of movement is experienced.
- With the α_2 section in a negative position, a lordosis is reinforced in the lumbar spine and the resistance to the patient flexing on the table is created by pressing into the lumbar curvature, creating distraction for the lumbar spine distal to the point of contact.
- Clinician is positioned with hands on the area to be treated. The table is activated (the speed and timer are set before activating the table) with the foot switch, and the arc of movement is started; the cycle of downward bending is performed 4 to 6 times.
- The cycle is followed by a rest period of a few seconds and then another cycle is undertaken, with the hands of the clinician in place to provide resistance on the patient. *(Table by Leander Health Technologies Corp., Port Orchard, Wash.)*

These characteristics lead to important differences between the two techniques. The creation of a lordosis while in the prone position does change the biomechanics of the vertebral motion segment unit, with less compression taking place toward the anterior of the disc. The fulcrum created in the lower back with the lordosis present moves from the L5-S1 level into the midthoracic spine and alters the mechanics of the tractive force. The use of lateral flexion with the cephalad section (α_1 and α_2) is also quite different from one table and technique to the other. Lateral flexion is more difficult for the clinician to perform and circumduction of the lumbar spine is impossible with the Leander table. When lateral flexion is performed, the release handle for lateral movement must be continually compressed by the clinician, and, on release of the handle, the table locks in that particular position until released again. The leverage for the clinician in lateral flexion (α_1 and α_2) is greatly altered and made more difficult on the Leander table. Additionally, the amount of excursion of the pelvic piece (β section) is greatly increased with the Leander table and the distance is constant. It therefore cannot be varied nor modified for individual patients.

APPLICATION OF THERAPY

The double-hand contact is established over the spinous process of the superior vertebral segment to be treated, and pressure is applied inferiorly to superiorly while the table is in downward motion. Pressure is released in the spine while the table is moving toward neutral in the y axis of the spine. As in all the traction techniques, the amount of pressure applied varies with conditions relating to the patient. With a patient who is in acute pain, osteoporotic, or very small (i.e., a child) or in the presence of certain other conditions, less pressure is required than with a healthy young male or female of moderate build. The double-hand contact will provide the clinician with a high level of leverage and control when applying force to the spine. This force can be regulated because the clinician has great potential for control with the use of two hands and the CPM mode.

With the Leander table, controls are necessary for speed, trajectory of the caudal (β) section (the distance of travel), and α lateral flexion. Control of the trajectory is achieved through positioning inside the motor housing and by adjusting the stroke through manipulating the height of the table, which will give more or less flexion or extension. Speed and the timer are controlled with a dial on the left lower level of the base of the table. For lateral flexion of the α section, controls are located under the arm rests. Lateral flexion in the α section is accomplished with the upper, or cephalad, section of the table while the table in the lower or β section is in motion. Laterally flexing the table (α section) increases the pull on the side opposite the flexion and can be enhanced by placing the hands as shown in Fig. 4-72 and holding with moderate pressure as the table completes its flexion of the β section during CPM in the spine. This table allows the clinician to provide treatment incrementally and allows gradual reduction of an abnormal position of a vertebra without using the rapid force of a short-lever, high-velocity technique.

The Leander technique is applied as follows:

1. A patient history is taken, the patient is examined, and additional studies, such as imaging, are performed as appropriate.
2. Once the problem is identified and an approach to treatment is determined, the patient is placed on the table.
3. Care is taken to place the patient correctly, with the crest of the ilium at the upper edge of the lower leaf, or β, section. The first time the patient is placed on the table the clinician is advised to stand near the patient, to be available should the patient need support.
4. The feet are observed and leg length is checked for a short leg on either side. If a short leg is observed, a challenge or other test may be in order to determine if there is pelvic (sacroiliac) involvement.
5. The patient's ankles can be secured to the table with the ankle straps; however, testing of the flexion-extension of the lower section should be performed initially with the ankle straps unattached, to determine tolerance of the traction effect, speed setting, and trajectory.
6. When tolerance has been established, traction in the β (-) direction can be initiated at the appropriate speed and depth for approximately 10 to 20 minutes of CPM.
7. The clinician contacts the patient with both hands. No power for the flexion-extension is provided by the clinician because the unit has motorized power for the distractive force. The contact is made by the clinician on the segment above the level of desired treatment.
8. Once a period of trial therapy has been completed using CPM on the Leander table, a full course can be scheduled, with periodic reevaluations and setting of new schedules according to progress of pain reduction and improvement in function.

SPECIAL TREATMENT

Treatment of scoliosis using the Leander table is advocated. A combination of body-restraining straps are used, with the patient in a prone position. Straps are secured over the upper thoracic (T3), midthoracic (T7), and upper lumbar (L1) spinal areas. An additional strap may be used at the lower pelvis, across the level of the sacrococcygeal area. Lateral flexing of the upper, or cephalad, section of the table is required to offset the curvature by flexing away from the curve, using the belt as a compensatory support mechanism. During treatment using the belts, CPM of the table is maintained for about 20 minutes. This procedure is repeated daily, 5 times per week for 14 to 20 weeks to affect the scoliotic curvature. No available data, however, supports the efficacy of this treatment.

Treatment of facet syndrome, spondylolisthesis, and other conditions is possible with this table. The power assist functions free both of the clinician's hands for treatment. The clinician can also treat extremities with a traction force applied with a combination of table flexion-extension (β [+/-]) and clinician holding and positioning of the extremity. As with any treatment, the relevant indications and contraindications must be understood and heeded.

PROTOCOL/REGIMEN

The Leander technique is based on the concept of CPM, which is applied with the patient lying prone on the table. Treatment is initiated following the usual chiropractic, orthopedic, and neurologic evaluation of the patient, as well as any necessary studies and tests. The patient is then started on a treatment plan that usually incorporates a trial period of therapy to determine how the patient will respond to the treatment. The treatment plan should reflect the severity of the condition and the state of the patient. The treatment is to be applied until the patient shows improvement, pain is eliminated or at least improved, and function is restored.

The treatment should relate to the patient's state; the more severe condition should receive a gentler application of treatment until the patient shows improvement. The table should always be started in the neutral position, with both upper sections parallel with the ground and the lateral flexion section set at neutral. The flexion control will not work unless the timer is set, and the speed of the flexion unit must be adjusted. Careful control of the speed and the timer is necessary to minimize potential danger to the patient as a result of too rapid speed or too much flexion (β [-]). With the Leander table, the depth of the flexion (β [-]) is difficult to control; therefore extra caution must be taken with the speed.

The response to treatment on this table should approximate that on other distraction tables, and the patient should demonstrate improvements in the capacity to function. The treatment will range from daily to 2 to 3 times per week. A treatment session lasts approximately 5 to 15 minutes. As the improvement becomes more apparent, the patient is seen on a diminishing schedule until completion of treatment.

GRAVITY-ASSISTED INTERMITTENT TRACTION (GAIT) (USING THE HILL INTERTRAC TABLE)

The motion-assisted distraction (MAD) technique performed on the Hill Intertrac table allows the patient to be treated in many positions while in traction, including the gravity-assisted position (GAIT), with the feet elevated above the level of the head. The Hill table, like the Leander table, is a MAD table with a motor that minimizes the manual effort required in adjusting patients. The Hill technique and table were developed by Thomas Hill of Lakefield, Ontario, Canada. In the process of exploring the methods traditionally used to perform distraction, Hill[24] developed a technique and a motion-assisted table on which to perform his manipulative steps. Through the use of their tables and techniques, others such as Cox and Leander have advocated moving the spine through an arc in the sagittal plane to accomplish a stretch in the lower back. The intermittent traction achieved on these tables repeatedly creates this arc as the patient is bent at the waist and the lower part of the body is alternately lowered and elevated (β [-] to neutral [0]) to achieve this arc.[24] The major emphasis and capability of the Hill table is the mechanized, or motion-assisted, traction of the patient in the y axis of the body. This is a direct approach to achieving traction of the spine because it involves a minimum fulcrum and causes a direct separation of the spine in an axial, or long axis, direction.

The practitioner should be familiar with the Hill Intertrac table and its operation and capabilities when attempting the various movements. The caudal section is capable of side-bending approximately 45 degrees to both the right and left. This movement, which can be locked in the full laterally-flexed position (β right or left) is also capable of simultaneous movement into flexion. Side-bending is possible with the β, or lower, section, in combination with the simultaneous distractive movement (MAD) of this section.

Recumbent motion assisted palpation (MAP) is possible using the Intertrac table. The extremely easy manual side-bending action of the caudal (β) section of the table allows the performance of MAP. This positioning allows for specific and easy "joint-play" examination of the sacrum, ilia, symphysis, hip, lumbars, thoracic spine, and ribs. Because MAP is performed with the patient recumbent, the technique is appropriate for any patient condition (acute, chronic, aged, obese, and so on) (see Chapter 6).

With the patient in the prone position, the clinician palpates the lumbar and thoracic spine. Side-bending the patient to the left will produce a convexity on the right side of the spine. By contacting the left side L5 level with the thumb, the clinician firmly forces the spinous process into the produced convexity. The clinician is thus assessing motion of the L5 spinous from its neutral position to its maximum deviation to the right. This assessment also can include quality of movement and the end-feel of motion.

As the motion-assisted palpation continues, each level of the spine is examined in the same manner. Each level of the spine is side-bent to either side, with one level immediately following the other.

This procedure allows the clinician to formulate an immediate assessment of adjacent articulations, one after the other. Motion-assisted palpation should be defined as part of the assessment or evaluation of the spine so that lack of motion or motion aberrations can be identified and marked for appropriate treatment. Related articulations must be compared at the same level (the facets), and the "fish tailing" of the lower section of the table allows for this motion-related comparison.[24]

The motion described by this side-bending is a combination of lateral flexion and rotation of the spine. Hill[24] contends that separation of the two actions during examination and treatment modes is not easily accomplished. He notes that the two actions are so coupled that to try to discern or correct alleged separate action is not worth the effort. Farfan[25] states as a further elaboration on this point that "Lateral bend without rotation or flexion appears possible only for small degrees of movement." Grieve[26] also relates his insights on side-bending, stating that "Side bending without rotation seems impossible, except for the first degree or two of motion only." We do not know if these biomechanics apply to the musculoskeletal system in a prone or a non–weight-bearing position without a lordosis formed.

The active sitting form of motion palpation of the lumbar spine has the practitioner examine for any aberration in the expected spinous movement into the concavity.[27] With the patient in the prone position, the examiner evaluates for any compromise in the anticipated spinous motion into the convexity. That spinous motion should be

to the concavity in the sitting position and to the convexity in the prone position represents a novel contradiction. Hill (Hill, unpublished data, 1978) indicates that he performed a radiographic study in 1978 to determine if radiographic findings would correlate with palpation findings where, in the prone position, the normal excursion is for the spinous to move into the convexity. Two students at Anglo-European Chiropractic College, in their jointly prepared thesis, studied this same area and reached the similar conclusion that the spinous processes in prone bending rotate to the same side as the concavity.[28] These findings suggest the axis of movement for axial rotation shifts with a change in lordosis.

The practitioner can test motion in the spine by laterally flexing the caudal section of the table alternately right and left and palpating for fixations, beginning at the L5 level and progressing up the spine (toward the head), through the thoracic vertebrae (until motion is no longer detectable). Placement of the patient for this procedure is with the ASIS of the pelvis positioned at the upper edge of the caudal section of the table.

The thoracolumbar junction requires special attention. Instead of palpating the area by stressing each spinous separately, the clinician should first stress left side-bending, using a three-finger contact on the left side of T11, T12, and L1, and then check right side-bending by stressing with three fingers on the right of T11, T12, and L1. It is well established that T12 is considered to be the transitional area between the more mobile lumbar spine and the less flexible thoracic spine. The clinician should assess the gradient of motion in this area by spanning the levels to avoid assuming that a fixation exists at the upper levels when only palpating a normal decrease in function (Fig. 4-94).

After the three-finger contact is made at this area and a feel for the usual motion decrease at the more cephalad levels is determined, single-finger contact can be made at each spinous to determine fixation at each specific level. The thoracolumbar junction is a difficult area to palpate and treat. It is, however, an area that requires thorough examination. In a study of 350 patients suffering with low back pain, Maigne[29] demonstrated that the low back pain of 40% of the subjects originated in the thoracolumbar junction and that treatment of this area alleviated their symptoms.

The Hill table is designed to duplicate the standing antalgia of the patient and then pull, or traction, the patient along the y axis of the body. There is no repeated flexion moment (β [-]). Hill[24] notes that there can be many causative factors in the spinal problems treated by chiropractors, including those that involve the disc directly or those that identify the facets or some other related structure of the spine and its biomechanics. Many of these problems present with an "antalgic signature," and the Hill Intertrac and other tables that provide for lateral flexion are designed to accommodate this resultant posture in its adaptable form. However, the Hill table is the only one that provides axial traction while the patient is laterally flexed. Moreover, although other tables (Cox, Lloyd, Barnes) produce linear distraction through manual or mechanical means, the Hill table is the only one that produces this movement of motorized cyclic action.

PATIENT POSITIONING

Consider, for example, the patient that presents with low back pain and sciatica that is aggravated by the erect position and further increased by extension. This patient is more comfortable in a flexed, or forward-bent, position and therefore requires distraction in flexion. The β section of the table can be moved downward (β [-]), negative from the horizontal to any point up to 22 degrees. This flexion is achieved through a mechanical actuator under the β section of the table and activated by a floor-mounted switch. The speed of distraction is controlled by a table-mounted rheostat that creates speeds ranging from 1 to 30 rpm. The rheostat is located under the β section of the table.

Some patients experience low back and sciatic pain that is aggravated by the forward-bent position. This case is often relieved by the extended position, and therefore traction should be applied in extension. The β section is extended into the β positive (+) position. The maximum extension is 12 degrees and can be set at any desired point in this arc, up to the maximum 12 degrees. Once in this position, the patient is exposed to intermittent traction along the axis of the β section. The patient therefore experiences distraction in extension, and there is no repeated flexion-distraction moment (β [-/+]) during the therapy (Figs. 4-76 through 4-78).

APPLICATION OF THERAPY

In gravity-assisted intermittent traction (GAIT), the parallel-to-the-ground position can be altered by tipping the Δ section of the table to an inclination of up to 30 degrees. Linear traction can be continued with the table in this tipped position, and either flexion or extension, as well as lateral flexion, can be applied simultaneously. The GAIT technique allows intermittent linear traction,

which is in the plane parallel to the y axis of the body and can be performed with the table in a tipped position (Figs. 4-79 and 4-80).

The positioning of the feet is facilitated by the use of an ankle strapping system, when appropriate, or the Distrac Wedge (a foam wedge) placed under the ankles. This ensures proper ankle placement and slightly enhanced traction without firmly fixing the patient's feet. In some cases, enhanced traction is appropriate but in others a slight amount is adequate (Fig. 4-89).

The Hill technique includes the following, performed with motion-assisted linear distraction:

1. Linear traction or distraction applied in the y axis of the body (Figs. 4-86 through 4-90).
2. Gravity-assisted intermittent traction (GAIT), which includes tipping of the Δ section of the table up to 30 degrees, with the full assist of the table for any combination of flexion, extension, and/or lateral flexion (Figs. 4-97 through 4-100).
3. Motion-assisted thrust technique (MATT) couples intermittent distraction with specific common chiropractic adjustive procedures (see Chapter 6).
4. Recumbent motion-assisted palpation (MAP) allows for motion palpation with the patient in the recumbent position, allowing for patient comfort and full control by the clinician (Figs. 4-93 and 4-94).
5. Intermittent cervical traction (ICT) involves the use of a mechanical harness or clinician hand contact to the patient's cervical spine (see Chapter 5).

This traction, used in a controlled manner, is intermittent and horizontal, introducing flexion, extension, or lateral flexion into the process, along with elevation of the table caudally. The clinician must exercise skill in diagnosis of the condition, identifying the proper level of disc or other involvement. The usual orthopedic and neurologic tests for the establishment of a diagnosis of a disc or other lesion must be performed (Figs. 4-75 through 4-100).

SPECIAL TREATMENT

Intermittent cervical traction (ICT) is also possible with the GAIT technique on the Hill Intertrac table. The traction can be performed either with a traction harness attached to the table or with the clinician's hands manually holding the head of the patient. With the assistance of the harness and the "pin" on the table, the traction position can be altered, with various angles possible. However, with the use of the clinician's hands, many positions are possible and are instantly alterable for

Text continued on p. 146

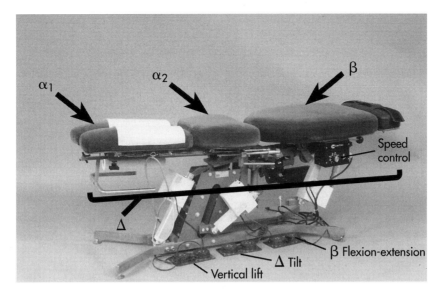

Fig. 4-75 Hill Intertrac in neutral position.
- The Hill Intertrac table is positioned in neutral.
- The α_1, α_2 and β sections are all neutral (0), parallel with the floor.
- The speed control and on-off switch are located on side of β section.
- Head, or α_1, section and α_2 sections do not move.
- Note foot switches located on floor to control elevation of whole table, Δ tilt, and positive and negative bending of β section. *(Table by Thomas Hill Tables, Lakefield, Ont.)*

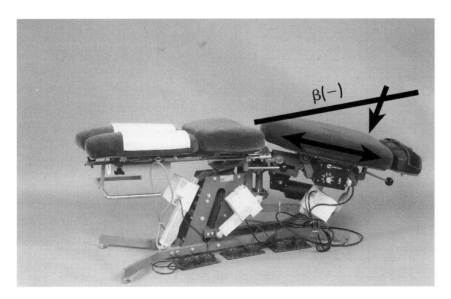

Fig. 4-76 Hill Intertrac table: Downward, or (-) negative bending of β section.
- The β section is positioned in β (-) position
- The remainder of the table is positioned in neutral, or 0, with no elevation. *(Table by Thomas Hill Tables, Lakefield, Ont.)*

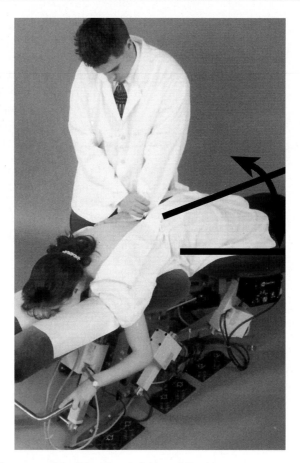

Fig. 4-77 Hill Intertrac table: Negative, left-lateral flexion.
- The β section is positioned in β (-).
- The β section is also positioned in left-lateral flexion, with no elevation. *(Table by Thomas Hill Tables, Lakefield, Ont.)*

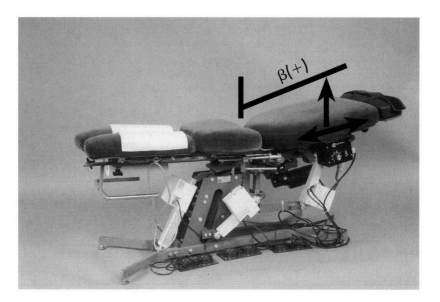

Fig. 4-78 Hill Intertrac table: Table is positioned β (+) positive.
- The β section is positioned in β (+).
- The remainder of the table is positioned in neutral, or 0, with no elevation. *(Table by Thomas Hill Tables, Lakefield, Ont.)*

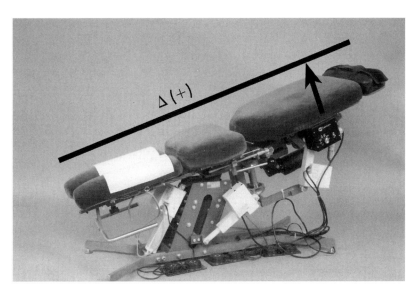

Fig. 4-79 Hill Intertrac table: Table is positioned Δ positive.
- The Δ section is positioned positive, with no elevation.
- Motion-assisted movement of β section is possible in this position. *(Table by Thomas Hill Tables, Lakefield, Ont.)*

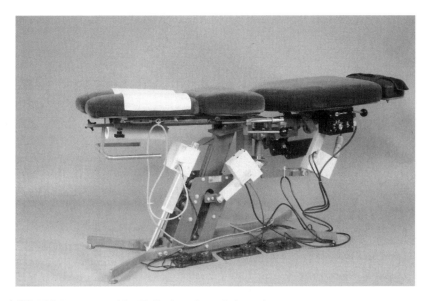

Fig. 4-80 Hill Intertrac table: Full elevation of Δ section.
- The Δ section is elevated fully to accommodate differences in working positions and height of clinicians.
- The other sections of the table are neutral and parallel to the ground. *(Table by Thomas Hill Tables, Lakefield, Ont.)*

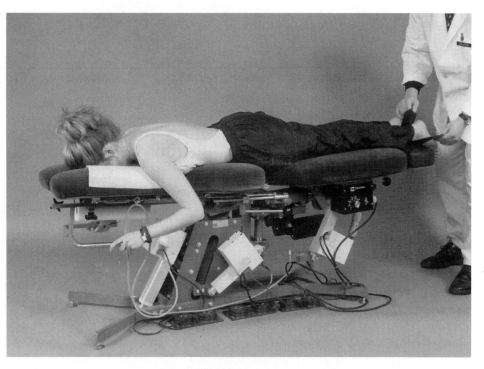

Fig. 4-81 Hill Intertrac table: Attaching ankle straps.

- Once the patient has been carefully assisted onto the table, the ankle straps can be attached. The ankle straps are used only when use is not uncomfortable in the traction and are attached before axial distraction is initiated.
- Patient is positioned with the crest of the ilium slightly on the α_2 section, and the legs are straight.
- The ankles are positioned so that the adjustable ankle rest is against the dorsum of the foot, creating slight ankle extension. *(Table by Thomas Hill Tables, Lakefield, Ont.)*

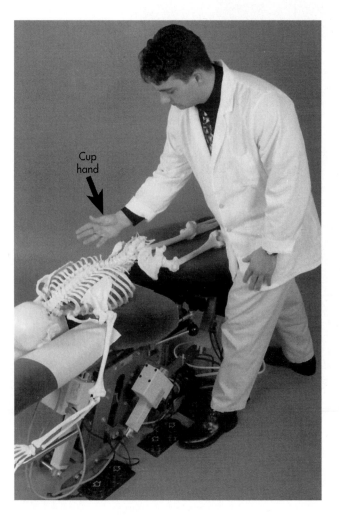

Cup
hand

Fig. 4-82 Hill Intertrac table: Position of patient (skeleton) and clinician's hand position.

- Patient is positioned on the table as shown, and clinician assumes a position adjacent on the right or on the left side.
- Clinician's hands are placed as shown, with the carpal tunnel of the hand over the spinous that is to be treated. *(Table by Thomas Hill Tables, Lakefield, Ont.)*

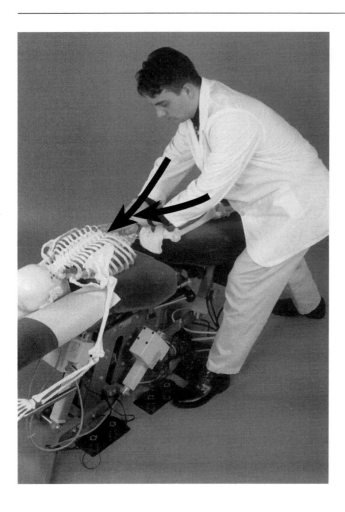

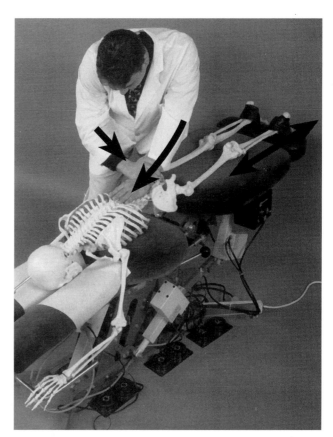

Fig. 4-83 Hill Intertrac table: Clinician's hand placement and stance.

- Clinician stands adjacent to the table during the application of the distractive motion of the table.
- Clinician's feet are placed approximately shoulder-width apart, and the table is raised to a position comfortable for the delivery of the manipulation.
- Clinician is standing on the side opposite that shown in the previous illustration. All else remains unchanged. *(Table by Thomas Hill Tables, Lakefield, Ont.)*

Fig. 4-84 Hill Intertrac table: Clinician's hand placement and stance.

- Clinician stands adjacent to the table during the application of the distractive motion of the table.
- Clinician's hands are placed as described at the appropriate level for treatment.
- In this illustration the entire table is in a neutral position, with the working surface elevated slightly. *(Table by Thomas Hill Tables, Lakefield, Ont.)*

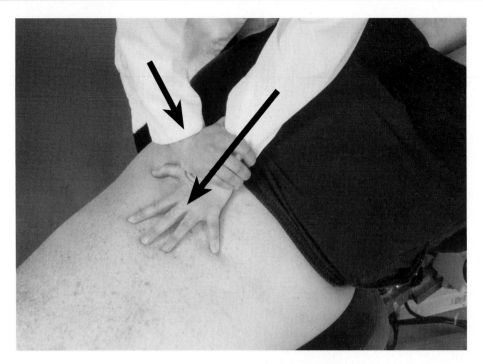

Fig. 4-85 Hill Intertrac table: Placement of clinician's treating hand.
- The hand of the clinician is positioned as shown in the illustration.
- The carpal tunnel of the treating hand is placed over the spinous of L5.
- The stabilizing hand is placed over the treating hand.
- The treatment provides a resistance I-to-S force on the table, providing axial distraction while the stabilizing hand provides P-to-A force to hold the treating hand in the appropriate position. *(Table by Thomas Hill Tables, Lakefield, Ont.)*

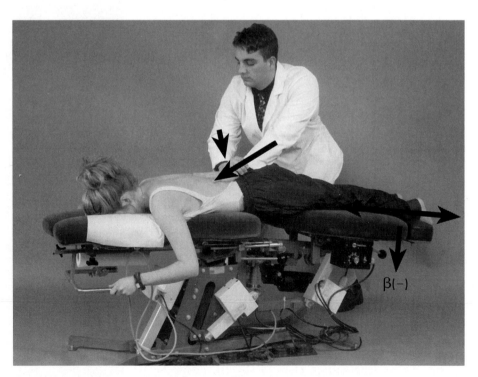

Fig. 4-86 See legend opposite page.

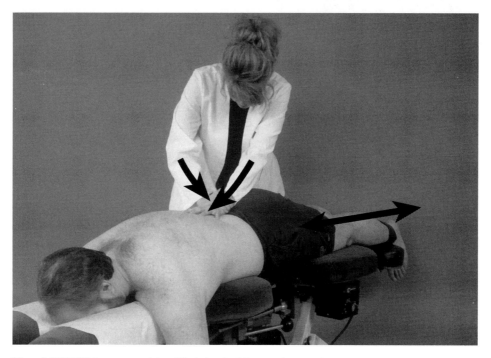

Fig. 4-87 Hill Intertrac table: Clinician holding resistance in lumbar spine in distraction.
- Clinician stands adjacent to patient, with treating hand on patient supported by opposite hand providing stabilization.
- Table is in $\beta(-)$ negative position and is activated to provide axial distraction.
- The speed of the table and the angle of the β section are set before clinician contact with the patient's spine.
- The treatment of distraction in an axial direction is implemented for several cycles at 2 to 3 vertebral levels in the area of concern.
- The procedure is to determine patient tolerance as the speed of the distraction is increased. The usual treating speed is approximately 10 to 15 rpm. *(Table by Thomas Hill Tables, Lakefield, Ont.)*

Fig. 4-86 Hill Intertrac table: Clinician applying distractive force in neutral position.
- Clinician is standing on the right side of patient. The patient is in a prone position on the table.
- The hand position is as described previously.
- Clinician is positioned to resist the traction of the table on the patient.
- Table is in a neutral position while it provides motorized traction to the patient in an axial direction.
- The patient's hands and arms are comfortably placed on the rests, and the ankles are strapped into the ankle rest. *(Table by Thomas Hill Tables, Lakefield, Ont.)*

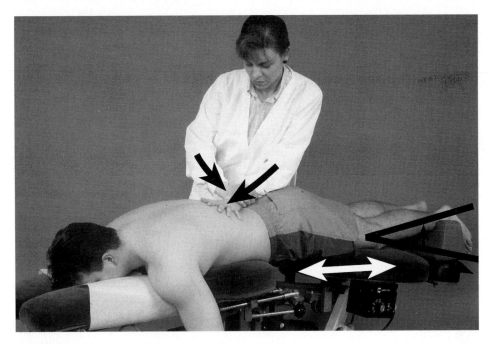

Fig. 4-88
Hill Intertrac table: Use of the Distrac Wedge.
- Patient is positioned in the prone position on the table.
- The Distrac Wedge is placed under the ankles, with the ankle support appropriately placed for the patient's height.
- The Distrac Wedge can replace the ankle straps to provide distraction to the patient unless the Δ is raised to (+) positive.
- The Distrac Wedge angles the lower leg into slight flexion (approximately 15 degrees) and reduces stress on the lower back. The Distrac Wedge can be used on other tables, as well. *(Table by Thomas Hill Tables, Lakefield, Ont.)*

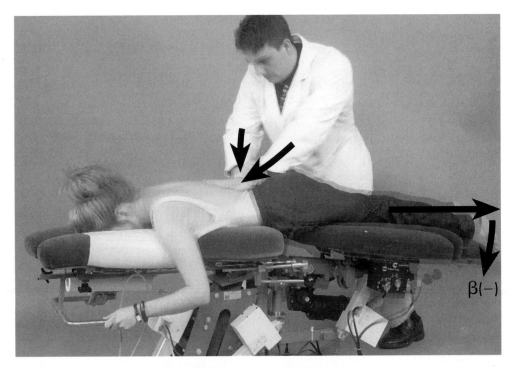

Fig. 4-89 See legend opposite page.

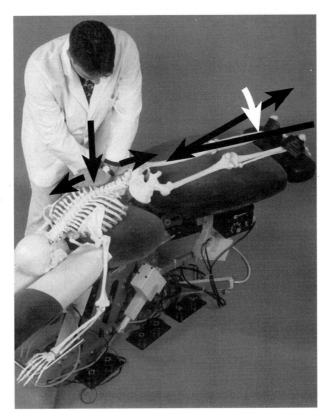

Fig. 4-90 Hill Intertrac table: Clinician hand position in lateral flexion of β section.
- Clinician stands adjacent to table, with patient (skeleton) in prone position.
- The ankles are strapped into ankle section β_1.
- Table in the β section is laterally flexed, with slight downward positioning; the patient is flexed downward and lateral.
- Both of the clinician's hands contact patient's body, applying slight pressure while the table provides axial distraction. The clinician's purpose is to keep the patient's lower body in close contact with the table while linear distraction is provided. *(Table by Thomas Hill Tables, Lakefield, Ont.)*

Fig. 4-89 Hill Intertrac table: Clinician applying distractive force, showing motion.
- Clinician stands adjacent to the patient and applies traction to the lower lumbar spine.
- Note the motion displayed as the β section in slight (-) negative moves, flexing the patient and distracting in an axial direction.
- The α and α_1 sections remained fixed, and no movement occurs in these areas. *(Table by Thomas Hill Tables, Lakefield, Ont.)*

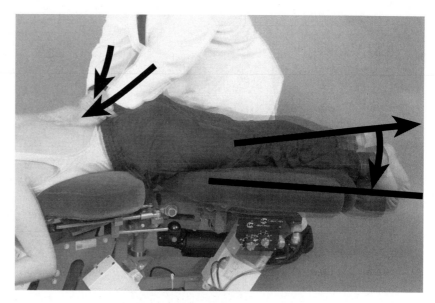

Fig. 4-91 Hill Intertrac table: Motion of the β section.
- Clinician stands adjacent, applying distraction with the contact hand.
- The motion is shown for the β section of the table.
- Oscillation is 12 to 15 rpm.
- Table is shown with slight downward bending (β [-]). *(Table by Thomas Hill Tables, Lakefield, Ont.)*

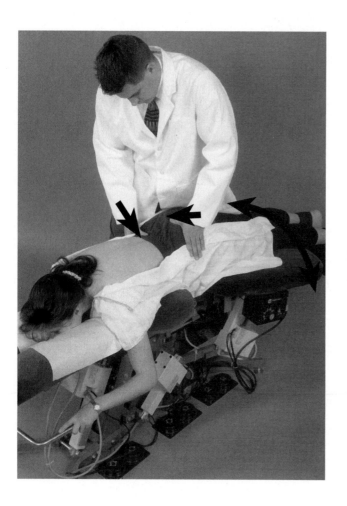

Fig. 4-92
Hill Intertrac table: Motion palpation of SI joints using table.
- Clinician contacts prone patient's SI joints on right side with right thumb.
- Left thumb contact is on coccyx on left.
- The β section in neutral is released and swung from side to side while motion is palpated.
- The motion is created by the clinician with a leg against the table, moving the β section.
- The motion detected should be against the thumb, moving laterally as sacral movement is detected.
- For opposite-side motion, the clinician should relocate to opposite side of table. *(Table by Thomas Hill Tables, Lakefield, Ont.)*

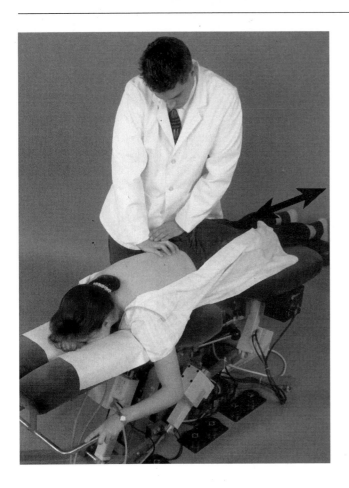

Fig. 4-93 Hill Intertrac table: Motion palpation of intersegmental movement.
- Clinician stands adjacent to patient in prone position, with β section slightly (-) negative.
- Clinician uses his fingertips to palpate intersegmental motion while table is in axial motion. *(Table by Thomas Hill Tables, Lakefield, Ont.)*

Fig. 4-94 Hill Intertrac table: Clinician maintains pressure over lumbar musculature with lateral flexion.
- Clinician maintains moderate pressure over the paraspinal musculature on the right side while the table, in slight β (-) and slightly laterally flexed, moves in distraction.
- Clinician's hand position is designed to provide stabilization over the patient's right side, preventing it from rising while distraction with lateral flexion is provided. *(Table by Thomas Hill Tables, Lakefield, Ont.)*

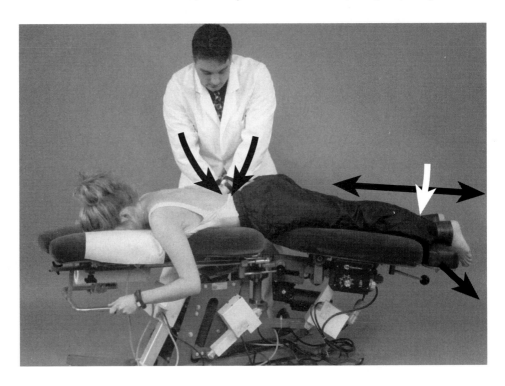

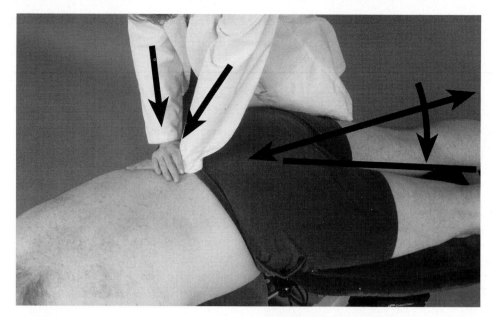

Fig. 4-95 Hill Intertrac table: Close-up of hand position.
- Note the position of the clinician's hands and the placement of the hands over the right paraspinal muscles.
- Table is left-laterally flexed and is providing distraction to the lower lumbar spine. *(Table by Thomas Hill Tables, Lakefield, Ont.)*

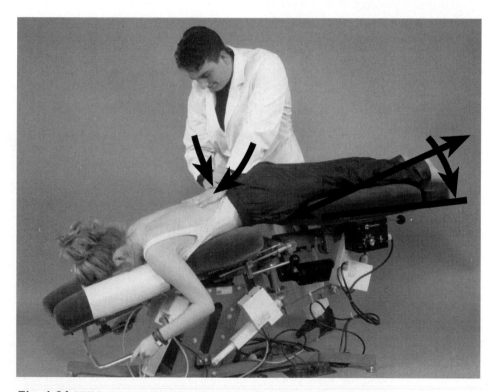

Fig. 4-96 Hill Intertrac table: Gravity-assisted position.
- Clinician positions table with Δ (+) and β neutral.
- Patient's ankles are strapped in to assist in distraction and to prevent slide as Δ is positioned (+) positive.
- Table is set to provide axial distraction at a speed of 12 to 15 rpm. *(Table by Thomas Hill Tables, Lakefield, Ont.)*

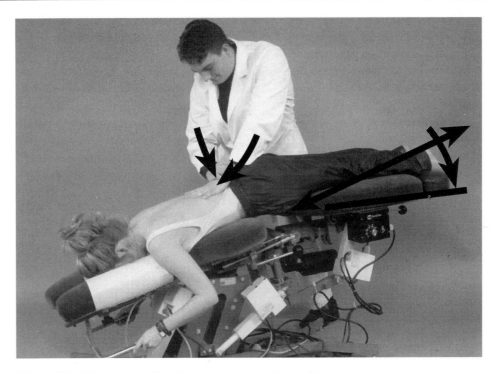

Fig. 4-97 Hill Intertrac table: Gravity-assisted position, β (-).
- Clinician positions table with Δ (+) and β (-).
- Patient's ankles are strapped in to assist in distraction and to prevent slide as Δ is positioned (+) positive. *(Table by Thomas Hill Tables, Lakefield, Ont.)*

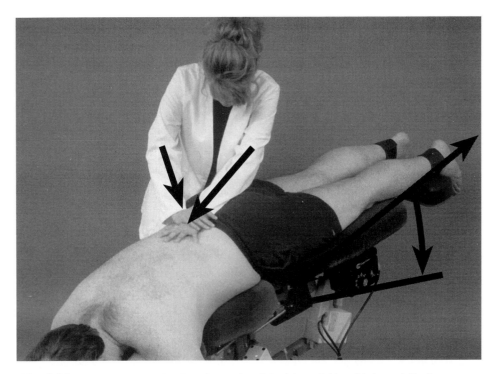

Fig. 4-98 Hill Intertrac table: Gravity-assisted position, β (-), with lateral flexion.
- The clinician positions table Δ (+), β (-), and laterally flexed to right.
- The patient's ankles are strapped in to assist in distraction and to prevent slide as Δ is positioned (+) positive. *(Table by Thomas Hill Tables, Lakefield, Ont.)*

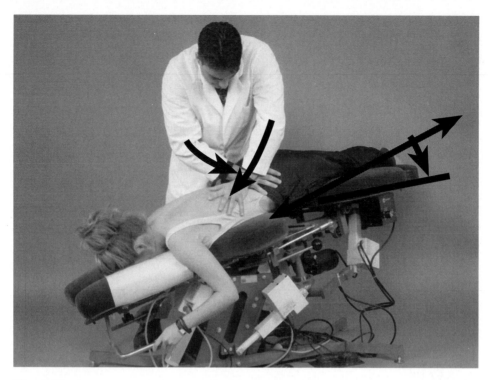

Fig. 4-99 Hill Intertrac table: Gravity-assisted position, β (-).
- Another view of gravity-assisted position with Δ (+) and distraction over the lumbar spine.
- Clinician positions table with Δ (+) and β (-). *(Table by Thomas Hill Tables, Lakefield, Ont.)*

patient comfort. The rheostat speed control on the table will control the speed of the lower portion of the unit. This approach to treatment is discussed in Chapter 7.

ADJUNCTIVE THERAPY

As in other techniques, adjunctive therapies can be applied while the patient is in treatment on the table, in this case while in axial traction. The patient, while prone or supine, can have other therapies, such as electrical stimulation, high- or low-volt galvanism, interferential current, microcurrent, ultrasound, or hot or cold packs, applied to the part under treatment. Under these circumstances, however, the table cannot be operating nor can it be connected to the electrical outlet while an electrical therapy is also connected to a power source. This is to prevent possible injury to the patient from an electrical source. Simultaneous use of the table and an electrically powered therapy is contraindicated. A device with a battery may, however, be used simultaneously. Microcurrent is usually battery powered and therefore can be considered for use with the Hill table. In all instances the patient must be protected from any potential harm by the treatment or therapy.

Acupuncture can be applied while the patient is in a distractive mode without affecting the tractive therapy. Obviously, when a tractive force is applied by and to the patient, acupuncture needles must be removed from the area(s) when hand contact is applied or where the needle may be affected by the table or its motion.

Deep muscle therapy, or deep massage, is compatible with the use of this table or others that are motion-assisted (motor driven) and can readily be applied while the table is in motion. The slow, rhythmic motion of the table coupled with deep muscle massage can be very helpful in relieving trigger points or other muscle complications related to the joint misalignments or fixations treated with the traction or other chiropractic adjustment.

PROTOCOL/REGIMEN

The Hill Intertrac table can be used after a patient health history has been taken and the usual orthopedic and neurologic procedures have been performed. Certain imaging studies, such as are performed in the application of other traction-based techniques, may be necessary for the clinician to have sufficient information for decision making. As with any treatment, the plan for treatment is based on the severity of the condition and the state of the patient. As with most manipulative treatment, GAIT

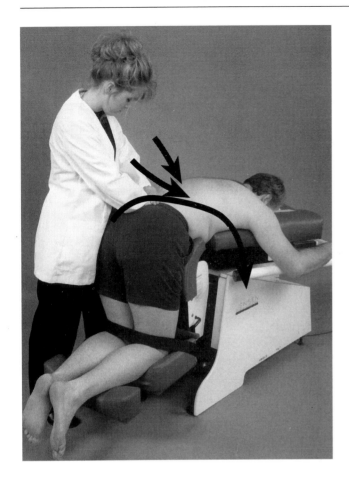

Fig. 4-100 Jensen table: The basic table with controls.

- The patient is positioned on the table in a kneeling position, with the ankle rest extended into a comfortable and supportive position.
- The table is initially positioned in Δ (0), with the circumduction set at a minimal level.
- The switches for control of the speed of the circumduction are positioned on the side of the table.
- The controls for the arc of circumduction and the angle of tilt of Δ are at the level of the clinician's feet on either side.
- Lateral flexion in a fixed position while circumducting is manually controlled by the clinician.
- A strap is placed over the posterior flexed knee of the patient to stabilize position.
- The knee support and the pelvic support are adjustable to accommodate patient size. (*Table by Annova, Alexandria, Minn.*)

must be applied until the patient improves, pain is reduced, and function returns.

In acute cases in which the patient is in great pain, the treatment is applied less vigorously, the motion applied more slowly, and the ankle straps should not be applied. The motion can be slowed to an almost imperceptible level, with no downward bending of the β section (thus minimizing stress on the lumbar spine). The clinician can gradually increase the speed of the distraction, along with ankle strapping and the angle of either upward or downward bending of the β section.

The position of the patient for treatment of the lumbar and thoracic spine is the prone position, with the arms resting on the hand/arm rests under the α_1 section. The period for the treatment, including any soft tissue work, should range from 5 to 15 minutes. While the table is in motion, microcurrent may be applied either passively from the modality directly or with one electrode on the clinician's treating hand and one on the patient. This approach delivers the electrical current through the hand of the clinician while some form of deep muscle therapy is applied.

At some point in the course of treatment, it may be desirable to manipulate the patient with a thrust procedure. This can be accomplished on the Hill table with the patient in a tractioned position. A side-posture position, with the patient on either the right or the left side, may be used with the traction activated. The ankle(s) may be strapped or not, as appropriate.

As with most approaches to treatment, a short trial period of therapy should be undertaken to determine how the patient will respond. Some positive response (reduction of pain and increase in patient comfort), even if small, is required for continuation of the treatment. If improvement is evident, the treatment can continue and, depending on the severity of the condition, the protocol can range from daily to a gradual decrease of frequency of treatment as the patient improves.

Improvement of the patient should be similar on this table to that on the other tables discussed. As a general rule, the patient should demonstrate a 50% improvement over no longer than 3 weeks. If this does not occur, the patient should be referred to another provider within chiropractic for an additional evaluation or outside for additional evaluation, including imaging.

CIRCUMDUCTION: CPM (JENSEN)

RATIONALE: THE CONCEPT

The Jensen technique, a motion-assisted distraction (MAD) technique, using the Jensen, or "J" table, involves passive motion that produces circumductive movement, traction, and compression. According to Jensen, the body incorporates the principle of circumduction in the process of achieving normal motion. With each step, a person in the process of walking moves in a motion approximating circumduction. Conceptually, the body achieves the motion with each step, as the arms swing and the hips gyrate. Jensen attempts to replicate this movement with the table, claiming that it is mechanically compatible with the motion of the body.[30]

The patient should be placed in a kneeling position, similar to the position on a knee-chest table, with the face and upper chest resting on a moveable chest support and the hands holding onto a rail that is attached to the table. This position allows the patient to maintain the normal lordosis in the lumbar spine, and the chest support can be repositioned to allow a shift to the right or left to accommodate an antalgic posture or aid in the reduction of a scoliosis. The advantage to the patient is a stable, comfortable position during the manipulation.

The clinician stands adjacent to the table, on either the right or the left, with the hands free to perform manipulations or administer therapy. This position allows the clinician to perform a dynamic adjustment through a stabilizing hand position, letting the table assume the circumductive mode. The clinician applies pressure to individual segments of the spine while the table is in motion. Curves in both the lumbar and cervical spine can be affected through this table motion and the segmental stabilization (Fig. 4-101).

Jensen claims that the table "enhances the relief of muscle spasms, dissipates blood and lymph in the surrounding tissue, and is thought to play a part in centralizing the nucleus pulposis in symptomatic disc bulges."[27] In her article on the Jensen technique and table, Liebl[30] quotes from several sources that support the theory behind the Jensen table. The theory suggests that compression-traction and loading-unloading of the disc achieves a pumping action, enhancing the biomechanics of the disc and returning it to a normal preinjury state.[31-33]

Patient treatment may include the use of other techniques and tables in this application. In some cases the pelvis must be adjusted with a thrust technique to accomplish the repositioning or reduction of a pelvic misalignment, and this is best performed on another table on which the appropriate positioning and thrusts can be applied. The Jensen technique and table appear to be best applied in the described circumduction movement, stretching and compressing the lumbar and cervical spine to create a pumping action in the spine. This technique should be applied for approximately 5 minutes at a time, sometimes supplemented by an additional table for performing another procedure (such as side-posture for manipulating the pelvis or a drop mechanism, such as in a Thompson table).

Jensen claims that the technique is appropriate for cases involving facet imbrication, disc bulges or herniations, spinal stenosis, dural tube and nerve root adhesions, myofascitis, and other related conditions of the spine in the cervical, thoracic, and lumbar spine. Leibl[30] and Markoff and Morris[31] identify a possible reparative mechanism resulting from the application of compression in manipulation of the spine. They claim that the method, if applied correctly, may be used on various types of cases and with a broad range of ages. They indicate that the circumductive motion can be introduced gradually during each session and that it can be regulated.[30] No data exists, however, that demonstrates the clinical efficacy for this procedure.

PATIENT POSITIONING

Indications and contraindications for the technique and use of the table are similar to those for other traction-distraction tables and techniques. Contraindications are minimal and, with careful application of the technique and the table, most of the population can be accommodated safely for most conditions. The primary area of concern is the use of the table in maximum circumduction, which could be quite uncomfortable for a patient with an acute disc and even dangerous for an older person with osteoporosis. The extreme movement and the stretching of the soft tissue, including the disc, would prove potentially uncomfortable to the patient with an acute disc. The danger for the geriatric patient with osteoporosis is bone stress, which could cause a possible fracture. Keeping the table under control, with consideration for patient comfort and the potential for bone stress where applicable, is of prime importance.

The Jensen table is most appropriate and useful when circumductive movement of the spine is desired, which is the case for most spine-related problems (Figs. 4-102, 4-103).

APPLICATION OF THERAPY

The technique as applied by this method and with this table involves several steps, including assisting the patient onto the table and adjusting the table to fit the patient, strapping the patient onto the table, and treating manually with positions of the hands and the motion of the table. The steps in the process of treatment on the table are as follows:

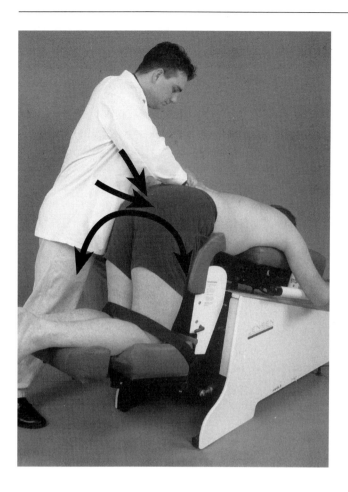

Fig. 4-101 Lumbar manipulation on the Jensen table.
- Patient is placed on the Jensen table in a prone position with the knees flexed (a knee-chest position), and the sections of the table are adjusted to fit the size of the patient.
- Patient's knees are strapped onto the table, and the circumductive arc is set by the clinician.
- Clinician stands adjacent to the patient.
- Clinician's hands are placed on the lumbar spine, with the spinous processes resting in the indentation at the level of the carpal tunnel on the active hand. The opposite hand acts as a stabilizer and is placed over the active, or treating, hand.
- Resistance is provided by the clinician as the table circumducts, creating traction with circumduction for the patient.
- The table can be positioned in a Δ (-) position and/or α lateral flexion right or left, as appropriate. *(Table by Annova, Alexandria, Minn.)*

Fig. 4-102 Lumbar manipulation on the Jensen table with Δ (-).
- Patient is placed on the Jensen table, with the α and Δ sections in a (-) negative position, and the β section is (+) positive, with circumduction at a moderate rate.
- The knees are strapped into the β section, which is extended to accommodate the size of the patient.
- Patient's arms are resting on the arm rest bar, with no lateral flexion of the α section.
- Clinician stands adjacent while distraction is applied with circumduction; the patient is in a Δ (-) position.
- Clinician's hands are positioned with an active, or treating, hand adjacent to the patient, with an overlying stabilizing hand.
- The stance of the clinician is with the feet sufficiently apart to provide a stable base and sufficient resistance for the traction. *(Table by Annova, Alexandria, Minn.)*

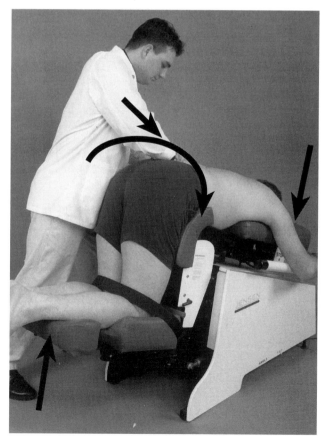

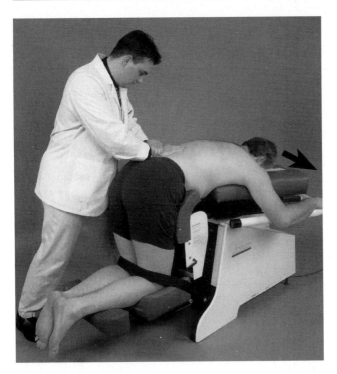

Fig. 4-103 Lumbar manipulation on the Jensen table, with slight Δ (-).

- Patient is placed on the Jensen table, with the α and Δ sections in a slight (-) negative position and the β section in a (+) positive position.
- The knees are strapped into the β section, which is extended to accommodate the size of the patient.
- Patient is positioned with slight right lateral flexion.
- Patient's arms are resting on the arm rest bar, with no lateral flexion of the α section.
- Clinician stands adjacent while distraction is applied with circumduction at a moderate rate while the patient is Δ (-).
- Clinician's hands are positioned with an active hand adjacent to the patient and an overlying stabilizing hand.
- The stance of the clinician is with the feet apart sufficiently to provide a stable base and sufficient resistance for the traction. *(Table by Annova, Alexandria, Minn.)*

1. The table is first adjusted to fit the patient. The β section can be adjusted to accommodate the height of the patient.
2. The patient is assisted onto the table and assumes a kneeling position, with the upper torso lying prone and the face placed in the split facepiece (the α section). The patient's arms rest on the side bars, with the hands grasping the bars securely.
3. The legs are strapped onto the lower, or β, section to provide a secure circumductive platform.

4. The table is switched on, and circumduction of the β section is initiated. This process starts with the table in neutral, and no real movement is initiated yet in the patient.
5. The amount of circumduction, the tilt of the table, and lateral flexion are all controlled by the clinician, with patient comfort in mind. The clinician uses foot levers to control the table settings.
6. The clinician applies treatment by positioning the hands on the patient, providing resistance to the circumductive movement of the β section of the table. The table can be adjusted for speed of circumduction, trajectory of movement in circumduction, and angle and lateral flexion of upper torso (α).
7. Treatment can be applied throughout the spine only with the patient in a prone position. The cervical, thoracic, and lumbar spine can be treated in this manner.

The Jensen table has several controls for activating the circumduction and for changing the position (attitude) of the table. The controls for positioning the angle of the table (for setting the angle of the Δ) and controlling the arc of circumduction are located on the side of the table, level with the clinician's feet. The switch for controlling the speed of the arc of circumduction and the on-and-off switch are located on the side of the table, at hand height.

SPECIAL TREATMENT

Treatment on the Jensen table for the cervical and lumbar spine is applied with the area in circumductive traction in CPM. One of the major differences in this technique compared with the others that use traction or distraction is that Jensen emphasizes the use of compression in the cervical and lumbar spine. This compression is applied while the table is in the circumduction (CPM) cycle, when the cervical and lumbar spine can be manually compressed on the "up stroke" of the table. The objective in this process is to reinstate the lordotic curve through repeated reinforcement of the spinal curvature by manual compression of the spine. This assumes that a lordosis of some magnitude in both these areas is normal and that the parameters for this have been established. Harrison[34] makes reference to the cervical lordosis and its role in normal biomechanics.

ADJUNCTIVE THERAPY

Adjunctive therapies, such as heat or cold, can be applied to the patient while the circumduction is operating. Other therapies can be applied but usually only microcurrent is advised, to prevent possible electrical shock. Protection of the patient is emphasized; therefore any therapy other than battery-operated electrical therapy is contraindicated, not just discouraged. Microcurrent is usually powered by batteries and can be used when an electrically powered table is operating.

Microcurrent can be used by manual applicators in the area of the focus, by surface electrodes attached to the skin of the patient, or with one electrode attached to the patient's skin and one to the dorsum of the clinician's hand. While the patient is circumducting, the current can be directed through the clinician's treating hand, thus offering treatment with a combination of pressure, kneading massage, and electrical stimulation.

The treatment time for using microcurrent is as recommended in the directions of the therapy equipment but can range up to 10 or 15 minutes, depending on the condition being treated and the patient's tolerance. The patient can also be treated on the table with other forms of electrical therapy, such as high-volt galvanism or ultrasound, but the table must be unplugged from the electrical outlet for safety.

PROTOCOL/REGIMEN

When using the Jensen table, the protocol of the usual chiropractic, orthopedic, and neurologic examinations must be performed before treatment. Certain imaging studies may also be required, to provide the clinician with necessary information. After the history and examination, the patient is placed on a treatment plan. The plan should reflect the severity of the condition and the state of the patient. The treatment must be applied until the patient improves, pain is reduced, and function returns.

In acute cases in which the patient is in great pain and has difficulty in posture and gait, a less vigorous treatment is used because of reduced tolerance. The table starts with zero motion (the table will return to neutral position after each treatment session), and motion is increased by the clinician. A gradual increase in the circumduction should continue for the first several sessions (3 to 6). Beyond this time, the circumduction, lateral flexion, and tilt of the table can be increased slightly, but optimal patient positioning may be reached before the maximum table position is achieved. This table is appropriate for treatment of patients able to assume the kneeling position. More patients may be capable of this position than the prone posture used in most chiropractic methods. If the patient cannot assume this position, another table and treatment technique may be appropriate.

Patient response on this table should be similar to response on other tables. That is, as the treatment progresses, the patient should show improvement and demonstrate additional capabilities as function returns. The treatment will range from daily, for a treatment session lasting 5 to 15 minutes, to sessions 2 or 3 times per week and then weekly, as the patient improves. To continue past the trial therapy of two or three visits, some improvement should be noted. If at least a 50% improvement does not occur over a 3-week period, the patient should be referred for further evaluation or treatment by another chiropractor or a practitioner outside the chiropractic system.

CONCLUSION

The techniques of MEAD and MAD are explored and the approaches to their use discussed in this chapter. Certain conclusions on the application of the technique and the appearance of the equipment can be drawn from the explanations. Actual use of the equipment, however, is necessary for a thorough understanding of the techniques and tables. The clinician must be sensitive to the response of patients to treatment with the equipment and techniques. In some cases the clinician will overtreat in the enthusiasm to make the patient well again; in other instances the clinician will undertreat. In all instances the welfare of the patient must be kept foremost in mind. The adage to "do no harm" while still being effective is the rule.

No data exists to demonstrate that any one chiropractic technique is better than another. Much research remains to be conducted in chiropractic before superiority can be claimed for any technique over another. Perhaps this need for further study will lead to a search for the best approach to treating problems of the body and especially of the musculoskeletal system. In the search for the best technique and equipment, clinicians should continue to apply the approaches to the improvement of the human frame in a responsible manner, bringing to practice the best that is available and offering patients the most appropriate and safest treatment.

REFERENCES

1. Kaltenborn FM. *Mobilization of the Extremity Joints.* 3rd ed. Oslo: Olaf Norlis Bokhandel; 1980.
2. Grieve GP. *Common Vertebral Joint Problems.* 2nd ed. London: Churchill Livingstone; 1988.
3. Mathews JA. Dynamic discography: a study of lumbar traction. *Ann Phys Med.* 1968;9:275.
4. Sheriff J. A flexible approach to traction. In: Grieve G, ed. *Grieve's Modern Manual of Therapy.* 2nd ed. Edinburgh: Churchill Livingstone; 1994.
5. Burton CV. Low back care: the gravity of the situation. In: Kirkaldy-Willis WH, Burton CV, eds. *Managing Low Back Pain.* 3rd ed. New York: Churchill Livingstone; 1992.
6. Hinterbuchner C. Traction. In Basmajian JV, ed. *Manipulation, Traction, and Massage.* 2nd ed. Baltimore: Williams & Wilkins; 1980.
7. Cyriax J. *Textbook of Orthopaedic Medicine.* 10th ed. London: Bailliere Tindall; 1980;2.
8. Anderson RT. *The Archives and Journal for the History of Chiropractic.* Baltimore: Association for the History of Chiropractic, Inc; 1983;3:1.
9. Peltier LF. A brief history of traction. *J Bone Joint Surg Am.* 1968;50:1603-1617.
10. Basmajian JV, ed. *Manipulation, Traction, and Massage.* 3rd ed. Baltimore: Williams & Wilkins; 1985.
11. Colachis SC, Strohm BR. Effects of intermittent traction of separation of lumbar vertebrae. *Arch Phys Med Rehabil.* 1969;50(5):251-258.
12. Lidstrom A, Zachrisson M. Physical therapy on low back pain and sciatica: an attempt at evaluation. *Scand J Rehabil Med.* 1970;2:37-42.
13. Dvorak J, Dvorak V, Schneider W. *Manual Medicine, 1984.* Berlin: Springer-Verlag; 1985.
14. Evjenth O, Hamberg J. *Muscle Stretching in Manual Therapy: A Clinical Manual—The Extremities.* Alfta Sweden: Alfta Rehab Forlag; 1984;1.
15. Nwuga V. *Manipulation of the Spine.* Baltimore: Williams & Wilkins; 1976.
16. Cantu RI, Grodin AJ. *Myofascial Manipulation, Theory, and Clinical Applications.* Gaithersburg, Md: Aspen; 1992.
17. Cox JM. *Low Back Pain: Mechanism, Diagnosis, and Treatment.* Baltimore: Williams & Wilkins; 1985.
18. Taylor H. The McManis table: professional papers. *ACA J Chiropr.* 1978;12:100.
19. McManis JV. *McManis Table Technic: Technic Instructions and General Information.* Kirksville, Mo: McManis Table Co; 1938.
20. McManis JV. A treating table innovation. *J Am Osteopathic Assoc.* July 1910;565-566.
21. Winter RB, Lonstein JE, Denis FD. Pain patterns in adult scoliosis. *Orthop Clin North Am.* 1988;19(2):339-345.
22. Eckard L. *Leander Technique Course Manual.* Port Orchard, Wa: Leander Research, Manufacturing, and Distributing, Inc.
23. Davis PT. GAIT (gravity-assisted intermittent traction): a motion-assisted form of distractive manipulation. *Chiropr Tech.* 1995;7:125-130.
24. Hill T. Privately published notes on the use of the Hill Intertrac table. Lakefield, Ont; undated.
25. Farfan HF. *Mechanical Disorders of the Low Back,* Philadelphia: Lea & Febiger; 1973.
26. Grieve GP. *Common Vertebral Joint Problems.* New York: Churchill Livingstone; 1981.
27. Grice A. Radiographic, biomechanical, and clinical factors in lumbar lateral flexion, I. *J Manipulative Physiol Ther.* 1979;2(1):26-34.
28. Khanchandani A, Mitchell P. *A Radiographic Study of Passive Lateral Bending in the Lumbar Spine in the Prone Position, with Reference to the Literature.* Bournemouth: Anglo-European College of Chiropractic; 1986. Thesis.
29. Maigne R. Low back pain of thoracolumbar origin. *Arch Phys Med and Rehabil.* 1980;61(9):389-395.
30. Liebl N. A new concept in technique using automated simulation of normal spinal biomechanics. *Chiropr Tech.* 1990;2:20.
31. Markoff KI, Morris JM. The structural components of the intervertebral disc. *J Bone Joint Surg Am.* 1974;56:675.
32. Virgin W. Experimental investigations into physical properties of intervertebral disc. *J Bone Joint Surg Br.* 1951;33:607.
33. Brown T, Hanson R, Yorra A. Some mechanical tests on the lumbo-sacral spine with particular reference to the intervertebral discs. *J Bone Joint Surg Am.* 1957;39:1135.
34. Harrison DD, Jackson BL, Troyanovich S, Robertson G, de George D, Barker WF. The efficacy of cervical extension-compression traction combined with diversified manipulation and drop table adjustments in the rehabilitation of cervical lordosis: a pilot study. *J Manipulative Physiol Ther.* 1994;17(7):454-464.

5

Traction-Distraction Techniques for Other Areas of the Body

THE CONCEPT

Concentration within the chiropractic discipline primarily has been on the spine; much less attention has been paid to the other articulations of the body. However, some authors have focused on the area of extremity adjusting or manipulation. Extremity manipulation has gradually become more common with the increase of understanding of the process and the accompanying publication of teaching manuals.[1-8] The attention of those interested in sports-related injuries and occupational injuries and illnesses is drawn to more detailed and credible analyses of the injuries.[9-13] Chiropractors are involved with many sports teams, treating injured athletes and acting in a proactive mode, enhancing the athlete's performance. The chiropractor is also involved in the workplace, caring for injured workers through the workers' compensation programs and assisting in rapid return to work, rehabilitation, and work-hardening. Although the lumbar spine is a common site for athletic and work injuries, the cervical spine and extremity joints are also frequently involved. Both the athletic field and the work environment are fertile areas for the practice of chiropractic.

Chiropractors often use some form of traction to treat injuries or other problems in the cervicothoracic spine and the extremities. Some traction is applied manually, with the patient lying prone or supine on the treatment table; other traction is performed with power-assisted equipment that applies the traction automatically. Other examples of traction are weight bags for cervical traction and automated intersegmental traction, in which rollers in the table are used on the spine of the supine patient.[1] Traction is also applied with the cervical collar or similar devices, which are discussed in Chapter 7.

The concept of motion-assisted distraction (MAD) is not new to chiropractic. An example of MAD is the use of the mechanically operated Leander table, which introduced to chiropractic the concept of spinal continuous passive motion (CPM). Leander Eckhard based his method of flexion-distraction on that of McManis. Clinicians have raised concerns about power-operated distraction and questioned its use because it requires less direct operator involvement and may endanger the patient. The problems with this method of distraction treatment, however, stem from a concern about clinician control of the equipment during its operation and how the equipment can be made to conform to the patient's needs. These concerns have been addressed in contemporary distraction equipment in the configuration of the table and provision for multiple positioning of the patient. Speed and trajectory of operation has also been controlled, and the table operates both manually and with power, with much better control than previously possible.

Some manual tables have been designed and redesigned to require much less effort in their operation and to allow clinicians and patients of most sizes to use them comfortably. The powered models, however, provide the greatest range of low-force (on the part of the clinician) devices available. One important difference and advantage of the powered table is that the clinician can use both hands to deliver manual treatment, instead of having to use one hand for powering the flexion action of the table. This increases the control of the treatment, a plus for the patient, and control of the required power, a plus for the clinician.

With any motion-assisting device of this type the clinician has considerable leverage and control over the patient and condition. This kind of adjusting and/or manipulation has the advantage of repetition of movement in a very controlled fashion, whereas a short-lever, high-velocity move tends to be of the "all or nothing" sort. When the thrust is made the segment either moves or does not move. Flexion-distraction or linear distraction, however, allows the clinician to apply an incremental manipulation for both a structural problem and its pathologic derivative.

Multiple positions of the patient are possible with this distraction equipment; therefore a common terminology is necessary for operation of the table and correct positioning of the patient. The various positions relate to the axes of movement of the human body. The treatment table may enhance body movement in the three axes of the body (x, y, and z), with possible positive or negative motion around or along the axis.

Treatment using multiple axes can be provided with the Hill Intertrac table or Chattanooga Ergotrac which provide linear distraction along the y axis and distractive motion in flexion (β [-] [+ θ x]) (assuming that the patient is positioned prone) in the lower (β) section of the table (Fig. 5-1). Table positions also allow for lateral flexion of the lower section. It can be moved to the right or left and noted as β *right* or *left lateral flexion (+ or - θ z)*. The entire table can also be tilted, with the head down and feet raised, which is described as Δ *positive (+)*.

This notation system provides the practitioner with a common method for understanding and noting the position of the table. When the patient is treated the clinician can note what adjustment or manipulation was performed, and the table position can be noted and replicated at a later date. In some cases it may be important to place the patient in the same relative position as when previously treated, because that will be the most comfortable position for the patient. Usually, a relative position in the same direction is sufficient. In addition, this notation system provides a quick and clear method for recording which table position was appropriate in a patient's treatment.

In all techniques, there are certain caveats that must be respected. Indications and contraindications for traction-distraction are well known and should be considered carefully. The cervical spine is to be treated with caution, and the first responsibility of the clinician is to do no harm. This is possible only if the clinician knows the technique well and has adequately practiced its application.[2,14]

The discussion in this chapter focuses on chiropractic treatment of the cervical and thoracic spine and the upper and lower extremities, using distraction equipment for performing Motion-Assisted Distraction (MAD) and Mechanically Assisted Distraction (MEAD). Techniques with no specific protocol for use in these areas are identified.

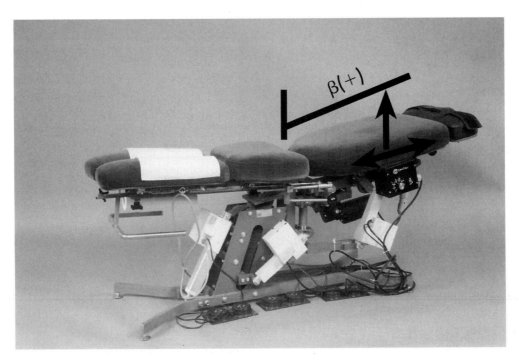

Fig. 5-1 Hill Intertrac table position (schematic).

Positioning on the tables under discussion is usually prone, with the exception of some of the Hill technique positions on the Hill Intertrac or Chattanooga Ergotrak table. When the patient is prone, the arms are supported by arm rests and the hands can either rest on the supports or provide resistance and enhance the distraction. Hand position depends on tolerance of the distraction by the patient.

TREATMENT OF THE CERVICAL SPINE

A patient history and an examination should be performed before any manipulation. This is particularly important in treatment of the cervical spine because of the greater degree of vulnerability (neurovascular) in the cervical spine compared with the thoracolumbar spine. The evaluation should include questions on recent experiences of dizziness or vertigo. The examination should continue with a test for vertebrobasilar insufficiency (the VBI test) (see discussion of the assessment of joint function in Chapter 3).[15] Although this approach does not guarantee patient suitability for the treatment proposed, the clinician should use good clinical judgment at all times, continually evaluating the patient for reactions to the treatment and modifying the approach to suit the circumstances. If the treatment is not successful within the usual time of the customary treatment for the problem, referral is a logical next step.

THE ALLOPATHS: CERVICAL SPINE

The allopaths, represented by clinicians such as Cyriax, have developed certain traction techniques for the cervical spine, but most of the procedures consist of mechanical traction of either a static/sustained or intermittent nature. Other uses of allopathic cervical traction include fracture repair and the use of mobile cervical traction harnesses, such as the halo brace. In addition, continuous traction is used on recumbent patients.

Cyriax[16] demonstrates techniques for the cervical spine that are applied primarily on a flat therapy table at approximately waist height, with the help of one or two assistants. Traction is applied to the cervical spine in positions of either straight traction or with lateral bending (lateral flexion). To facilitate this process the clinician cradles the patient's skull in an unbending y axis, with lateral bending as required. The assistants provide the resistance force by holding the patient against the distraction of the clinician. Cyriax also injects tender intraarticular joints with a steroid as an adjunctive procedure.

Other allopaths emphasizing manipulation include Basmajian, Dvorak, Greenman, Mennell, and Janda. Prominent therapists who use manipulation (and who have written on the subject) include Maitland (physiotherapist), Cantu (physical therapist), Lidstrom (physical therapist), Nwuga (physical therapist), and Evjenth (manual therapist). These practitioners developed special characteristics for the techniques they use to treat musculoskeletal problems. Some of these techniques are for treatment of the bony structure of the skeleton and its joints, whereas others are for treatment of the soft tissues, the myofascial components.[6,17-26] Most who have written about the various forms of manipulation include the application of distraction techniques.

Rogoff[27] describes the use of mechanical traction devices for the cervical through lumbar areas of the spine. These traction devices are used with both manual and mechanical methods, with variations in the forces applied to the spine. He notes that the cervical spine is an easier area for traction than the lumbar spine, because it is less bulky and less encumbered by musculature. Other authors describe similar orientations with the use of mechanical traction and accompanying devices. The cervical spine often is treated with a home halter device that hangs on the patient's bedroom door, subjecting the patient to a sustained traction force dependent on the amount of water or other material placed in the weight bag.[6,28,29]

THE MCMANIS TABLE: CERVICAL SPINE

McManis' technique is applied to the trunk of the body. The only part of the table that relates specifically to the head is the facepiece, which is split, allowing for face and head comfort with the patient lying prone or supine. Taylor's article on the use of McManis' table focuses on its use in treating the low back. Because of this focus on the thoracolumbar spine the McManis table is not considered a device for treating the cervical spine, although it certainly could be used for performing cervical adjusting or manipulation on a prone or supine patient, depending on the needs of the patient and the skills of the clinician.

THE MECHANICALLY ASSISTED DISTRACTION (MEAD) TECHNIQUES: CERVICAL SPINE
The Zenith-Cox Table: Cervical Spine
The headpiece of the Zenith-Cox table allows a specific distraction adjustment in the cervical spine in multiple axes. Other tables of the same type have a cervical head-

piece that allows the clinician to provide a separate distraction process in the cervical spine, apart from the trunk. The adjustment can be performed with the patient prone, and the movement duplicates that of the lower part of the table. The distraction is carried into the cervical spine and performed in the same manner as it is performed in the thoracolumbar spine. These tables allow only a sustained flexion or an extension position. The headpiece provides positioning, and the lower section of the table provides flexion and subsequent distraction, with the hand of the clinician stabilizing and resisting in the cervical spine.

The Zenith-Cox headpiece provides a multiplanar distraction capability for the patient, with the clinician treating at the head of the table. The distraction is initiated at the cervical spine with manual positioning of the α_1 section in flexion-extension, lateral flexion right or left, and/or rotation right or left. The clinician attaches the tensioning strap or cord and then releases the mechanism and performs the desired distraction (Figs. 5-2, 5-3, and 5-4).

The protocol for use of the Cox technique on the Zenith-Cox table in the cervical spine includes the following steps described by Cox[14]:

1. For the tolerance test for cervical flexion-distraction, the patient is positioned prone on the table, with the area to be distracted placed over the divide between the cervical and thoracic sections of the table.

2. Testing for flexion-distraction tolerance is performed using the segment below the segment to be treated (in contrast to the flexion-distraction method for the lumbar spine, which uses the segment above the desired distraction point). No strapping is done nor is any specific pressure applied initially, because the objective is to test the body's ability to tolerate only the weight of the head. The testing is performed three levels above and below the level of the intended distraction treatment.

3. No discomfort is to be felt by the patient in the neck, shoulder, arm, or thoracic spine while the distraction is tested. Palpation is performed to identify muscle spasms. If muscle spasm is found, it should be reduced or eliminated manually before mechanically assisted distraction is applied.

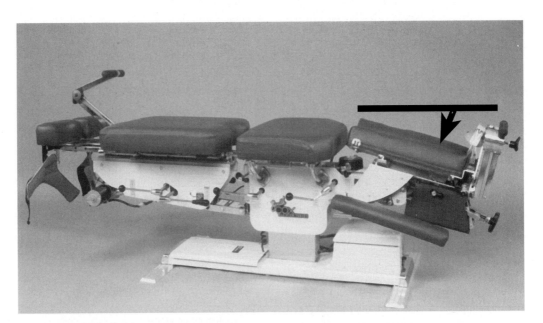

Fig. 5-2 Zenith-Cox table with cervical distraction headpiece (in flexion).
- Table is in neutral position, except α_1, which is in slight flexion.
- Note the headpiece, with the patient to be positioned prone.
- The headpiece has the capability of flexion and extension, lateral flexion, and rotation in the cervical spine.
- All of the controls are located on the headpiece, including the balancing adjustment to accommodate for the weight of the patient's head.

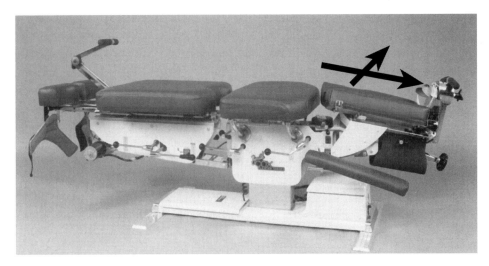

Fig. 5-3 Zenith-Cox table with cervical headpiece in left lateral flexion and slight flexion (β, [+]), with the rest of the table in neutral position.

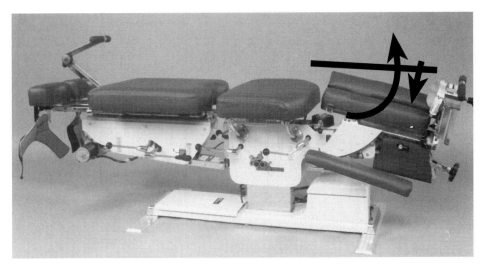

Fig. 5-4 Zenith-Cox table with cervical headpiece in right rotation and slight flexion (β, [+]), with the rest of the table in neutral positions.

4. The flexion halter can be applied if no pain is elicited in the initial testing. The halter is attached to the patient as shown in Figs. 5-5 and 5-6. Comfortable fit of the halter is critical for both the patient and the practitioner. The strap is loosened at the very top of the headpiece, the cups are positioned on the small ropes and then applied to the posterior aspect of the occiput, the small ropes are then connected to the brackets on the headpiece, and the strap is then tightened and locked before the clinician uses the flexion-distraction function.

5. The positions of the headpiece can then be assumed, but within the elastic ranges of motion of the joints of the cervical spine, which, according to Cox,[14] will minimize joint dysfunction. These positions include flexion, extension, lateral flexion (right and left), rotation (right and left), and circumduction (right and left). The process is to "apply the distraction slowly until a gentle separation and distraction of the spinous processes and paravertebral muscles is felt." (Figs. 5-5 through 5-10.)

On the Zenith-Cox table, the α_1 section (headpiece) is the table section used for cervical distraction, which begins in a neutral position (α [0]), as shown in Fig. 5-5. This table allows the positions of α_1 neutral, α_1 flexion, α_1 extension, α_1, lateral flexion R/L (right/left), α_1 R/L rotation, and α_1 circumduct. With these positions it is also possible to achieve combinations of positioning, such as α_1 (-) R lateral flexion.

Cervical motion palpation can also be performed while using the flexion-distraction headpiece. This can be carried out with an emphasis on flexion, lateral flexion, or rotation.

The value of using this device for motion palpation is its relative control over specific and defined movement of the cervical spine. The clinician has total control of the patient's head, and the amount of leverage applied requires that the spine be treated with care because leverage is great.

Other Mechanically Assisted Distraction (MEAD) Approaches: Cervical Spine

The Chattanooga table is an example of tables that perform manual cervical distraction. It has power assistance in elevation and in adjustment for the weight on the

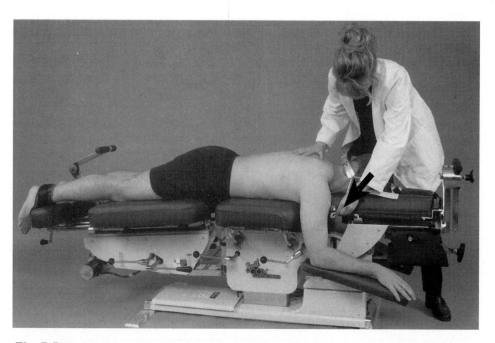

Fig. 5-5 Zenith-Cox table: Attaching the occipital cups.
- All locks are to be secured on the α headpiece before positioning patient on the table.
- Face paper is placed on the facepiece before placement of the patient.
- Patient is placed on the table before the occipital cups are attached, with special attention to placement of the face on the headpiece.
- The face is placed over the indentations on the bilateral face cushions that are located toward the caudal end of the headpiece.
- The occipital cups are placed over the base of the patient's occiput.
- The cords are released to create slack and attached to the headpiece.

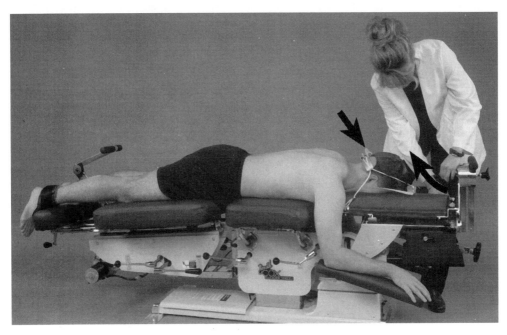

Fig. 5-6 Zenith-Cox table: Attaching the occipital cups (continued).
- The cord is drawn through a tensioning clamp, and the occipital cups are firmly attached to the base of the occiput.
- With tensioning, the face is pulled into the facepiece, and the positioning is complete.

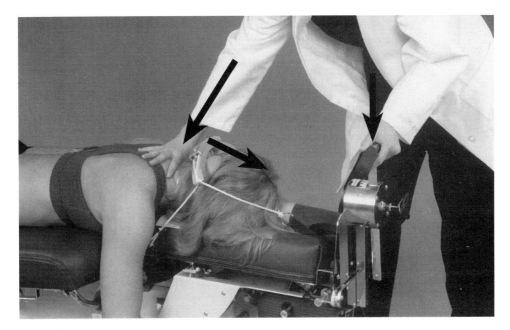

Fig. 5-7 Zenith-Cox table: Start of traction.
- Traction is initiated by the clinician placing the treating hand over the vertebra below the site of disc involvement or below the site of discomfort.
- The opposite hand contacts the handle on the α headpiece to initiate action.
- The lock(s) should be released before treatment is initiated.
- Flexion ($+ \theta$ x) is shown in this illustration.

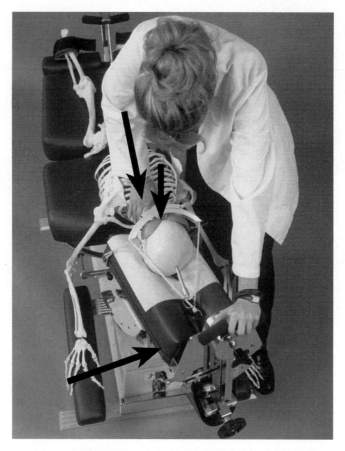

Fig. 5-8 Zenith-Cox table: Skeleton in lateral flexion.
- Patient is positioned prone on the table; in this case the ankle straps are fastened to provide additional distraction.
- The α and β sections may be in neutral (0).
- The treating hand contact is made below the level of the problem, as noted in this illustration. That is, for disc or joint dysfunction between C4 and C5, C5 or distal is contacted.

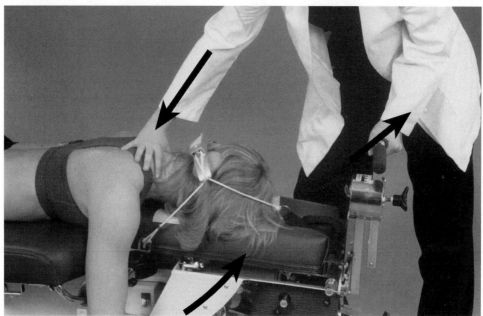

Fig. 5-9 For legend see opposite page.

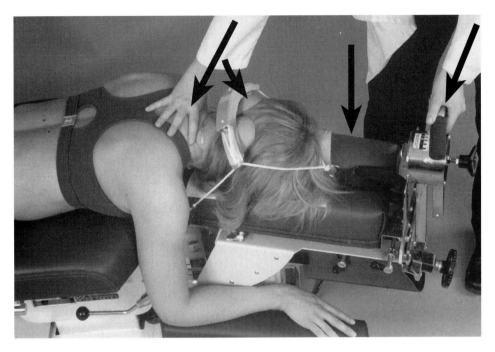

Fig. 5-10 Zenith-Cox table: Close up of rotation.
- Patient is positioned prone on the facepiece (α section), with the occipital cups positioned and tensioned as noted.
- The lock(s) on the headpiece is released to allow the function desired.
- Clinician places one hand on the area to be treated and the opposite hand on the handle, creating distraction and initiating the rotation.
- Clinician's hand on the handle creates the distraction to the cervical spine.
- Rotation ($+ \theta y$) is initiated by the clinician, with consideration of patient tolerance of the position and force applied.
- From this position, circumduction may be applied using the handle to create the motion, with all headpiece locks released.

Fig. 5-9 Zenith-Cox table: Close-up of lateral flexion.
- Patient is positioned prone on the facepiece (α section), with the occipital cups positioned and tensioned as noted.
- The lock(s) on the headpiece is released to allow the function desired.
- The clinician places one hand on the area to be treated and the opposite hand on the handle, creating distraction and initiating lateral flexion.
- Clinician's hand on the handle creates the distraction to the cervical spine.
- Lateral flexion ($- \theta z$) is initiated by the clinician, with consideration of patient tolerance of the position and force applied.

lower section of the table. The table is manually operated, requiring the clinician to use one hand to depress the β section, while the other hand delivers distraction into the cervical spine on the prone patient (Figs. 5-11 and 5-12). The clinician can apply additional distractive adjustment and manipulation with the patient supine by applying traction into the cervical spine or delivering a high-velocity thrust as described in Chapter 6. (Figs. 5-13 through 5-17.)

The Lloyd, Spinalight, and other tables are capable of performing the same kind of distractive adjustments. The mechanically assisted tables (manual tables), however, require the use of one hand to provide the distractive force and the other hand to stabilize the section of the spine, thus limiting the distractive treatment.

THE MOTION-ASSISTED DISTRACTION (MAD) TECHNIQUES: CERVICAL SPINE

The Jensen Table: Cervical Spine

The Jensen technique and table differ considerably from the methods and tables discussed previously. This table is designed for a kneeling patient position for the circumductive movement produced by the table. Jensen advo-

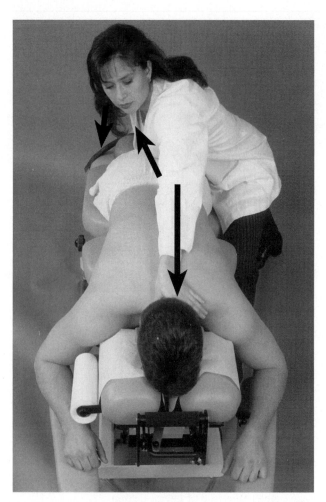

Fig. 5-11 The Chattanooga table: Cervical distraction on prone patient.
- Patient lies prone on the table, with or without ankles strapped.
- Clinician stands adjacent to the table and applies distractive force to the cervical spinal segment above the level to be distracted.
- Distractive force is applied by the clinician's power hand, creating trunk traction by down-bending the β section.

cates a compressive cervical manipulation adjustment that is performed when the table is in the rising portion of the circumductive stroke. Compression in the cervical spine is achieved by the clinician holding the top of the skull with one hand and, as the stroke progresses, molding the cervical spine with the other hand, lightening the hold on the skull after the compression is completed. An incremental manipulation is possible, gradually increasing and decreasing the pressure on the skull and the spine.[30] (Figs. 5-18 through 5-22.) (Jensen R. Seminar notes. Seminar NWCC; 1993.)

This cervical manipulation can be performed in either the Δ (0) or Δ (+) position, without elevation of the β sec-

tion and lowering of the α section, maintaining the ability to perform circumductive motions and the resultant compression to the cervical spine and the molding of the cervical lordosis.

In the process of this manipulative approach, the cervical spine should assume a lordosis. Most chiropractors agree that this is desirable, but little evidence exists that this is indeed correct or even necessary to the normal functioning of the spine. Others will explore this concept and produce extensive information on how to achieve the lordotic state, but little research exists to confirm the assumption that is made about the value of the curve. This is discussed further in Chapter 7.

Text continued on p. 169

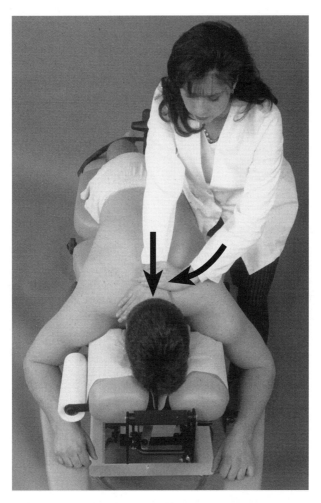

Fig. 5-12 The Chattanooga table: Cervical distraction on prone patient.
- Patient lies prone on the table, with or without ankles strapped.
- Clinician stands adjacent and applies traction with both hands against distractive force of the downward-bent β section.
- The presence of both of the clinician's hands on patient's cervical spine ensures that the distractive force is relatively continuous.
- All sections of the table are positioned in neutral (0), with the possible exception of the α_1 section that could be flexed (negative [-]) or extended (positive [+]).

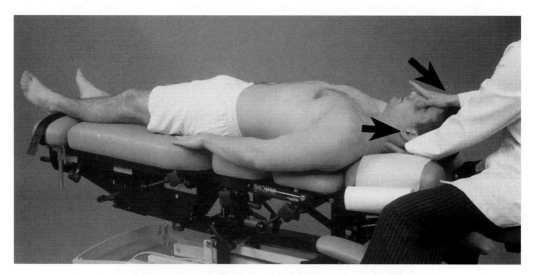

Fig. 5-13 The Chattanooga table: Cervical distraction on supine patient.
- Patient lies supine on the table, with or without ankles strapped.
- Clinician sits at the head (α) end of the table and cradles the patient's head.
- Distraction is provided by the clinician pulling steadily in the y axis with both hands.
- No deviation is made in any direction.

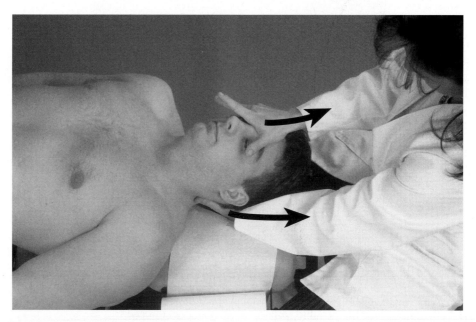

Fig. 5-14 The Chattanooga table: Cervical distraction on supine patient (continued).
- Patient lies supine, with clinician positioned at the head (α) end of the table.
- Clinician's hands are positioned on the patient's head and neck to provide distraction.
- Distraction of the cervical spine is maintained for up to 10 seconds and then slowly released. The distraction is initiated several times (approximately 5 times), then the patient is allowed to rest.

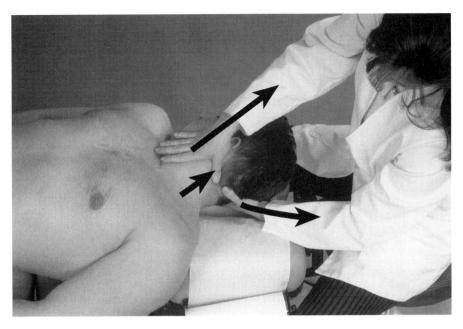

Fig. 5-15 The Chattanooga table: Cervical distraction on supine patient (continued).
- Patient lies supine, with the clinician positioned at the head (α) end of the table.
- Traction of the patient's cervical spine is initiated and then the spine is rotated to the left or right.
- Traction is maintained in this position for up to 10 seconds and is repeated on each side 2 to 3 times, with the clinician attempting each time to increase the rotation.

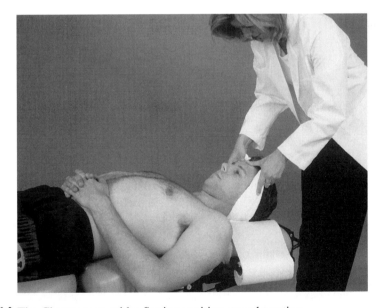

Fig. 5-16 The Chattanooga table: Supine position, towel traction.
- Patient is positioned supine.
- Towel is applied to occiput for high cervical traction.
- Traction is applied manually.
- This method can be applied on other tables employing MAD/MEAD techniques, including Hill Intertrac or Chattanooga Ergotrak with linear distraction.

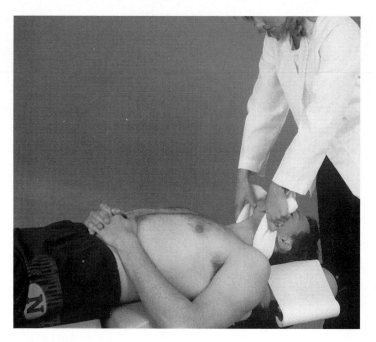

Fig. 5-17 Chatanooga table: Supine position, towel traction.
- Patient is positioned supine.
- Towel is applied to the midcervical spine for traction of lower cervical area.
- Posterior-to-anterior prestress is applied first to induce the cervical curve.
- Traction is applied manually.

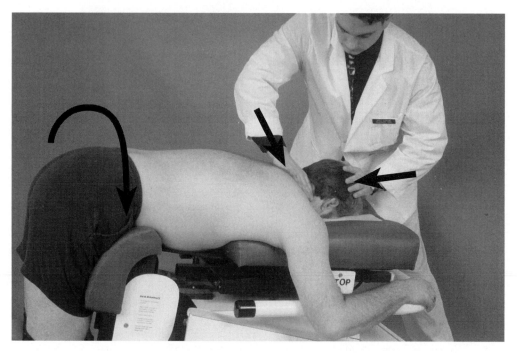

Fig. 5-18 For legend see opposite page.

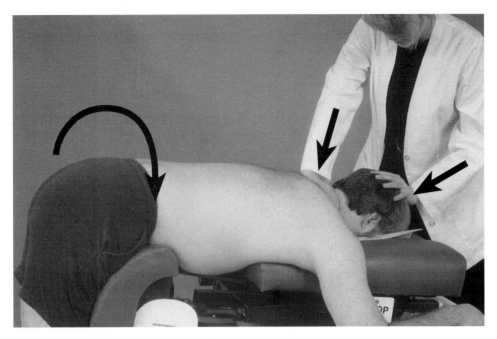

Fig. 5-19 Jensen table: Adjusting the cervical spine.
- Clinician resisting-hand position preparatory to distraction.
- Patient positioned with clinician treating hand on cervical spine during upstroke of circumduction.

Fig. 5-18 Jensen table: Patient prone, with clinician at a section applying compression.
- Patient is positioned prone and kneeling, with arms on arm rests and the table is oscillating through circumductive arcs.
- Clinician stands adjacent to the α section and stabilizes the cervical spine while blocking the forward motion of the skull, creating a compressive stroke to the cervical spine.
- The objective is to reinforce the cervical lordosis by molding the spine with one hand while the other blocks the forward trajectory of the head.
- The α section is neutral, the β is neutral to positive (+), and the Δ is negative (-) to positive (+) with some degree of circumduction.

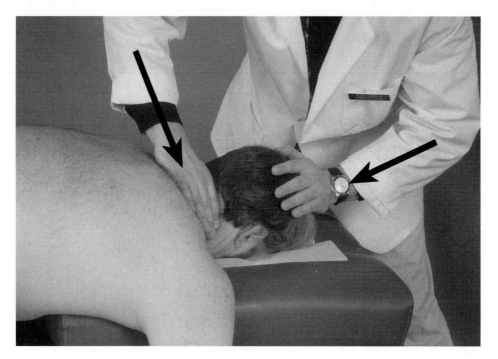

Fig. 5-20 Jensen table: Adjusting the cervical spine (continued).
- Close up of compression stroke on cervical spine of patient.

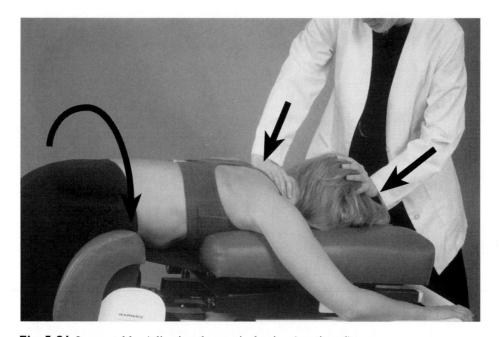

Fig. 5-21 Jensen table: Adjusting the cervical spine (continued).
- Patient and clinician positions for compressive stroke on cervical spine.

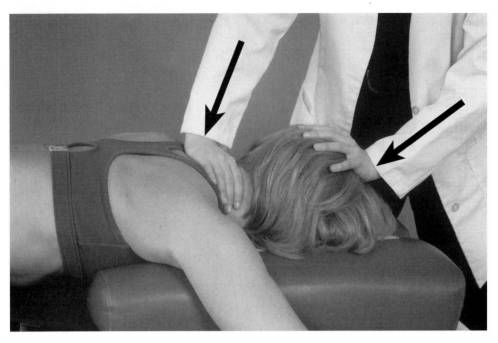

Fig. 5-22 Jensen table: Adjusting the cervical spine (continued).
- Close up view of patient and clinician positions for compressive stroke on cervical spine.

The Hill Table: Cervical Spine

The Hill technique and table are different from other cervical techniques and equipment because they allow the patient to be treated in either a prone or supine position. This table performs axial, or long axis, distraction instead of flexion-distraction. The patient is positioned with the head completely over the headpiece; the clinician may be either seated or standing at the head of the table. In all cervical manipulation on the Hill Intertrac table the treatment is manual with a traction assist and the patient is not required to be strapped to the table during treatment. The clinician's hands perform the manipulation by their position on the cervical spine. The clinician may decide to make a purely traction adjustment or a thrust with or without rotation. The table provides the mechanical or motion-assisted traction, and the manual therapy is applied by the practitioner. Control of each position is accomplished entirely by manual hand position, with the table providing axial distraction to the trunk. (Hill T. Privately published notes on the use of the Hill Intertrac table. Lakefield, Ont; undated.)

Because the head is not strapped or harnessed, it can assume positions of flexion, extension, lateral flexion, and rotation. The clinician provides much of the traction stabilization with a single hand, using the other hand as needed. The major tractive force, however, is provided by traction to the lower body. With the second hand, the clinician can apply surface or deep massage to the soft tissues of the cervical spine and shoulder girdle while traction is underway. As with the Jensen table, a compression stroke of the table allows the cervical structure to be molded and the lordosis of the neck reinforced. Cervical spine compression in the supine position allows for a posterior-to-anterior translation movement to be applied, producing a "stair-stepping" effect.

The outstanding difference between the action of this table and that of the others is that the patient is supine rather than prone during treatment because the distraction is performed axially. Both of the clinicians hands are free, and the cervical spine is under the direct control of the clinician at all times. If more traction or another position is desired (e.g., change from lateral flexion to flexion), the clinician releases the hands and repositions them to create a different traction moment vector of force (Figs. 5-23 through 5-30).

Text continued on p. 174

Fig. 5-23 Hill table: Cervical spine distraction (skeleton).
- Patient is positioned prone on the table, with arms resting on the arm and hand support.
- Table is in a neutral position, except for the β section, which is in slight negative (-).
- Clinician stands adjacent, with the treating hand contacting the cervical spine segment(s) to be distracted.
- The speed of the table is relatively slow (8 to 10 rpm) when this distraction is undertaken.
- Care must be taken to monitor and respond to the patient's sensitivity in the cervical spine.

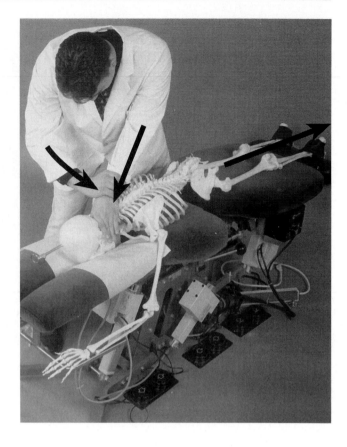

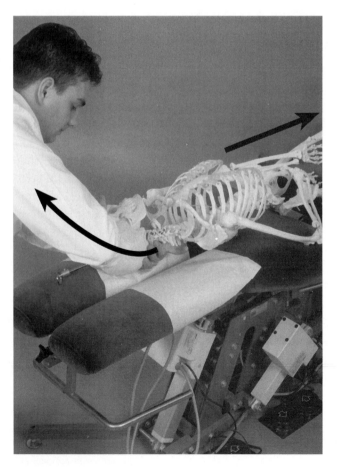

Fig. 5-24 The Hill table: Patient positioned supine (skeleton).
- Patient is positioned supine on the table, and the clinician is standing at the head (α) of the table.
- The treating hand and the support hand are placed at the part of the cervical spine that is to be treated.
- The spinal section is held while distraction is performed.

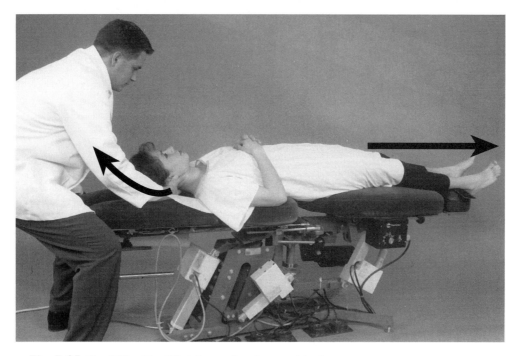

Fig. 5-25 The Hill table: Clinician and patient positioning.
- Patient is positioned supine on the table, with the β section and the Δ in neutral (0).
- Clinician is positioned at the end of the α section and cradles the patient's head while providing the distractive hand position.
- The β section provides the distractive force for treating the patient.
- Table is positioned at a height comfortable for the clinician. The clinician may enhance the position by sitting on a stool at the α section.
- The speed of distraction of the table is relatively slow (approximately 8 to 10 rpm).

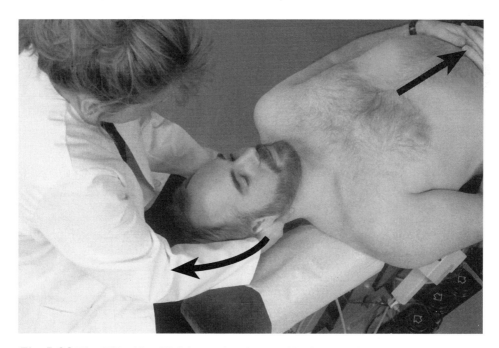

Fig. 5-26 The Hill table: Clinician and patient positioning (continued).
- Patient is positioned supine on the table, with head on the α section.
- Clinician is positioned at the end of the α section.
- Clinician's hands are positioned to cradle the head and create traction on the posterior elements as the table distracts the trunk.

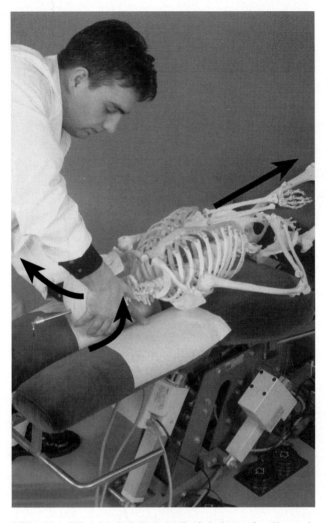

Fig. 5-27 The Hill table: Clinician holding skull of skeleton for distraction.
- Clinician stands at the head of the table and cradles the head in both hands, creating traction in the cervical spine as the table distracts the trunk.
- The entire table is kept in a neutral (0) position as the distraction progresses.
- Straight traction in the y axis and traction with lateral flexion and/or rotation are possible (left rotation and left lateral flexion are shown).
- The speed of distraction of the table is relatively slow (approximately 8 to 10 rpm).

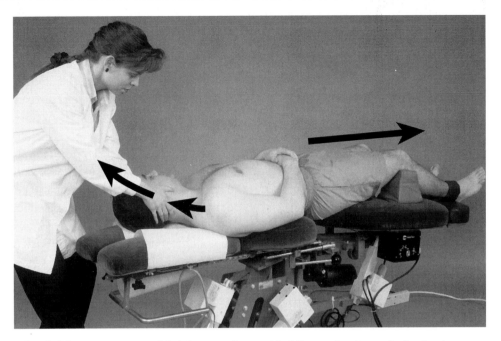

Fig. 5-28 The Hill table: Clinician standing and holding patient's cervical spine in rotation and lateral flexion.
- Patient is supine on the table, with the knees supported and the ankles strapped.
- Clinician stands at the head (α) of the table, supporting the patient's head.
- The table is in motion during the distractive process (8 to 10 rpm).
- The head is deviated to a position in rotation and/or lateral flexion (left rotation, left lateral flexion).
- The process is performed for approximately 3 repetitions on the side of treatment and may be performed bilaterally.

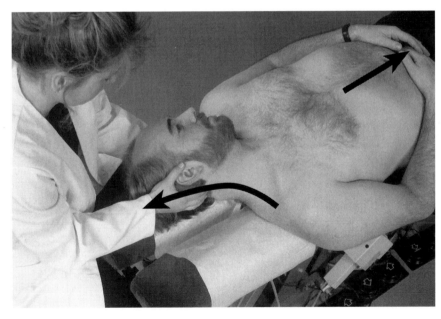

Fig. 5-29 The Hill table: Close-up of lateral flexion.
- Clinician stands or sits at head of table.
- Patient is supine, with hands resting on abdomen.
- The patient's head is supported by the clinician's hands and is flexed and/or rotated and/or laterally flexed (left lateral flexion shown).
- Patient comfort and tolerance of the procedure is important.

The Leander Table: Cervical Spine

The Leander technique and table have no specific protocol for use in the treatment of cervical spinal problems; however, provision is made in the design of the table for distraction of the neck. The headpiece can be moved in flexion or extension, which is noted as α_1 in the α (+) or (-). There is no specific lateral movement of the cervical section of the table. Because of the configuration of the Leander table, the cervical spine is usually adjusted with the patient prone if CPM of the spine is used (Fig. 5-31). Doctor's stance and hand position are the same as for prone distraction on the Hill Intertrac table (Fig. 5-23). However, it is possible to create distractive motion in the cervical spine with the patient in a supine position; extension distraction is applied to the low back to create distraction in the cervical spine (Fig. 5-32). If this section is not engaged, any other cervical adjustment can be executed in either prone or supine positions, and the table will be comparable to any other stationary table with an adjustable headpiece. The α section of the table has the capability of lateral flexion in the y axis of the body, but only as a full a section, including the upper trunk. This probably will not facilitate manipulation of the cervical spine because the axis of lateral flexion is located at approximately L4-5 or L5-S1.[31] (Figs. 5-33 and 5-34.)

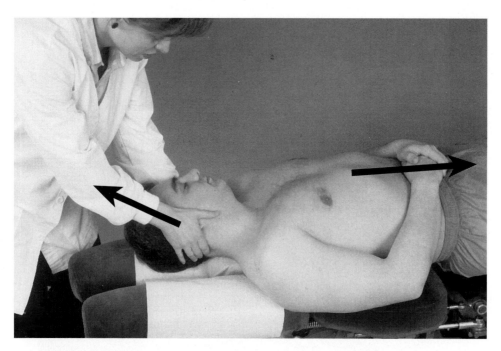

Fig. 5-30 The Hill table: Close-up of distraction.
- Clinician stands at head of table.
- Clinician cradles patient's head while table distracts lower trunk.
- Patient tolerance of distraction should guide clinician in amount of force used.

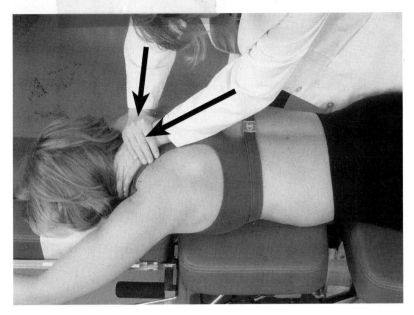

Fig. 5-31

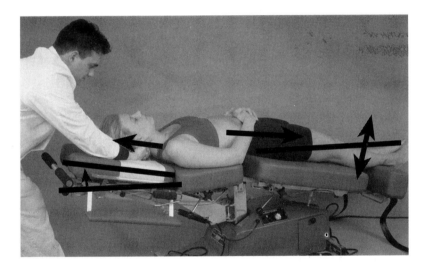

Fig. 5-32

Fig. 5-31 The Leander table: Cervical distraction on prone patient.
- Patient is prone on the table, with or without the ankle straps fastened.
- Clinician stands adjacent to the table.
- The treating hand of the clinician contacts the patient's cervical spine at the level of desired treatment.
- Table is set in motion with flexion of the patient's lower trunk, creating distraction in the cervical spine.
- Resistance to the distraction is maintained for three or four repetitions, and pressure is released between tractions.
- The α_1 and α_2 sections are maintained in neutral (0) position.
- The speed of flexion of the table is relatively slow.

Fig. 5-32 The Leander table: Cervical distraction on supine patient.
- Patient is positioned supine, with no ankle strapping.
- Clinician stands at the head (α) of the table, cradling the patient's head.
- The α_1 section is elevated (α_1, [+]) slightly to aid in flexing the patient's cervical spine.
- Table is set to distract by moving downward in the β section, creating extension in the lower trunk of the patient.
- The α_2 section is positioned neutral.
- The table is set for a relatively slow speed, and the distractive cervical adjustment should consist of three to four repetitions, with the hands of the clinician distracting the cervical spine.

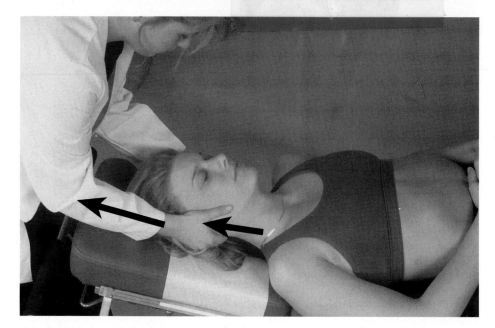

Fig. 5-33 The Leander table: Patient supine, straight distraction, slight flexion.
- Patient is positioned supine on the table, with or without distraction to the lower trunk.
- Patient's skull is cradled by the clinician's hands.
- The α_1 section is positioned in slight flexion.

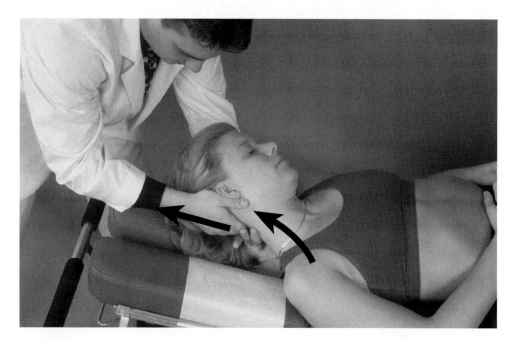

Fig. 5-34 The Leander table: Cervical adjusting, lateral flexion.
- Patient is positioned supine, with extension in the lower trunk or with table used as a flat table with no extension.
- Clinician stands at head of the table and cradles the patient's head.
- Traction, which may or may not be motion-assisted, is applied to the cervical spine.
- The cervical spine is flexed and/or rotated and/or laterally flexed (left lateral flexion shown).

TREATMENT OF THE THORACIC SPINE

THE ALLOPATHS: THORACIC SPINE

The allopaths, for example, Cyriax, demonstrate several manipulations for the thoracic spine. Cyriax uses some form of manual traction, with the help of assistants, in the process. Instead of having distraction applied mechanically, the thoracic spine is manipulated by assistants pulling manually on either end of the patient while the clinician provides the thrust or rotational stretch.[16,24]

Other allopaths who perform manipulation in the thoracic spine include Basmajian, Dvorak, Greenman, Mennell, Janda, and Travell and Simons. Prominent therapists who use manipulation in the thoracic spine (and who have written on the subject) include Maitland (physiotherapist), Cantu (physical therapist), Lidstrom (physical therapist), Nwuga (physical therapist), and Evjenth (manual therapist). These practitioners have developed unique techniques for treatment of musculoskeletal problems. Some of these techniques are for treatment of the bony structure of the skeleton and its joints, some are for treatment of the soft tissues (the myofascial components), and others are a combination of the two approaches. Few of the techniques promoted by these authors provide a distractive approach to manipulation of the thoracic spine, relying instead on pressure and thrust to accomplish the particular treatment.[6, 18-26]

THE MCMANIS TABLE: THORACIC SPINE

Thoracic manipulation can be performed on the McManis table. This table can be used in the same fashion as other manual distraction tables that allow the clinician to depress the lower, or β, section and hold the spinous process superior to the point to be distracted. Pressing of the β section (-) negative applies traction to the prone patient. There is no protocol for the application of this distraction, but it can be anticipated from the information available.[32] The patient's position and clinician's stance and hand contacts would be the same as for producing segmental distraction in the lumbar spine (see Chapter 4).

THE MEAD TECHNIQUES: THORACIC SPINE

Cox and other MEAD Techniques: Thoracic Spine

All of the MEAD techniques and the tables used in their application are similar in that they are manual and the power for the distraction is provided by the clinician's hand. The clinician's other hand can be used for the treatment of the patient. A single hand contact will provide only traction. A distractive adjustment of the thoracic spine can be made by performing the usual flexion maneuver with the power hand (the hand operating the table), while the other hand provides a tractive stabilization against the vertebrae being distracted. In the thoracic spine the adjusting hand contacts the vertebra above the joint being treated. While the table is depressed in flexion the joint held by the opposite hand will receive the distraction, and separation can occur at the disc level and at the facet joints below the point of contact. In this manner, muscles, ligaments, and tendons will be tractioned and taken to the outer limits of the elastic range. This distractive process in the thoracic spine is similar to that described for the lumbar spine, which uses the hand positions of Cox (the spinous process contact is on the surface of the hand over the carpal tunnel) or Markey (the spinous process contact is on the palmar web of the hand, between the thumb and the second digit). (Markey P. Privately published notes for Markey Technique Seminar; undated.)

THE MAD TECHNIQUES: THORACIC SPINE

The Leander Table: Thoracic Spine

The Leander table is motion-assisted and uses, through its motorized operation, the concept of continuous passive motion (CPM). Use of this technique in the thoracic spine allows both hands to be free to provide the treatment and allows appropriate adjustment of the speed on the table for the condition being treated. To enhance the distractive effect, traction can be provided by a contact hand and a supporting hand.

The table can be raised or lowered for the clinician's comfort. The patient is positioned prone on the table, with the feet over the ankle rest (β_2); ankle strapping is optional. The α and α_1 sections of the table are held in neutral, while the lower, or β, section is allowed to slowly flex when distraction of the thoracic spine is initiated. The β section cycles between β (0) and the full β (-) along the y axis of the body until the distraction is complete. The table should cycle through 3 to 4 downward-bending positions of the β section, with the treating and supporting hands in place over the area to be treated. The patient should rest briefly, and the 3 to 4 cycles of the β section should be repeated.

The Leander table allows lateral flexion of the α section around the z axis of the body while the β section moves through a full negative (-) cycle, producing linear distraction along the y axis. In the thoracic spine, this provides additional traction to the right or the left side, depending on the position of lateral flexion.

The Hill Table: Thoracic Spine

The patient is positioned on the Hill table, with all table sections in neutral (0). The table can be flexed slightly (to patient tolerance) in the β section, and this section can be laterally flexed. The ankle straps can be placed on the patient if more traction is desired, and the ankle rest adjusted for the patient's height. The table can be raised to a height comfortable for the clinician. For thoracic spine manipulation the table uses axial traction in the y axis of the body, set at a speed of approximately 10 rpm. The β section also can be β (-) (set in a downward bend) and/or slightly laterally flexed. (Hill T. Privately published notes on the use of the Hill Intertrac table. Lakefield, Ont; undated.)

The full table or Δ portion of the table may remain at Δ (0) or may be placed in a degree of Δ (+) for the adjustment of the thoracic spine. The hand contact can be at any location on the thoracic spine, depending on the location of the patient's problem. One or both hands may be used, depending on the desired contact. The two-hand contact is possible with an axial distraction table because the power comes from the motor in the table. The upper, or α, section does not move during the traction process, remaining in neutral (0) position and providing the stable base against which the table pulls in the tractive process.

The Jensen Table: Thoracic Spine

With the Jensen table, the thoracic spine can be distracted using the motion of the β section. The patient is assisted into a kneeling position on the table, with the β section adjusted for the patient's size and the leg straps in place. The patient's head is placed in the headpiece, which is covered with paper, and hands are placed on the handles on either side of the table. This type of adjustment may be performed with a variation in the angle of approach to the spine and/or the position of the clinician toward the head or the feet of the patient, as shown in Fig. 5-19. (Jensen R. Seminar notes. Seminar NWCC. 1993.)

The positions of the Jensen table are similar to those described earlier, in which the head and chest, or α, section slides slightly when the table circumducts with the cycling of the β section, with the patient kneeling and the straps attached at the knees. The full table or Δ portion of the table may remain at Δ (0) or may be placed in a degree of Δ (+) for the adjustment of the thoracic spine.

The cycling of circumduction may be increased or kept at a minimum for the thoracic adjustment; however, it may be advantageous to use only a slow circumductive movement for the thoracic adjustment, because the lumbar spine may be affected as much as the thoracic spine if the movement is too vigorous. The α section is capable of lateral flexion around the z axis from 0 degrees to about 15 to 20 degrees either right (R) or left (L). For sufficient leverage when treating the thoracic spine the clinician can use a 3- to 8-inch high stand to be raised above the area being treated.

TREATMENT OF THE EXTREMITIES

THE UPPER EXTREMITY:
WRIST, ELBOW, AND SHOULDER

By manually creating traction in an extremity, the extremity can be treated on most of the distraction tables from almost any position. However, some positions are more advantageous to both the clinician (for leverage) and the patient (for comfort). The purpose of treating the upper extremities with traction is to separate and stimulate the joints. Furthermore, soft tissue massage can be applied on taut and tender fibers and on trigger points. To maintain sufficient pull on the limb for treatment requires sustained or clinician-generated intermittent traction, which can be a great physical strain on the clinician. A traction device that provides some of the tractive force can be of benefit.

The Allopaths: Upper Extremity

The allopaths do perform extremity manipulation; however, the use of distraction does not appear to figure greatly in the allopathic literature. Much of the manipulation is of the thrust type or is involved with soft tissues. Some, such as Cyriax, use an assistant in treatments to the extremities, to provide manual traction as the clinician performs manipulations. Some, such as Cyriax and Travell, provide adjunctive injections with the manipulation.[16,26] Greenman and others advocate the use of thrusting maneuvers in the upper extremity, using only the hands.[6]

The McManis Table: Upper Extremity

The McManis table also can be used for the treatment of the upper extremity. This table is manual and requires the action of a clinician's hand to provide distraction. The lower section is depressed (β [-]), which precludes one operator providing both the tractive force and the holding of the limb. Two persons can operate the table, creating distraction of the limb, with the clinician concentrating on treatment while the other is providing the necessary distractive force.[32]

The MEAD Technique: Upper Extremity

The Zenith-Cox Table: Upper Extremity. Cox advocates the use of his table for the tractive process in treating the upper limbs. This is a manual table, however, and requires the clinician to be the source of power. The primary tractive force comes from the clinician, and the table serves as a stable platform for the application of a manual tractive force originating with the clinician. The whole table is maintained in Δ (0), but a slight β (-) (downward bend) will enhance the distraction. Mild linear distraction can be provided with the manual crank at the distal end of the table while the patient is fastened in the ankle straps, a process that probably requires two operators for the table. Two persons are preferred because successful traction requires that the shoulder, elbow, or wrist be maintained in traction while the β section is distracted manually.

The application of this technique on tables other than Zenith-Cox, such as Chattanooga, Lloyd, and so on, is much the same as on the Zenith-Cox, and the application of the force is not greatly different. The preference of one table over another is based on clinician perception of the action of the table with a patient in distraction. The table is used as a stable platform on which all surfaces, α and β, are in neutral (0), and the joint (the wrist, elbow or shoulder) is manually distracted, perhaps with the β section providing a mild axial distractive force.

The MAD Techniques: Upper Extremity

These techniques provide a motion-assist to the clinician in delivering the adjustment to the patient. The two techniques that allow distraction to the extremities with motion-assist are the Leander and Hill techniques applied on their respective tables. Each provides a different approach to the distractive process; the Hill technique and table provide linear, or axial, distraction and the Leander technique and table provide distraction movements of the pelvic section (β [+] and [-]) with flexion and extension. The Hill technique applied on the Hill table is the only approach that lends itself well to the distraction of extremities. Other equipment can perform the distraction, but the process is not well suited to the extremity because the tractive process is either in the wrong plane or the table requires the clinician to use one hand to power the table. This renders distraction of the extremity difficult or impossible and the table useful only as a flat surface on which to work.

The Leander Table: Upper Extremity. The patient can be positioned prone on the Leander table, and the β section set in motion while the clinician holds the upper extremity during the distractive process. Flexion-distraction in CPM provides a traction process for the upper extremity coupled with the flexion of the lower back over the fulcrum at the pelvis. Distraction can thus be applied to the wrist, elbow, and/or shoulder of the patient. As the clinician holds the extremity, the table exerts a slow pumping distraction on the joint. The angle of treatment can be altered by the clinician's stance and position at the head of the table. The cycles, although undefined specifically by the technique, can be five to six, followed by a rest with no traction on the extremity, and then repeated one or two additional times.

The Hill Table: Upper Extremity. The Hill table has a different action than the tables described previously. The linear, or axial, distractive force is in the y axis of the body, which, with some variations in the planes of the adjacent structures, provides a separating force within the elastic range. The y axis is the axis that produces the most predictable results, because it parallels two central planes of the body (coronal and sagittal). Extremities that are distracted in the y axis will receive an even tractive force that usually will separate the joint surfaces, pumping synovial fluid through the joint and reapproximating the surfaces, which helps correct misalignment of joint surfaces and restore normal movement. The Hill table can perform this task with the patient prone or supine.

The limb and joint are held by the clinician while the table slowly distracts the joint with a pumping action. The trajectory of the table is about 3 inches, and to increase the tractive force, the patient's ankles can be fastened into the ankle rest on the β section of the table. The length of time for this process depends on the patient's tolerance for the treatment and the clinician's clinical judgment. Generally, the process can provide a tractive force to the joint for five or six cycles, then rest for one or two cycles, and then be repeated for another series of three to four cycles. Three or four of these complete distractive cycles should be a full treatment for the joint at each session. The joint, particularly the wrist or shoulder, can be repositioned to accommodate a slightly different distractive angle that focuses on a movement component of the joint. The low back also is tractioned with this method; if this is not desired, an alternative position is appropriate. (Hill T. Privately published notes on the use of the Hill Intertrac table. Lakefield, Ont; undated.)

The alternative position has not yet been fully tested on the table, but the approach has been used previously. If it is desirable to isolate the particular joint, then a strap and holder can be provided for the table and used independently of low back axial distraction. The table is positioned in α, β, and Δ (0) while the distraction is applied to the seated patient. Soft tissue deep massage and/or trigger point work may be applied while the extremity is in distraction, but the clinician is less directly involved and less

directly in control than with the patient lying on the table. (Figs. 5-35 through 5-42.)

The Jensen Table: Upper Extremity. The Jensen table, which has a power operation that creates MAD, provides a source other than the clinician for producing traction. The prone position of the patient slightly limits the use of the table for this type of traction of an upper limb. However, the limb can be stabilized while in the traction cycles, producing a stimulating effect and an increase in the range of motion of the shoulder. In this instance the α section should be in neutral (0) and the β section in limited circumduction, sufficient to provide a tractive force for the distraction of the joint (wrist, elbow, or shoulder). (Jensen R. Seminar notes. Seminar

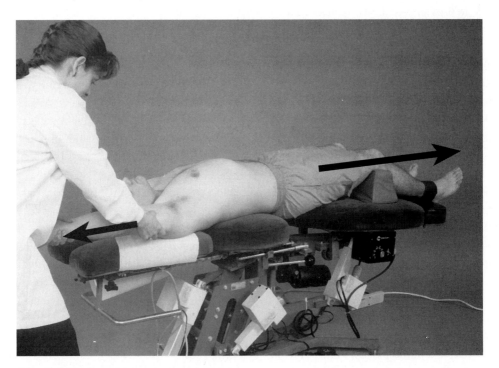

Fig. 5-35 The Hill table: Shoulder distraction.
- Patient is positioned supine on the table, with knees on the Distrac Wedge cushion for support.
- The ankle straps may be fastened, to create the necessary distraction for the shoulder.
- Clinician stands at the head of the table, holding the arm on the side to be treated.
- Clinician contacts the wrist with one hand and the nearer shoulder with the other; the table provides the motion-assisted distraction (MAD).
- Clinician maintains hold on the arm while the table distracts; hold is relaxed while the table moves in a nondistractive direction.

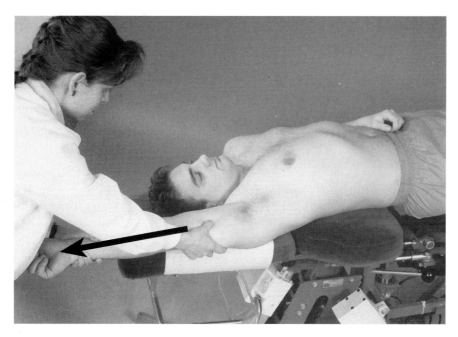

Fig. 5-36 The Hill table: Close-up of shoulder distraction.
- The patient, clinician, and table are positioned the same as in Fig. 5-35.
- Traction is provided both from the clinician holding the arm and from the distractive force of the table moving.
- The distraction is maintained with the table moving at 8 to 12 rpm for three to five repetitions and two to three applications per session to patient tolerance.

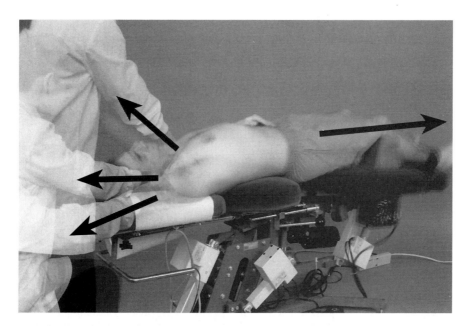

Fig. 5-37 The Hill table: Multiple views of distraction process.
- Patient is positioned prone on the table.
- Clinician holds the patient's shoulder and wrist while the table distracts and the clinician holds the position.
- Multiple positions are shown, to demonstrate the start and the increase introduced in the positioning of the arm as more distraction is applied.
- The shoulder can also be placed in 90 degrees of abduction or 90 degrees of forward flexion to produce inferior glide of the glenohumeral joint.

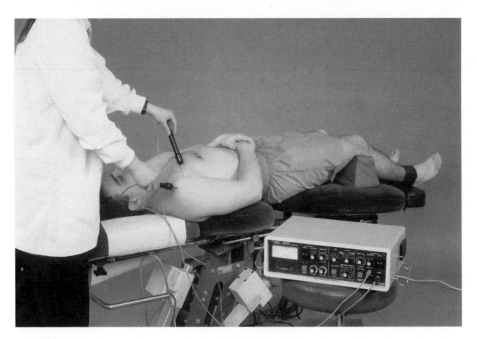

Fig. 5-38 The Hill table: Applying microcurrent to the shoulder.
- Patient is positioned supine on the table; all table sections are neutral (0), the ankles are strapped, and the knees are supported.
- The microcurrent unit is applied with dual probes or pads to the area to be treated.
- Microcurrent is direct current and can be applied while the table is performing distraction under power.

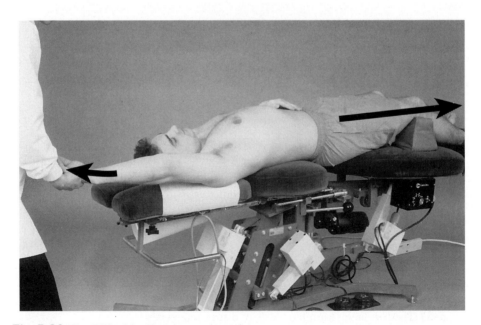

Fig. 5-39 The Hill table: Traction to the wrist.
- Patient is positioned supine on the table, with the ankles strapped and the knees supported.
- Patient's wrist is grasped by the clinician as the table distracts.
- The process is similar to that for the shoulder.
- General distraction to the wrist can be applied or specific contacts can be established over each carpal or metacarpal to focus the distraction force.

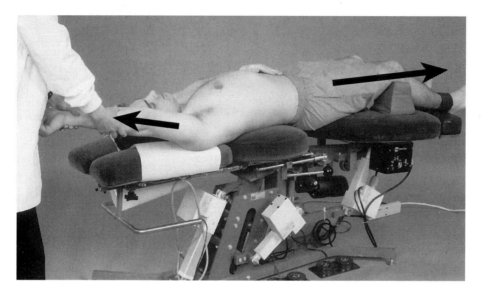

Fig. 5-40 The Hill table: Traction to the elbow.
- Patient is positioned supine on the table, with the ankles strapped and the knees supported.
- Patient's elbow is grasped by the clinician as the table distracts.
- The process is similar to that for the shoulder.
- The elbow may be placed in pronation or supination.

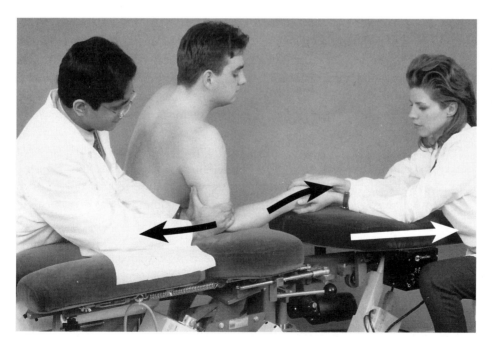

Fig. 5-41 The Hill table: Traction of the wrist (assisted).
- Patient is positioned adjacent to the table while the clinician and an assistant provide support for distraction.
- Clinician's elbows are supported on the β section while grasping the wrist.
- The same protocol is followed as for the other positions and for the shoulder.

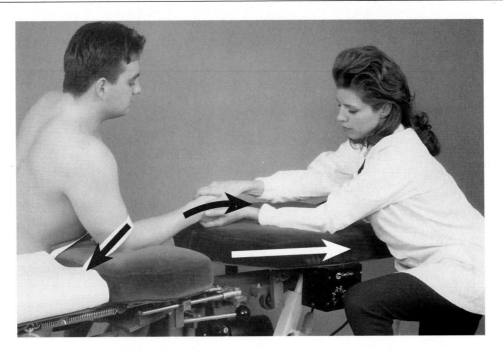

Fig. 5-42 The Hill table: Traction of the wrist (strap).
- Patient is positioned adjacent to the table, with the wrist to be treated resting on an elbow on the α_2 section.
- The elbow is strapped onto the α_2 section, and the clinician grasps the wrist to be treated.

NWCC; 1993.) The limb can then be positioned manually to effect the maximum distraction of the joint during the cycle. The difference between the Jensen table and the manual distraction tables is that the Jensen table supplies a portion of the force.

THE LOWER EXTREMITY: HIP, ANKLE, AND KNEE
The Allopaths: Lower Extremity

Most allopathic approaches to manipulation of the lower extremity are performed manually, with little involvement of the table or platform to enhance the process. The clinician provides most of the force, and the limb is perhaps incidentally tractioned. As noted earlier, the major use of traction by the allopaths is in the trunk, primarily the low back. Little traction is used outside the lumbar and cervical spine, except in the correction of fractures of the extremities or the spine. Cyriax uses traction in his approach to treatment of the lower extremities, and both Cyriax and Travell use injections of medications at the site of muscular involvement, along with their particular manipulation of both bony joints and soft tissue, to improve the patient's condition.[6,16,26]

The McManis Table: Lower Extremity

The McManis table is presented as primarily for treatment of the low back. Other positions can be assumed, the treatment can be performed as on other flat tables, and traction can be initiated manually.

The MEAD Technique: Lower Extremity

The Zenith-Cox Table: Lower Extremity. Cox advocates the use of his table for the tractive process in the lower limbs. This is a manual table, however, and requires the clinician to be the source of power. The primary tractive force comes from the clinician, and the table is used incidentally as a stable platform for the application of a manual tractive force originating with the clinician. Mild linear distraction could be provided with the manual crank at the distal end of the table, with the patient fastened in the ankle straps. The lower limb (ankle, knee, and hip joints) can be maintained in traction while the β section is distracted manually. The hip can be distracted by contacting the pelvis superior to the acetabulum, and the β section can be lowered, creating distraction of the area. This can be performed with the

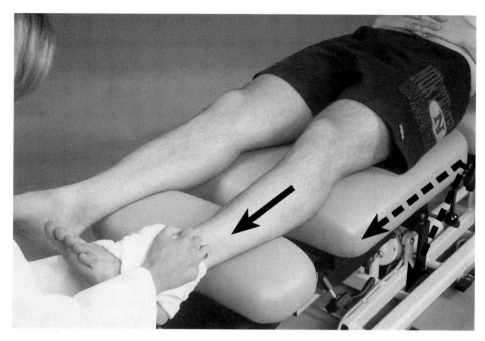

Fig. 5-43 Chattanooga table: Towel traction of lower extremity.
- Patient is positioned supine on the table.
- Clinician uses a towel wrapped around the ankle to provide a traction hold for the extremity.
- Clinician grips the towel with both hands to provide the tractive force.
- The same technique can be used on a linear distraction table, such as the Hill Intertrac.

patient prone or supine. This move requires a manual distractive process, and the clinician must use both hands, one for the power of the distraction and the other to stabilize the area.

The application of distraction on this table or on others, such as Lloyd, Chattanooga Spinalator, and so on, is much the same, and the application of the force is similar. (Fig. 5-43) The table is used as a stable platform in which all surfaces, α, β, and Δ are neutral (0), and the joint of the lower extremity is manually distracted, perhaps with the lower β section providing a mild axial distractive force.

The MAD Techniques: Lower Extremity

The Leander Table: Lower Extremity. The Leander table is motion-assisted and, with its power distraction, is an example of continuous passive motion (CPM). Use of this technique in the lower extremity allows both hands to be free to provide the treatment and allows adjustment of the speed on the table for the type of condition being treated.[31] The pelvis can be stabilized, and the hip, knee, or ankle can be distracted on a prone patient. This tech-

nique can be applied using motion-assisted distraction to free the hands for stabilization of the area under treatment. The β section can be set to cycle slowly, allowing the clinician to adjust contact and achieve the appropriate distractive force and position.

The Hill Table: Lower Extremity. With the Hill table, the axial approach to distractioning in the upper extremity is also appropriate in the lower extremity. The ankle, knee, and hip can all undergo distractive forces. A major value of the axial approach to distraction of the extremities and trunk is that this direction is in line with the major supportive column of the body. The Hill table, which provides tractive force for distraction, can be adjusted in speed and direction of travel through lateral flexion and downward bending of the β section. The ankles can be strapped to accentuate certain forces in the distraction process. (Hill T. Privately published notes on the use of the Hill Intertrac table. Lakefield, Ont; undated.)

The limb and joint that are being distracted are held by the clinician while the table slowly moves the joint with a pumping action. It may be necessary to strap the ankles to achieve the necessary tractive force. Generally,

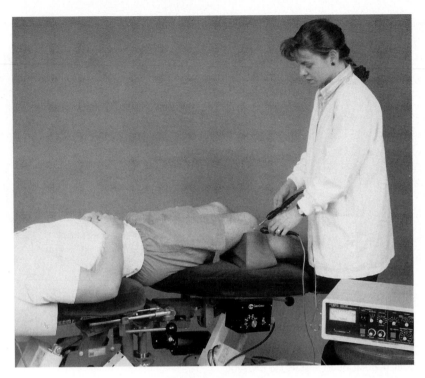

Fig. 5-44

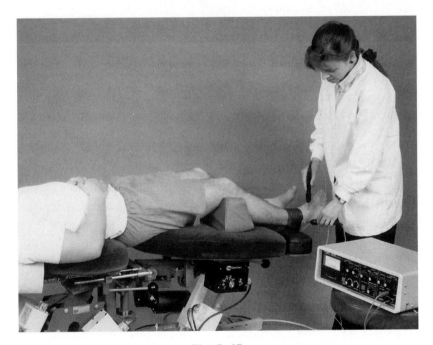

Fig. 5-45

Fig. 5-44 The Hill table: Distraction of the knee or hip.
- Patient is positioned supine on the table, with the knees supported on the Distrac Wedge.
- Table is positioned with all sections in neutral (0).
- The ankle is strapped, and the knee is distracted.
- Microcurrent is applied to the knee as distraction progresses.
- The same protocol applies as in the upper extremity.

Fig. 5-45 The Hill table: Distraction of the ankle.
- Patient is positioned supine on the table, with the knees supported on the Distrac Wedge.
- Table is positioned with all sections in neutral (0).
- The ankle is strapped, and the ankle is distracted.
- Microcurrent can be applied to the ankle as distraction progresses.
- The same protocol applies as in Fig. 5-44.

the process provides a tractive force to the joint for three to five cycles, followed by a rest for one or two cycles and another series of three to five cycles. Three or four of these complete distractive cycles should be a full treatment for the joint at each session. The low back also is tractioned with this method; however, if this is not desired, an alternative position is more appropriate. As always, the patient's tolerance to the distractive force should be considered and monitored carefully. (Figs. 5-44 and 5-45.)

CONCLUSION

Forms of manipulation and mobilization have been described and used for all articulations and supportive soft tissues of the musculoskeletal system. An often mentioned procedure to the extremity joints is long axis distraction. Mechanically assisted or motion-assisted procedures and equipment can be used to supply some of the tractive force in the long axis of the joint. This is a relatively new concept that should be clinically studied. Although it holds promise and is based on sound principles, no clinical data exists to support effectiveness or efficiency.

REFERENCES

1. Burns, JR. *Extremities: Adjusting and Evaluation* Davenport, Iowa: self published; 1984.
2. Christensen KD. *Illustrated Manual of Common Extremity Adjustments.* 2nd ed. Milwaukee, Ore: self published; 1980.
3. Gertler L. *Illustrated Manual of Extra-Vertebral Technic.* 2nd ed. San Francisco, Calif: Oak Bay Chiropractic; 1978.
4. Kirk CR, Lawrence DJ, Valvo NL. *States Manual of Spinal, Pelvic and Extra-Vertebral Technic.* 2nd ed. Baltimore: Waverly Press; 1985.
5. Schafer RC, Faye LJ. *Motion Palpation and Chiropractic Technic: Principles of Dynamic Chiropractic.* Huntington Beach, Calif: Motion Palpation Institute; 1989.
6. Greenman PE. *Principles of Manual Medicine.* Baltimore: Williams & Wilkins; 1989.
7. Kaltenborn FM. *Mobilization of the Extremity Joints: Examination and Basic Treatment Principles.* 3rd ed. Oslo: Olaf-Norlis-Bokhandel; 1980.
8. Wadsworth CT. *Manual Examination and Treatment of the Spine and Extremities.* Baltimore: Williams & Wilkins; 1988.
9. Broersen JP, Weel AN, van Dijk FJ, Verbeek JH, Bloemhoff A, Duivenbooden JC. The atlas of health and working conditions by occupation, II: a comparison with the "atlas of health and working conditions in the construction industry." *Int Arch Occup Environ Health.* 1995;67(5):337-342.

10. Andersson GB. Factors important in the genesis and prevention of occupational back pain and disability. *J Manipulative Physiol Ther.* 1992;15(1):43-46.

11. Pustaver MR. Mechanical low back pain: etiology and conservative management. *J Manipulative Physiol Ther.* 1994; 17(6):376-384.

12. Tuchin PJ, Bonello R. Preliminary findings of analysis of chiropractic utilization and cost in the Workers' Compensation System of New South Wales, Australia. *J Manipulative Physiol Ther.* 1995;18(8):503-511.

13. Shekelle PG, Hurwitz EL, Coulter I, Adams AH, Genovese B, Brook RH. The appropriateness of chiropractic spinal manipulation for low back pain: a pilot study. *J Manipulative Physiol Ther.* 1995;18(5):265-270.

14. Cox JM. *Neck, Shoulder, Arm Pain: Mechanism, Diagnosis, Treatment.* Fort Wayne, Ind: self-published; 1991.

15. McGregor M, Haldeman S, Kohlbeck FJ: Vertebrobasilar compromise associated with cervical manipulation. In: S Haldeman, ed. *Topics in Clinical Chiropractic.* Gaithersburg, Md: Aspen; 1995.

16. Cyriax J. *Textbook of Orthopedic Medicine.* 10th ed. London: Bailliere Tindall; 1975;2.

17. Lidstrom A, Zachrisson M. Physical therapy on low back pain and sciatica: an attempt at evaluation. *Scand J Rehabil Med.* 1970;2:37-42.

18. Basmajian JV, ed. *Manipulation, Traction and Massage.* 3rd ed. Baltimore: Williams & Wilkins; 1985.

19. Dvorak J, Dvorak V, Schneider W. *Manual Medicine 1984.* Berlin: Springer-Verlag; 1985.

20. Nwuga V. *Manipulation of the Spine.* Baltimore: Williams & Wilkins; 1976.

21. Cantu RI, Grodin AJ. *Myofascial Manipulation: Theory and Clinical Application.* Gaithersburg, Md: Aspen; 1992.

22. Evjenth O, Hamberg J. *Muscle Stretching in Manual Therapy: A Clinical Manual—The Extremities.* Alfta, Sweden: Alfta Rehab Forlag; 1984.

23. Janda V. *Muscle Function Testing.* London: Butterworths; 1983.

24. Maitland GD. *Vertebral Manipulation.* 5th ed. London: Butterworths; 1986.

25. Mennell JM. *Back Pain: Diagnosis and Treatment Using Manipulative Techniques.* Boston: Little, Brown; 1960.

26. Travell JG, Simons GS. *Myofascial Pain and Dysfunction: The Trigger Point Manual.* Baltimore: Williams & Wilkins; 1983.

27. Rogoff JV. *Motorized Intermittent Traction.* Baltimore: Williams & Wilkins; 1985.

28. Sherriff F. A flexible approach to traction. In: Boyling JD, Palastanga N, eds. *Grieve's Modern Manual Therapy.* 2nd ed. Edinburgh: Churchill Livingstone; 1994.

29. Basmajian JV, Nyberg R, eds. *Rational Manual Therapies.* Baltimore: Williams & Wilkins; 1993.

30. Liebl N. A new concept in technique using automated simulation of normal spinal biomechanics. *Chiropr Tech.* 1990;2(1):20.

31. Eckard, L. *Leander Technique Course Manual.* Port Orchard, Wash: Leander Research, Mfg. and Distr., Inc.

32. McManis JV. *McManis Table Technic: Technic Instructions and General Information.* Kirksville, Mo: McManis Table Co; 1938.

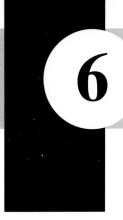

6

Motion-Assisted Thrust Technique (MATT)

The majority of chiropractic technique systems were started by practitioners who noticed a consistent pattern in their results and began to ask why those results occurred. The impetus to gain and disseminate new knowledge was largely self-driven.[1] Historically and traditionally the form of manual therapy identified with the chiropractic profession is the high-velocity, low-amplitude thrust applied to a short lever of a spinal segment or extremity joint. However, many of the technique systems do not use the high-velocity, low-amplitude thrust procedures. One reason for the development of nonthrust techniques is that certain patient presentations (e.g., the elderly or patients with osteoporosis, patients with extremely acute pain conditions, patients in later stages of pregnancy, and so on) are either a nonindication or a contraindication for the use of a thrust technique. Another reason may be a clinician's inability to produce a thrusting force sufficient to produce a change in a joint's mechanics. If the practitioner's size, strength, or ability to develop the needed speed is inadequate to produce the appropriate force, another type of technique application is necessary. Motion-assisted procedures can provide additional force to assist in the application of thrust techniques.

Any manipulative procedure that uses a thrust is considered to be a physical application of a well-directed, specific force to the body. It is therefore necessary to describe and, ideally, measure the magnitude, duration, direction, and variability of the thrusting forces.[2] Certainly, there is a critical force and energy that must be supplied by the clinician to bring a synovial joint to cavitation and influence its structural and functional relationship. The development of this force is dependent on many factors, including stiffness of the joint and patient, elasticity of the joint and patient, the proportion of energy entering the joint and patient, and the amount of joint distraction at which cavitation takes place. These parameters are governed by properties of the patient, clinician, joint, and adjustive process.[3] The average adjustive force produced by spinal manipulation can be expressed as the *impact kinetic energy* (mass and velocity) of the clinician and the *combined mechanical resistance to deformation* (stiffness and elasticity) of both clinician and patient.[4] Nonetheless, to produce the necessary force (F) for a manipulative thrust, a certain amount of mass (m) must travel a short distance quickly (acceleration – a). This represents Newton's second law of motion: $F = ma$. Herzog[5] identifies four external forces that must be considered in the performing of a thrusting technique. They are the weight force at the clinician's center of gravity and three contact forces (force that occurs where the clinician is in contact with the environment). Herzog modified the equation by including the weight force of the clinician (W) and the force of the ground acting on the clinician's left and right foot (R1, R2) to obtain $F = ma - W - R1 - R2$. He points out, however, that in the application of these equations, the model of the thrusting procedure is the impact of a free-falling clinician against a stationary patient, which is not a realistic picture. Furthermore, any forces acting internal to a system (e.g., muscular forces in the clinician) do not enter into these equations.[6] Nonetheless, critical forces must be produced by the clinician to develop the thrusting mechanism for joint separation or cavitation.

When tension is applied to the joint and causes a separation, the elastic barrier is engaged. With further tension, especially when applied quickly, a point is reached at which the joint surfaces "jump apart," coinciding with a cracking noise. The process of joint separation and cavitation can be accomplished in the plane of the joint, at right angles to the plane of the joint, or with joint distraction, any of which may produce an audible joint pop, or click. Heilig[7] believes that the high-velocity, low-amplitude manipulative technique is important because it produces the effect of joint separation, or gapping, and the possible momentary restoration of involuntary movement, or joint-play. To produce the high-velocity, low-amplitude thrust, the clinician must be able to develop the critical force to produce joint separation. This necessitates acquiring reflex contractile speed and stabilizing contractions of specific muscles (triceps and pectorals), as well as having sufficient body weight or mass for the maneuver. Mechanical assistance can augment these physical attributes.

One of the primary psychomotor skills necessary to generate the force for a thrusting joint manipulation is the speed or quickness to overcome inertia. Overcoming inertia requires the development of a high velocity over a short time. Sufficient speed developed over a short time is thought to facilitate joint isolation by causing the contact segment to reach maximum joint distraction before a noncontacted segment can be set in motion.[8] Haas,[8] however, suggests that if sufficient countertension can be produced (i.e., tension in the opposite direction of the thrust), distraction or cavitation can be accomplished with less speed.

Another important psychomotor skill is the ability to control the depth of the thrust. A short amplitude protects the joint from distension past the limit of anatomic integrity and protects adjacent motion segments from unwanted and unnecessary distraction by isolating the joint of interest.[8,9] Amplitude is controlled by regulating the duration and velocity of the thrust. The use of preadjustive tension can limit the dissipation of energy that occurs because of damping forces. Preloading the joint limits further motion during the thrust so that force and energy are not lost to other areas.[8] Use of a preliminary distraction means that the thrust must supply only the remainder of the force necessary for joint cavitation, diminishing the amount of physical exertion required of the clinician. The resulting enhanced efficiency facilitates a gentler adjustment, with less exertion by the clinician.[8] Moreover, if preadjustive tension and countertension can be produced by a mechanical device (adjusting table), even less force, speed, and energy will be required from the clinician.

Using a specially designed force transducer, Wood and Adams[10] demonstrate that for a specific type of lumbar adjustment a rather high force is generated (182.2 plus or minus 66.6 Newton) for a short duration (434 plus or minus 249 ms). Furthermore, these results carry a fair degree of reproducibility across male and female chiropractic clinicians possessing similar practice experience but of different strengths, ages, and body weights. This represents at least a preliminary study demonstrating consistency amongst clinicians to be able to generate similar high-velocity, low-amplitude thrusts on segmental contact points in the lumbar spine. In contrast, Hessel et al[11] conducted a study to quantify the forces exerted during spinal manipulations. The force characteristics were analyzed with respect to preloading force, peak force, duration of manipulation, impulse of manipulation, and point of application of peak force. The results demonstrate some common characteristics (e.g., preload force always followed by a large thrusting force) but mainly demonstrate major differences between manipulators. The values for the preload force, peak force, duration and impulse were found to have large standard deviations for a given adjuster and between patients.[11] This was a small study, limiting generalizations, but reasonable speculation may be made that the magnitude of force and impulse generation will vary among chiropractors and among patients.

To produce a joint separation sufficient to bring about a cavitation response a specific force is necessary. Because of the variation in patient characteristics and clinician size and capabilities, it may be difficult to produce the critical force. Therefore consideration should be given to the use of a device to assist in the development of the force. Adjusting tables have manual and motorized mechanical assistance components. One such modification is the drop-section mechanism, which represents a form of manual mechanical assistance. Another modification is a moving table section, which represents a form of motorized mechanical assistance.

DROP SECTION
MANUAL MECHANICAL ASSISTANCE

The first drop headpiece was introduced in chiropractic in 1952. B.J. Palmer stated that the principle behind the drop headpiece is one of the greatest advancements in chiropractic.[12] Grice[13] states that a free-fall headpiece may be used with a setspring reset-release to take up part of the force. This also allows counterresistance of the fixed vertebra when a recoil adjustment is applied in a specific direction, with a specific depth, high velocity, and low amplitude. In 1957, Dr. J. Clay Thompson developed adjusting tables with cervical, thoracolumbar, and pelvic drop pieces, to provide a mechanical advantage for producing a high-velocity, low-amplitude adjustment, with minimal observed discomfort for the patient. Thompson developed the mechanical drop-section table that, on delivery of a chiropractic thrust, allows a table section to drop a small distance and then stop suddenly. He believes this procedure incorporates Newton's laws of motion to develop kinetic energy not seen in other forms of chiropractic technique. He theorizes that the mechanical drop mechanism reduces the muscular effort required for the clinician to produce the adjustive thrust; therefore the muscular strength of the clinician is not a limitation in providing manipulative therapy. Moreover, it is thought that when the drop piece releases, the amount of force exerted on the joints is minimal and therefore more comfortable for the patient. Finally, because the patient cannot resist the effects of the drop sections, it is reasoned that joint movements will be more easily achieved. No studies have been conducted that support these contentions.[14] Theoretically, with the tension for the drop sections properly set, every patient can receive a consistent and measurable thrust. The drop table technique emphasizes high-velocity, low-amplitude adjusting and presumably reduces stress on the clinician, requires less force be generated by the clinician, and allows for a predictable thrust (Box 6-1).[15]

The forces involved in applying a drop-table thrust were measured by Wood and Adams,[10] who found that men applied stronger thrusts than women, clinicians could not accurately estimate the amount of force they were generating, and handedness did not seem to be a factor in determining the forces generated. These tests, however, were performed on the surface of the table, and therefore the results are difficult to apply to the technique performed on a patient in a clinical situation.

APPLICATION OF DROP SECTION TECHNIQUES

The basic procedure for applying a thrust that is augmented by a drop section table piece is as follows:

- Position the body part over the drop section
- Cock the drop section, checking its tension
- Establish contacts over the part to receive the thrust
- Generate a thrusting action to make the section drop
- Repeat the thrust procedure for a total of 3 times

Tables equipped with drop section mechanisms have levers to set each drop section in a "cocked up" position (Fig. 6-1). See Box 6-2 for a key to abbreviations and symbols used in several of the figures. Some tables use a pneumatic cocking mechanism that is operated by a foot pedal, freeing the clinician's hands. The patient is positioned on the table, with the segment to be adjusted posi-

---

> **BOX 6-1**
>
> **THE PRIMARY FUNCTIONS AND ADVANTAGES OF DROP SECTION TECHNIQUES**
>
> 1. Reduces wear and tear on the clinician
> 2. Enables low-force adjustments to be delivered safely and effectively
> 3. Permits fine tuning of the forces applied through adjustment of the tension on the drop pieces.

From Cooperstein R. Thompson technique. *Chiropr Tech.* 1995; 7(2)60-63.

> **BOX 6-2**
>
> **KEY TO ABBREVIATIONS AND SYMBOLS**
>
> PP: Patient position: The placement of the patient before delivery of the thrust
>
> DP: Doctor position: The clinician's stance and position in relation to the adjusting table and patient
>
> CH: Contact hand: Designates which hand is the thrusting hand, the specific area of the hand that is used, and the part of the patient that is contacted
>
> IH: Indifferent hand: Specifies which hand is used to stabilize the patient or reinforce the contact hand
>
> LOD: Line of drive: Direction of the adjustive thrust
>
> P: Procedure: The steps in establishing the contacts, including tissue pull and prestress leading to the thrust procedure
>
> Direction of thrust, stabilization, and/or prestress
>
> Drop piece direction

---

tioned on the drop section. The tension for the drop section must be set so the patient's body weight will not cause the section to drop. There are specific considerations for each joint, such as the segmental contact point, vector of thrust, and clinician position. Specific procedures for each joint are described and demonstrated elsewhere.[16] A representative sample is considered here.

SACROILIAC ARTICULATION

Treatment of the sacroiliac articulation is typically accomplished with the patient lying in the prone position. Contacts are established over the bony landmarks of the pelvis, including the posterior superior iliac spine (PSIS), sacral base, sacral apex, and ischial tuberosity. The com-

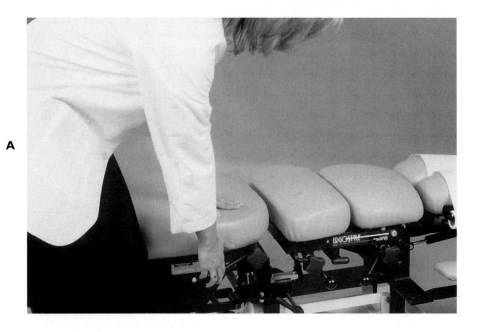

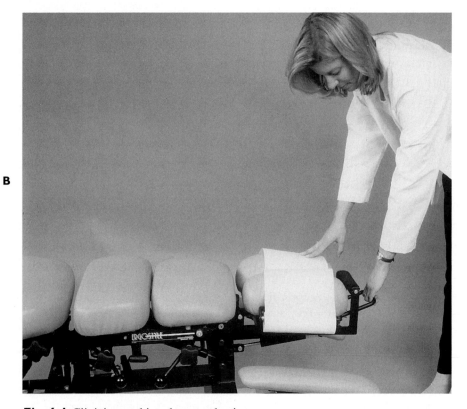

Fig. 6-1 Clinician cocking drop mechanism.
A.   Clinician lifting up on lever to cock the pelvic drop mechanism.
B.   Clinician lifting up on lever to cock the cervical drop mechanism.

bination of contacts influences the specific direction of the thrust and movement of the joint. A posterior-to-anterior thrust applied over the PSIS, with a counterthrust against the sacral apex, develops extension movement in the sacroiliac joint, with the innominate moving anterior (Fig. 6-2). A posterior-to-anterior and lateral-to-medial thrust against the lateral aspect of the sacral apex, with a stabilizing counterthrust over the opposite sacral base and PSIS, produces an extension of the sacroiliac joint, with the sacral base moving posterior and superior (Fig. 6-3). A posterior-to-anterior and inferior-to-superior thrust against the ischial tuberosity develops flexion movement in the sacroiliac joint, with the innominate (PSIS) moving posterior (Fig. 6-4).

LUMBAR SPINE

Treatment of lumbar spine dysfunction is accomplished with the patient lying in either the prone or side-posture position. Contacts are established over the bony landmarks of the lumbar spine, including the mammillary process and the spinous process. The contact point influences the specific direction of the thrust and movement of the joint. A posterior-to-anterior, lateral-to-medial thrust applied over the spinous process of the prone patient develops rotation and ipsilateral lateral flexion movement (Fig. 6-5). A posterior-to-anterior thrust against the mammillary process on the patient in the side-posture position produces rotation and contralateral

lateral flexion (Fig. 6-6). Although not demonstrated, flexion and extension malpositions or restrictions can also be influenced. The patient is prone and contacts established over the posterior-inferior aspect of the spinous process to apply a thrust mostly inferior to superior to create flexion. With the patient prone, contacts are established over the posterior aspect of the spinous process or both mamillary processes to apply a thrust mostly posterior to anterior to create extension.

THORACIC SPINE

Treatment of thoracic spine dysfunction is accomplished with the patient lying in either the prone or supine position. Contacts are established over the bony landmarks of the thoracic spine, including the transverse process, spinous process, and rib angle. The contact point influences the specific direction of the thrust and movement of the joint. A posterior-to-anterior thrust applied over the transverse processes of two adjacent vertebral segments on the prone patient develops rotation (counterrotation) (Fig. 6-7). A posterior-to-anterior thrust with torque against the transverse processes of the same vertebral segment produces rotation and contralateral lateral flexion on the prone patient (Fig. 6-8). A posterior-to-anterior thrust applied with torque over the spinous process on the prone patient develops rotation and ipsilateral lateral flexion movement (Fig. 6-9). A drop-section thrust can also be used in the cervicothoracic junction for rotation and lat-

Text continued on p. 201

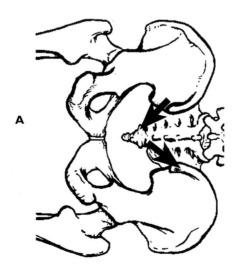

Fig. 6-2, A Diagrammatic representation of the contact points for a right posterior inferior innominate (PI), right flexed ilium, and right upper ilium fixation. *(Modified from Medical Illustration Library: General Anatomy. Baltimore: Williams & Wilkins; 1994;1.)*

Continued

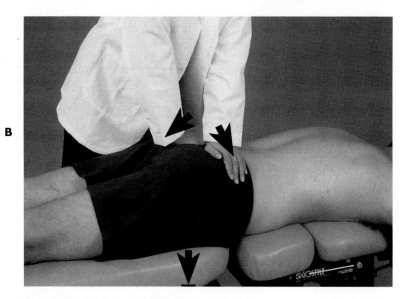

Fig. 6-2, *B* Clinician demonstrating the procedure for a right posterior inferior innominate (PI), right flexed ilium, and right upper ilium fixation.

PP: Patient lying prone on table, with ASISs on pelvic drop section.

DP: Clinician standing at the side opposite the posterior innominate, in a stance square to the table (e.g., right PI: stand on left side).

CH: Cephalad hand establishes a pisiform contact over the posterior inferior aspect of the PSIS (e.g., left pisiform, right PSIS).

IH: Caudal-hand pisiform contact against the contralateral aspect of the sacral apex (e.g., right pisiform, left sacral apex).

LOD: Cephalad hand posterior-to-anterior and medial-to-lateral; caudal hand mostly posterior-to-anterior.

P: With the pelvic drop section set with the appropriate tension, two to three thrusts are performed.

Fig. 6-3 Diagrammatic representation of the contact points for a right rotation of the sacral base (posterior sacral base), left lateral flexion of sacrum, and right upper or left lower sacral fixation accomplished using the following:

PP: Patient lying prone on table, with ASISs on pelvic drop section.

DP: Clinician standing at the side of posterior sacral base, in a stance square to the table (e.g., right posterior sacrum: stand on right).

CH: Cephalad-hand pisiform contact over the PSIS and sacral base, with fingers pointing footward (e.g., right pisiform, right PSIS and sacral base).

IH: Caudal-hand pisiform contact against the ipsilateral aspect of the sacral apex (e.g., left pisiform, right sacral apex).

LOD: Cephalad hand posterior-to-anterior and medial-to-lateral; caudal hand mostly lateral-to-medial.

P: With the pelvic drop section set with the appropriate tension, two to three thrusts are performed. A modification is a crossed-hand contact in which caudal hand contacts sacral base/PSIS, and cephalad hand contacts sacral apex. (*Modified from* Medical Illustration Library: General Anatomy. *Baltimore: Williams & Wilkins; 1994;1.*)

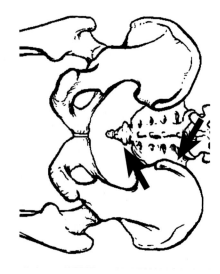

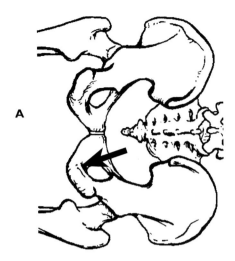

Fig. 6-4, A Diagrammatic representation of the contact points for a right lower ilium fixation, right anterior superior ilium (AS), and right extended ilium. (*Modified from* Medical Illustration Library: General Anatomy. *Baltimore: Williams & Wilkins; 1994;1.*)

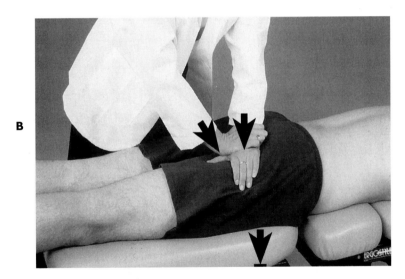

Fig. 6-4, B Clinician demonstrating the procedure for a right lower ilium fixation, right anterior superior ilium (AS), and right extended ilium.

PP: Patient lying prone on table, with ASISs on pelvic drop section.

DP: Clinician standing at side of table, facing cephalad in a fencer's stance (lunge), typically on the side opposite the AS ilium (e.g., right AS ilium: stand on left side of table).

CH: Cephalad hand establishes a knife-edge, or soft pisiform (hypothenar), contact over the posterior aspect of the ischial tuberosity (e.g., left knife-edge: right ischial tuberosity).

IH: Caudal hand reinforces the contact hand (e.g., right hand).

LOD: Posterior-to-anterior.

P: With the pelvic drop section set with the appropriate tension, two to three thrusts are performed.

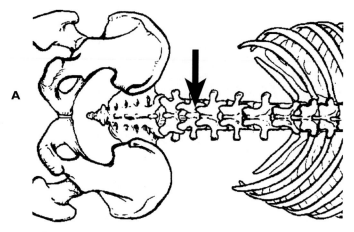

Fig. 6-5, A Diagrammatic representation of the contact points for a right rotated and/or right laterally flexed malposition and/or left rotational and/or left lateral flexion restriction L4-5. (*Modified from* Medical Illustration Library: General Anatomy. *Baltimore: Williams & Wilkins; 1994;1.*)

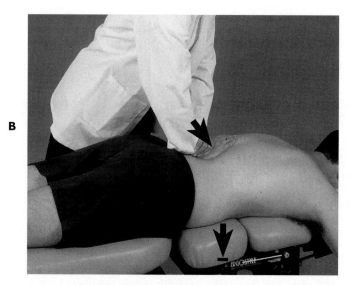

Fig. 6-5, B Clinician demonstrating a procedure for a right rotated and/or right laterally flexed malposition and/or left rotational and/or left lateral flexion restriction L4-5.

PP: Patient lying prone on table, with lumbar motion segment on the lumbar drop section.

DP: Clinician standing on side of table in a stance square to the table (e.g., right rotated, right laterally flexed L4-5 [PLS; RPI] or a left rotational restriction and a left lateral flexion restriction L4-5: stand on left side).

CH: Caudal-hand pisiform contact against the lateral aspect of the spinous process (e.g., right pisiform, left side of L4 SP).

IH: Cephalad hand reinforces contact hand (e.g., left hand).

LOD: Both hands thrust posterior-to-anterior and lateral-to-medial.

P: With the lumbar drop section (lumbar and pelvic sections for lower lumbars) set with the appropriate tension, two to three thrusts are performed. Alternatively, procedure can be performed on patient in side-posture position, as in Fig. 6-6.

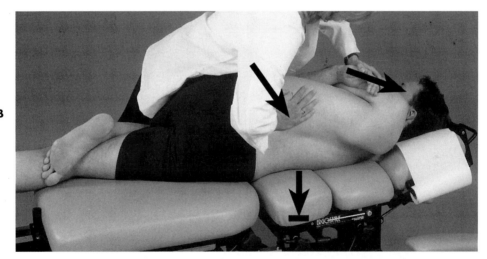

Fig. 6-6, *A* Diagrammatic representation of the contact points for a right rotated and/or left laterally flexed malposition and/or left rotational and/or right lateral flexion restriction L3-4. (*Modified from* Medical Illustration Library: General Anatomy. *Baltimore: Williams & Wilkins; 1994;1.*)

Fig. 6-6, *B* Clinician demonstrating the procedure for a right rotated and/or left laterally flexed malposition and/or left rotational and/or right lateral flexion restriction L3-4.

PP: Patient lying in the side-posture position, with the lumbar motion segment on the lumbar drop section (e.g., right rotated, left laterally flexed L3-4 [PLI-M, RPS], left rotation restriction, right lateral flexion restriction L3-4).

DP: Clinician standing at side of table, facing the patient at right angles; caudal foot off the floor, with a lateral knee-to-knee, thigh-to-thigh contact over the patient's flexed thigh.

CH: Caudal-hand pisiform contact over the mammillary process (e.g., right pisiform, left MP L4).

IH: Cephalad hand grasps the lateral aspect of the upper humerus over the deltoid tubercle (e.g., left hand, patient's left humerus).

LOD: Posterior-to-anterior.

P: With the lumbar drop set with the appropriate tension, remove slack with CH, IH, and thigh; IH stabilizes in cephalad direction; CH thrusts MP anterior or directs thrust superior and inferior for the appropriate listings (torque); two to three body-drop thrusts are performed. Alternatively, procedure can performed on patient in prone position, as in Fig. 6-5.

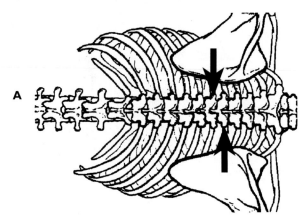

Fig. 6-7, A Diagrammatic representation of the contact points for a right rotational malposition and/or left restriction T5-6. (*Modified from* Medical Illustration Library: General Anatomy. *Baltimore: Williams & Wilkins; 1994;1.*)

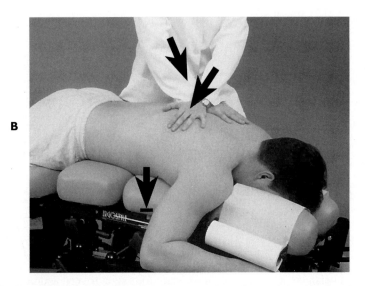

Fig. 6-7, B Clinician demonstrating the procedure for a right rotational malposition and/or left restriction T5-6.

PP: Patient lying in prone position, with the thoracic motion segment on the thoracic drop section.

DP: Clinician standing at side of table, facing the patient at right angles (e.g., right rotated T5-6 [PL, RP], left rotation restriction T5-6: stand on left side).

CH: Cephalad-hand pisiform contact over transverse process of upper vertebrae (e.g., left pisiform, right TP T5).

IH: Caudal-hand pisiform contact over transverse process of lower vertebra (e.g., right pisiform, left TP T6).

LOD: Posterior-to-anterior.

P: With the thoracic drop section set with the appropriate tension, two to three thrusts are performed to produce a counterrotation between T5-6.

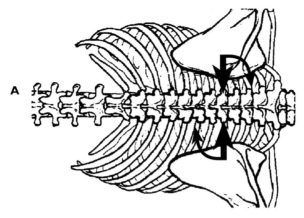

Fig. 6-8, A Diagrammatic representation of the contact points for a right rotation, left lateral flexion malposition and/or left rotational, right lateral flexion restriction T5-6. (*Modified from* Medical Illustration Library: General Anatomy. *Baltimore: Williams & Wilkins; 1994;1.*)

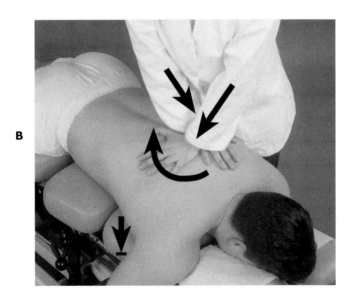

Fig. 6-8, B Clinician demonstrating the procedure for a right rotation, left lateral flexion malposition and/or left rotational, right lateral flexion restriction T5-6.

PP: Patient lying in the prone position, with the thoracic motion segment on the thoracic drop section.

DP: Clinician standing at side of table, facing the patient at right angles (e.g., right rotated, left laterally flexed T5-6 [PLI-T, RPS], left rotational, right lateral flexion restriction T5-6: stand on left side).

CH: Cephalad-hand pisiform contact over transverse process of upper vertebra (e.g., left pisiform, right TP T5).

IH: Caudal-hand pisiform contact over transverse process of lower vertebra (e.g., right pisiform, left TP T5). To develop counterrotation the caudal-hand pisiform contact can be established over the transverse process of the lower vertebra (e.g., right pisiform, left TP T6).

LOD: Posterior-to-anterior, clockwise torque.

P: With the thoracic drop section set with the appropriate tension, two to three thrusts are performed. Alternatively, procedure can be accomplished for the same dysfunction with clinician on the other side of table.

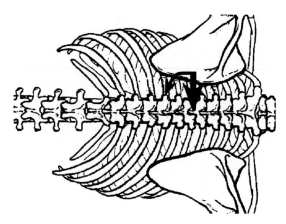

Fig. 6-9 Diagrammatic representation of the contact points for a right rotation, right lateral flexion malposition and/or left rotational, left lateral flexion restriction T5-6.

PP: Patient lying in the prone position, with the thoracic motion segment on the thoracic drop section.

DP: Clinician standing at side of table, facing the patient at right angles (e.g., right rotated, right laterally flexed T5-6 (PLS, RPI), left rotational, left lateral flexion restriction T5-6: stand on left side).

CH: Cephalad-hand pisiform contact over spinous process of upper vertebra (e.g., left pisiform, left side of SP T5).

IH: Caudal-hand pisiform in snuff box of CH for reinforcement (e.g., right pisiform in left snuff box).

LOD: Lateral-to-medial (left-to-right), posterior-to-anterior, counterclockwise torque.

P: With the thoracic drop section set with the appropriate tension, two to three thrusts are performed. (*Modified from* Medical Illustration Library: General Anatomy. *Baltimore: Williams & Wilkins; 1994;1.*)

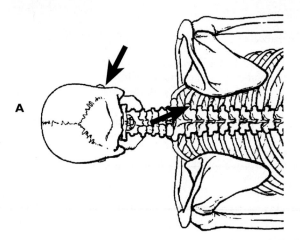

Fig. 6-10, A Diagrammatic representation of the contact points for a right rotation, left lateral flexion malposition and/or left rotational, right lateral flexion restriction T1-2. (*Modified from* Medical Illustration Library: General Anatomy. *Baltimore: Williams & Wilkins; 1994;1.*)

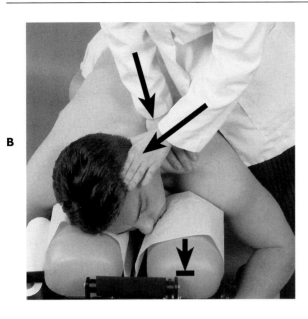

B

Fig. 6-10, B, C Clinician demonstrating the procedure for a right rotation, left lateral flexion malposition and/or left rotational, right lateral flexion restriction T1-2.

PP: Patient lying in the prone position, with the thoracic motion segment on the thoracic drop section.

DP: Clinician standing at side of table, facing the patient at right angles (e.g., right rotated, left laterally flexed T1-2 (PLI-T, RPS), left rotational, right lateral flexion restriction T1-2: stand on left side).

CH: Caudal-hand pisiform contact over transverse process of lower vertebra (e.g., right pisiform, left TP T2).

IH: Cephalad-hand thumb contact under base of occiput, palmar and finger contact on side of face and head (e.g., left hand, left side of head).

LOD: Posterior-to-anterior.

P: With the thoracic drop section set with the appropriate tension, cephalad traction, rotation, and lateral flexion prestress is developed between CH and IH; two to three body-drop thrusts are performed.

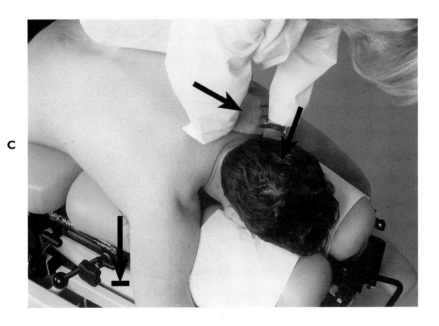

C

eral flexion dysfunction (Fig. 6-10). Although not demonstrated, flexion and extension malpositions or restrictions can also be influenced. With the patient prone, contacts are established over the posterior-inferior aspect of the spinous process to apply a thrust mostly inferior to superior to create flexion. With the patient prone, contacts are established over the posterior aspect of the spinous process or both transverse processes to apply a thrust mostly posterior to anterior to create extension.

CERVICAL SPINE

Treatment of cervical spine dysfunction is accomplished with the patient lying prone or, for the upper cervical spine, in the side-posture position. Contacts are established over the bony landmarks of the cervical spine, including the articular pillars (spinolaminar junction) and spinous processes in the lower cervical spine and the transverse processes of atlas. The contact point influences the specific direction of the thrust and movement of the joint. A posterior-to-anterior thrust applied over the articular pillars on the prone patient develops rotation and contralateral lateral flexion (Fig. 6-11). Although not demonstrated, flexion and extension malpositions or restrictions can also be influenced. With the patient lying in a prone position, contacts are established over the posterior-inferior aspect of the spinous process to apply a thrust mostly inferior to superior to create flexion. With the patient lying prone, contacts are established over the posterior aspect of the spinous process or both articular processes to apply a thrust mostly posterior to anterior to create extension. A lateral-to-medial thrust against the transverse processes of the atlas on a patient lying in the side-posture position produces lateral glide and the possibility of rotation and flexion-extension (Fig. 6-12).

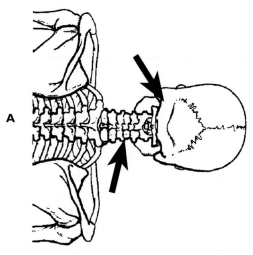

Fig. 6-11, A Diagrammatic representation of the contact points for a right rotation, left lateral flexion malposition and/or left rotational, right lateral flexion restriction C4-5. (*Modified from* Medical Illustration Library: General Anatomy. *Baltimore: Williams & Wilkins; 1994;1.*)

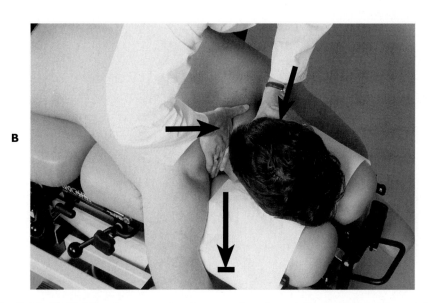

Fig. 6-11, B Clinician demonstrating the procedure for a right rotation, left lateral flexion malposition and/or left rotational, right lateral flexion restriction C4-5.

PP: Patient lying in the prone position, with the cervical motion segment on the cervical drop section.

DP: Clinician standing at side of table, facing the patient at right angles (e.g., right rotated, left laterally flexed C4-5 [PLI-L, RPS], left rotational, right lateral flexion restriction C4-5: stand on left side).

CH: Caudal-hand index (metacarpophalangeal joint) contact over articular pillar (e.g., right index, right AP C4).

IH: Cephalad-hand thumb contact under base of occiput, palmar and finger contact on side face and head (e.g., left hand, left side of head).

LOD: Posterior-to-anterior, lateral-to-medial (right-to-left).

P: With the cervical drop section set with the appropriate tension, cephalad traction, rotation, and lateral flexion prestress is developed between CH and IH; two to three thrusts are performed. Alternatively, clinician can stand on opposite side of table.

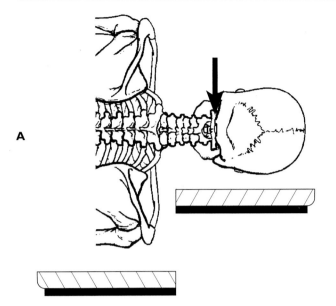

A

Fig. 6-12, *A* Diagrammatic representation of the contact points for a left laterolisthesis malposition and/or left to right lateral glide restriction C1-2 and/or C0-1. (*Modified from* Medical Illustration Library: General Anatomy. *Baltimore: Williams & Wilkins; 1994;1.*)

EXTREMITIES

Treatment of extremity joint dysfunction can also be accomplished using the mechanical assistance of drop sections. The extremity joint to be adjusted is positioned over the drop section of the table or on a portable drop mechanism. Contacts are established over the bony landmarks of the extremity joints to influence the specific direction of the thrust and movement of the joint. A representative sample is presented here. A posterior-to-anterior (dorsal-to-palmar) thrust can be applied over the lunate to create glide movements at the joints between the lunate and the radius, scaphoid, triquetrum, and capitate (Fig. 6-13). An anterior-to-posterior thrust can be applied over the fibula to produce glide movement at the proximal tibiofibular joint (Fig. 6-14). A posterior-to-anterior thrust can be applied over the proximal femur to create glide movement of the hip joint (Fig. 6-15).

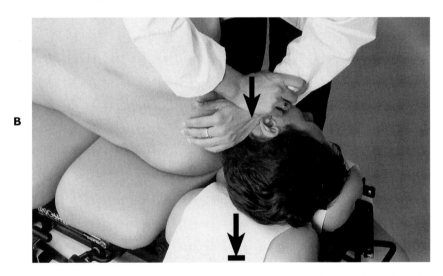

B

Fig. 6-12, *B* Clinician demonstrating the procedure for a left laterolisthesis malposition and/or left to right lateral glide restriction C1-2 and/or C0-1.

PP: Patient lying in the side-posture position, with the head on the cervical drop section.

DP: Clinician standing at side of table, facing the patient at right angles (e.g., left laterolisthesis C1-2 [ASL, LL], left-to-right lateral glide restriction C1-2: stand on left side, patient lies on right side).

CH: Cephalad-hand pisiform contact over lateral aspect of transverse process of atlas (e.g., left pisiform, left side of TP C1).

IH: Caudal-hand pisiform in snuff box of CH for reinforcement (e.g., right pisiform in left snuff box).

LOD: Lateral-to-medial (left-to-right), torque can be applied for flexion-extension.

P: With the cervical drop section set with the appropriate tension, two to three thrusts are performed. Alternatively, a single recoil type of thrust can be applied.

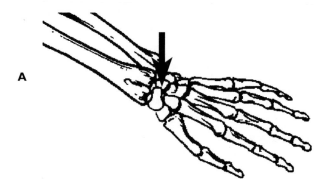

Fig. 6-13, *A* Diagrammatic representation of the contact points for a dorsal malposition and/or dorsal to palmar glide restriction of the left lunate. (*Modified from* Medical Illustration Library: General Anatomy. *Baltimore: Williams & Wilkins; 1994;1.*)

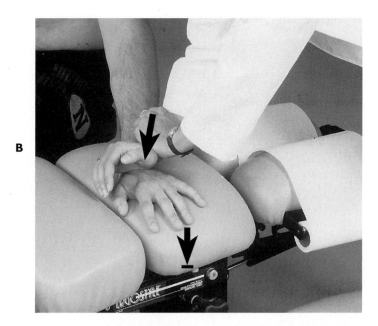

Fig. 6-13, *B* Clinician demonstrating the procedure for a dorsal malposition and/or dorsal-to-palmar glide restriction of the left lunate.

PP: Patient is seated at side of table to position affected wrist over a drop section of the table or on a portable drop mechanism.

DP: Clinician standing at side of table.

CH: Either hand, pisiform contact established over posterior (dorsal) aspect of lunate (e.g., right pisiform, left lunate).

IH: Other hand pisiform in snuff box of CH for reinforcement (e.g., left pisiform in right snuff box).

LOD: Posterior-to-anterior (dorsal-to-palmar).

P: With the drop section set with the appropriate tension, two to three thrusts are performed.

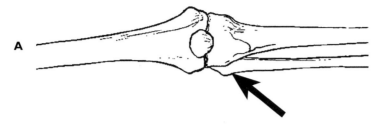

Fig. 6-14, A Diagrammatic representation of the contact points for an anterior malposition and/or anterior-to-posterior glide restriction of the right proximal fibula. (*Modified from* Medical Illustration Library: General Anatomy. *Baltimore: Williams & Wilkins; 1994;1.*)

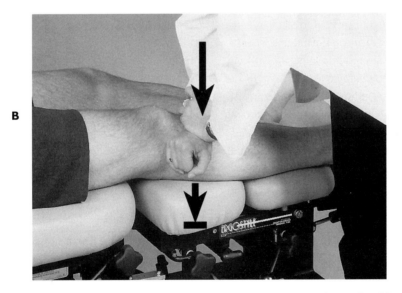

Fig. 6-14, B Clinician demonstrating the procedure for an anterior malposition and/or anterior-to-posterior glide restriction of the right proximal fibula.

PP: Patient lies or sits on table to position affected knee over a drop section of the table or on a portable drop mechanism.

DP: Clinician stands at side of table, facing headward.

CH: Caudal-hand pisiform contact established over anterior aspect of the proximal fibula (e.g., right pisiform, right fibula).

IH: Cephalad hand pisiform in snuff box of CH for reinforcement (e.g., left pisiform in right snuff box).

LOD: Anterior-to-posterior.

P: With the drop section set with the appropriate tension, two to three thrusts are performed.

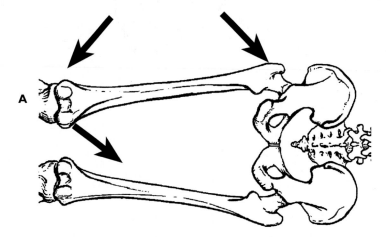

Fig. 6-15, A Diagrammatic representation of the contact points for a posterior malposition and/or posterior-to-anterior glide restriction of the left hip joint. (*Modified from Medical Illustration Library: General Anatomy. Baltimore: Williams & Wilkins; 1994;1.*)

MOTORIZED MECHANICAL ASSISTANCE

The motion that occurs as the pelvic unit moves away from the occiput at full distraction is referred to as *long axis distraction* or *long axis extension.* This is a translational movement occurring along the y axis. Spinal long axis distraction is difficult to evaluate and yet is considered an important component of spinal joint movement. A long axis distraction movement of joint-play occurs at every synovial joint.[17] In the extremity joints, considerable importance is placed on evaluation and manual treatment of loss of long axis distraction and its role in producing joint dysfunction.[18,19] In the spine, however, this important joint movement is generally ignored or not considered clinically for normal function of the spinal joints. Perhaps this is because long axis distraction of the spinal joints is difficult at best to elicit manually.

The use of a motorized distraction table enables the clinician to evaluate for a loss of long axis distraction on a segmental basis. Motion-assisted palpation (MAP) is possible using the Hill Intertrac table, Chattanooga Ergotrak table, or any table that produces linear distraction. Tables that produce motorized flexion movement (β [-]) also can be used. However, the linear-distracting pelvic piece allows specific and easy joint-play examination for long axis distraction of the sacrum, ilia, hip, lumbar spine, thoracic spine, and cervical spine. MAP is performed with the patient recumbent; therefore consideration must be given to any patient condition or characteristic (e.g., acute, chronic, aged, obese, and so on) before

the treatment is performed. MAP repeatedly stretches and compresses the patient, allowing long axis movement (translation along the y axis) to be determined. The evaluation of long axis distraction is difficult when performed on stationary benches or tables. Regardless of the degree of pain the patient may be experiencing the examination usually can be performed without discomfort. For this maneuver the patient is positioned prone on the Hill Intertrac or Chattanooga Ergotrak table, with the lumbosacral junction at the separation of the table. The pelvic section of the table (β) is switched on and set to reciprocate at about 15 cycles per minute (cpm) (modifying the speed for patient comfort and tolerance), exposing the patient to a push-pull force of gentle long axis oscillations. The patient is therefore being tractioned and compressed alternately along the y axis.

With the table functioning to create long axis distraction, the clinician pulls the pelvis caudally, placing digital contacts in the interspinous spaces (Fig. 6-16). As the table produces distraction, the clinician should be able to feel separation of the spinous processes (Fig. 6-17). If separation is not perceived, this indicates a loss of long axis distraction. Overpressure in long axis distraction can also be performed. As the motorized table provides prestress in long axis distraction, the clinician can apply inferior-to-superior overpressure, checking for the springing joint-play or end-feel movements of long axis distraction (Fig. 6-18).

Evaluation for segmental lateral flexion movement also is easily accomplished by releasing the caudal section, allowing it to swing from side to side. As the clini-

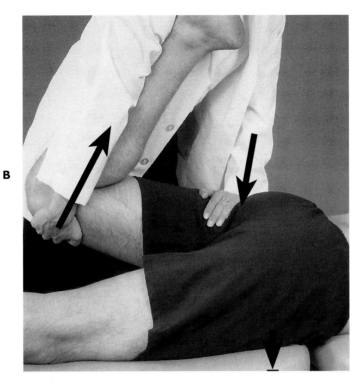

Fig. 6-15, *B* Clinician demonstrating the procedure for a posterior malposition and/or posterior-to-anterior glide restriction of the left hip joint.

PP: Patient lying in the prone position, with affected hip over the pelvic drop section.

DP: Clinician standing at side of table, facing headward (e.g., left hip: stand on left side).

CH: Cephalad-hand pisiform/knife-edge contact established over posterior aspect of the proximal femur (e.g., left pisiform/knife-edge, left femur).

IH: Caudal hand grasps distal femur of the patient's flexed knee on the anteromedial aspect affected side (e.g., right hand grasps left knee).

LOD: Posterior-to-anterior.

P: With the drop section set with the appropriate tension, the thigh is extended by the IH while the CH begins posterior-to-anterior pressure to apply prestress; two to three thrusts are performed.

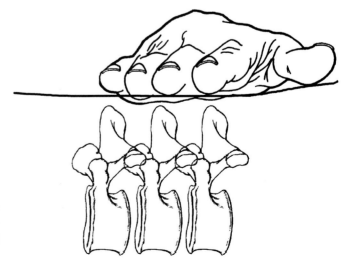

Fig. 6-16 Diagrammatic representation showing the starting relationship between the clinician's finger and the spinous processes of the patient's lumbar spine for determining the presence of intersegmental long axis distraction.

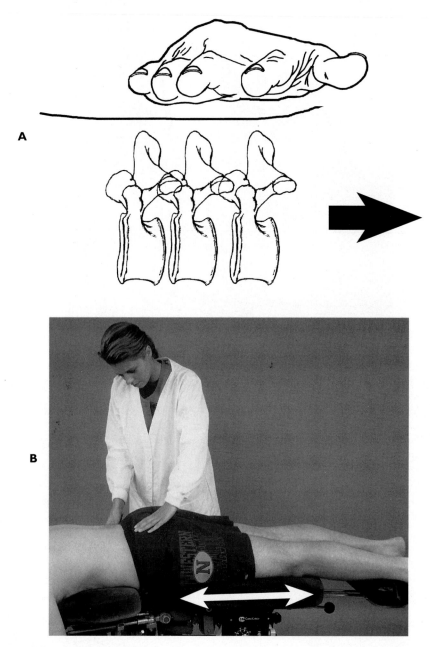

Fig. 6-17 A motorized, linear distraction table can be used to assess long axis (y axis) movement in the spinal joint.

A.   Diagrammatic representation of separation of the clinician's fingers as the distractive force of the pelvic section creates intersegmental long axis distraction between L4-5.

B.   Clinician palpating the spinous process in the lumbar spine; as the pelvic section distracts, passive separation representing long axis distraction (y-axis translation) can be felt.

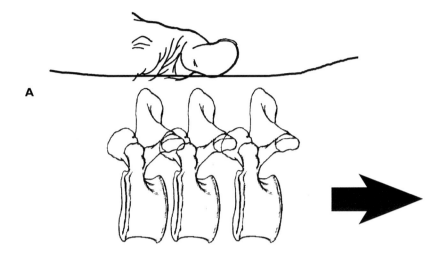

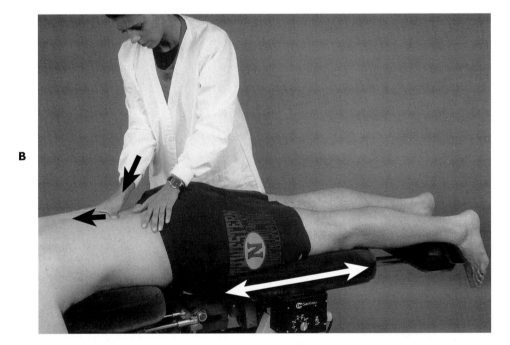

Fig. 6-18 Overpressure also can be used while the spine is passively distracted to evaluate end-feel in the long axis (y axis) of the spine.

A.   Diagrammatic representation of the clinician's thumb applying resistive overpressure to the L4 spinous process to identify the presence of end-play or joint-play in long axis distraction.

B.   Clinician using the right thumb to apply inferior-to-superior overpressure to the L4 spinous process while the table's pelvic section provides passive distraction in the long axis (y-axis translation).

cian moves the caudal section, palpation of the spinous processes in the lumbar and lower thoracic vertebra is performed to determine if proper lateral flexion between segments is occurring. Because coupling of rotation and lateral flexion takes place throughout the spine, information about rotation movement can also be obtained. However, the coupling pattern in the lumbar spine is affected by the extent of the lumbar lordosis. When the lordosis is maintained, coupling results in lateral flexion occurring with contralateral rotation, which is the expected relationship. When the lordosis is lost, coupling results in lateral flexion occurring with ipsilateral rotation, as it does in the cervical spine. Caution must be used in interpreting the findings for coupled rotation with lateral flexion movements in the lumbar spine with the patient in the prone position because the lordosis may be lost.

Motion evaluation of sacroiliac joints also can be performed with motion assistance, using different contacts. In performing this move the clinician has a double-hand contact on the pelvis. The left thumb and fingers have a firm contact along the crests of the left and right ilia respectively. The left hand then contacts both ilia and spans the sacrum. Although the left-hand contacts do press anteriorly, most of the pressure is toward the caudal direction. The right thumb and fingers contact the right lower angles of the sacrum. This location is where the sacrum narrows before attachment to the coccyx. The

right-hand contacts push slightly to the anterior but primarily toward the head (Fig. 6-19).

The pressure of the two examining hands is toward each other. This pressing together is correlated with the footward movement of the table. As the patient is stretched, the hands and their contacts are forced together. As the caudal body section pulls the legs and thighs footward, there is also a pull on the ilium. This causes a slight but discernible caudal movement of the ilium on the sacrum. The left-hand contacts push on the ilium to augment this movement and assess its presence. The sacrum, through its attachment to the spine and thoracic cage, is in contact with the stationary head section of the table. The sacrum is therefore pulled in a headward direction as the ilia are pulled footward. The right-hand contacts force the sacrum headward as the caudal body section pulls the ilium footward.

The result is that the caudal section uses the legs as pistons to produce a consistent and repetitive pull-push effect on the ilium. This pull-push effect causes a footward-to-headward, or long axis (y-axis translation), movement of the ilium on the sacrum. The contact hands actually push their respective contacts together only as the table stretches the patient. When the caudal section moves headward, the contact hands relax. The clinician should first push together with the thumbs to feel the y-axis movement at the left sacroiliac joint. This can be

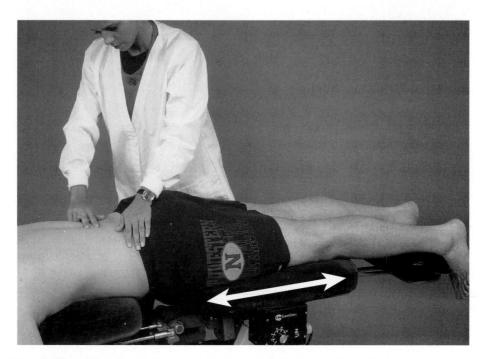

Fig. 6-19 Clinician palpating the sacroiliac articulations to identify separation movement while the pelvic section of the table produces distraction.

done through several cycles of the table. The fingers can push the respective right pelvic contacts together to determine the presence or absence of movement at the right sacroiliac joint. The side of the dysfunctional sacroiliac articulation will exhibit a hard end-feel. The ilium cannot be felt to move in a footward direction on the sacrum. Usually the contacts on the side of fixation are tender, as well.

Motion-assisted thrust technique (MATT) is a manual correction that uses a high-velocity, low-amplitude thrust applied to a dysfunctional joint while the individual spinal motion segment is placed in continuous passive motion (CPM) (long axis distraction) on a motorized distraction table. This therefore couples intermittent traction with the high-velocity, low-amplitude thrust of common and traditional chiropractic techniques. The thrust is applied while the patient is in traction, which allows joint distraction to be achieved through mechanical assistance. This is thought to make the thrust more easily applied by the clinician and received by the patient. A thoracic or lumbar thrust is delivered while the caudal section stretches. The intermittent distraction separates the involved motion segment producing an open-pack condition, greatly facilitating the adjustment and reducing the amount of force required for the thrust. In this tractive state the thrust can be delivered, requiring less exertion by the clinician and still resulting in cavitation and the audible release. As the moving table creates distraction of the patient, the force of the treating hands is applied primarily in the headward direction. A pull-push effect is thus created along the y axis, facilitating the repositioning of the joint and restoration of long axis distraction movement, which are critical in the normal functioning of the joint. Additionally, repeated pressure can be applied instead of a thrust, producing focused mobilization or incremental movement of the dysfunctional joint and its supporting soft tissues.

Considerable evidence exists for the use and value of CPM in the early stage of joint and soft tissue repair.[20,21] The use of a motorized distraction table will provide a form of CPM. CPM is developed through a motorized caudal section of the table that creates intermittent long axis traction to the spine, allowing the spinal tissue to relax and stretch. Motorized long axis distraction is thought to provide a smooth, predictable, and repetitious motion, both in distance and frequency. This motion theoretically allows the patient to relax, providing the clinician an opportunity to develop less force to specific spinal motion segments as necessary for an appropriate spinal correction.

Mechanized long axis distraction is believed to accomplish the following:

1. Increases the intervertebral disc space, potentially removing annular distortion in the pain-sensitive peripheral annular fibers
2. Allows the nucleus pulposus to assume its central position within the annulus and relieve irritation to the pain-sensitive fibers
3. Restores vertebral joints to more normal physiologic relationships
4. Improves posture and motion while relieving pain and improving body function
5. Produces repetitive loading and unloading of the disc and facet joints, causing imbibition of the fluids necessary for repair

APPLICATION OF MOTORIZED MECHANICAL ASSISTANCE TECHNIQUES

The segments of the spine and the extremity joints can be manipulated during the motion-assisted process, theoretically with less corrective force required of the clinician. Tissue pull and contacts are established in the same fashion as in an adjustment given on any table. However, the addition of the long axis distraction of the mechanized table provides a great amount of prestress. Additional prestress is applied through the clinician's contacts; however, much less prestress is required. A high-velocity, low-amplitude thrust can be applied at full excursion of the mechanized table. Again, less exertion should be required of the clinician to develop the force necessary to create the desired joint movement and alignment changes. Moreover, traction maneuvers produce long axis distraction in the joint to which they are applied. The movement of long axis distraction (y-axis translation) in spinal segments is not clinically addressed with most other manipulative approaches.

This technique is designed to provide a motion-assisted approach to treating the manipulable lesions of the spine and extremities. The technique involves using linear axial distraction, focusing on the long axis of the body. The Hill Intertrac table and Chattanooga Ergotrak table, motion-assisted treatment devices, allows the application of recumbent motion-assisted palpation (MAP), motion-assisted thrust technique (MATT), and gravity-assisted intermittent traction (GAIT).[22] For spinal joint dysfunction the patient is positioned so that the pelvis is on the pelvic section of the table. All recumbent positions (prone, supine, side-posture) can be used. With linear distraction as an enhancement to the clinician's physical application, virtually all recumbent techniques can be performed. There are specific considerations for each joint to be adjusted, such as the segmental contact point, vector of thrust, and clinician position. Specific procedures not using motion assistance are described and demonstrated elsewhere.[23] A representative sample is considered here, demonstrating the addition of motion assistance to typical adjustive technique procedures.

SACROILIAC ARTICULATION

Motion-assisted manipulation can be applied to the sacroiliac articulation in the prone or side-posture position. When performed on a patient lying in the prone position, contacts and thrust direction are the same as when using a drop-section table. However, the mechanical assistance comes from the linear distraction produced by the moving pelvic section (β section) (Fig. 6-20). When performed on a patient lying in the side-posture position, contacts and thrust direction are the same as for manipulative procedures performed on a patient in the typical side-posture (lumbar roll) position. However, mechanical assistance is provided by the moving pelvic section to apply long axis distraction, creating a separating prestress in the sacroiliac articulation (Fig. 6-21).

LUMBAR SPINE

Motion-assisted manipulation for the lumbar spine is performed with the patient in the side-posture position, using contacts and thrust directions similar to those used with the typical side-posture manipulative procedures (lumbar roll) (Fig. 6-22, A). The addition of the long axis distraction (y-axis translation) developed by the moving pelvic piece (β section) provides separation between the vertebra to be manipulated (Fig. 6-22, B and C). Theoretically, when facet joint and disc space separation occurs with the prestress produced by the table, movement of the joint in rotation, lateral flexion, or flexion-extension should be more easily accomplished (Fig. 6-22, D). Therefore motion-assisted techniques can be performed to influence lumbar intersegmental rotation (Fig. 6-23), lateral flexion (Fig. 6-24), and a combination of rotation and lateral flexion (Fig. 6-25). Intersegmental flexion and extension movements can also be accomplished using MATT (Fig. 6-26).

THORACIC SPINE

Motion-assisted manipulation for the thoracic spine is performed on a prone patient, using contacts and thrust directions in the same fashion as in typical high-velocity, low-amplitude thrust techniques performed on prone patients. The addition of the long axis distraction (y-axis translation) developed by the moving pelvic piece (β section) provides separation between the vertebra to be

Text continued on p. 221

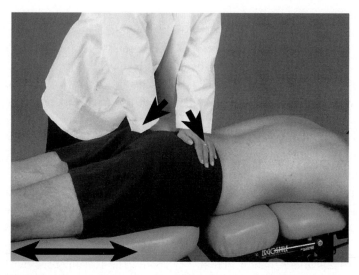

Fig. 6-20 Clinician demonstrating motion-assisted thrust technique for a right posterior innominate (flexed ilium, upper ilium fixation), with pisiform contacts on the right PSIS and left sacral apex; the pelvic section of the table is set in motion, producing linear distraction at a rate of 10 to 15 cpm. The thrust is applied in a posterior-to-anterior direction, at the peak of long axis distraction.

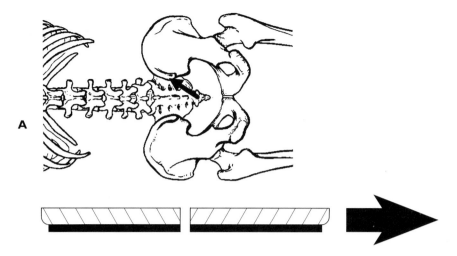

Fig. 6-21, A Diagrammatic representation of the contact point for a right posterior innominate (right flexed ilium, right upper ilium fixation). (*Modified from* Medical Illustration Library: General Anatomy. *Baltimore: Williams & Wilkins; 1994;1.*)

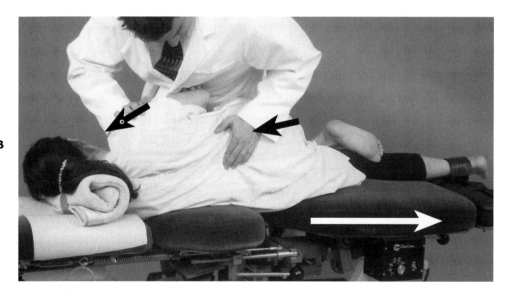

Fig. 6-21, B Clinician demonstrating the procedure for a right posterior innominate (right flexed ilium, right upper ilium fixation).

PP: Patient lying in the side-posture position, with the lower leg strapped to the footpiece.

DP: Clinician standing at side of table, facing the patient at right angles; caudal foot off the floor, with a lateral knee-to-knee, thigh-to-thigh contact.

CH: Caudal-hand pisiform contact over the PSIS (e.g., left pisiform, right PSIS).

IH: Cephalad hands grasps the lateral aspect of the upper humerus over the deltoid tubercle (e.g., right hand, patient's right humerus).

LOD: Posterior-to-anterior, medial-to-lateral, inferior-to-superior.

P: With the pelvic section distracting in the long axis at a rate of 10 to 15 cpm, remove slack with CH, IH, and thigh; IH stabilizes in cephalad direction against the distraction provided by the pelvic section, CH thrusts PSIS anterior at the peak of distraction.

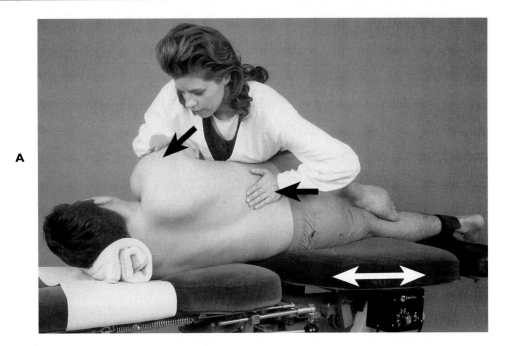

Fig. 6-22, *A* Clinician demonstrating a typical side-posture lumbar manipulative procedure using a pushing posterior-to-anterior thrust applied to a mammillary contact.

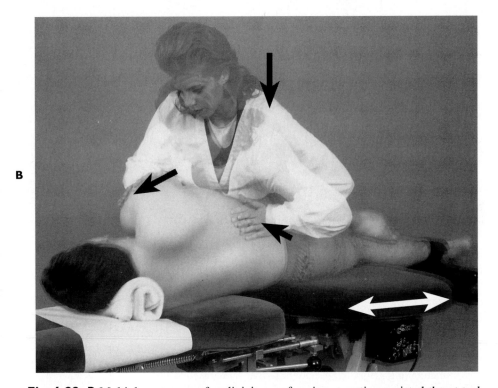

Fig. 6-22, *B* Multiple exposure of a clinician performing a motion-assisted thrust technique (MATT) using a pushing posterior-to-anterior thrust applied to a mammillary contact, with the assistance of the moving pelvic piece providing long axis distraction.

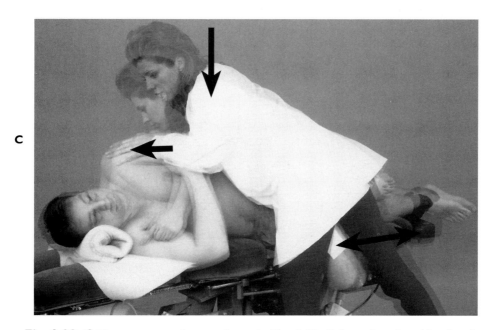

Fig. 6-22, C The same procedure as shown in Fig. 6-22, *B*, from the other side, showing the clinician's stance and body drop with motion assistance from the pelvic section.

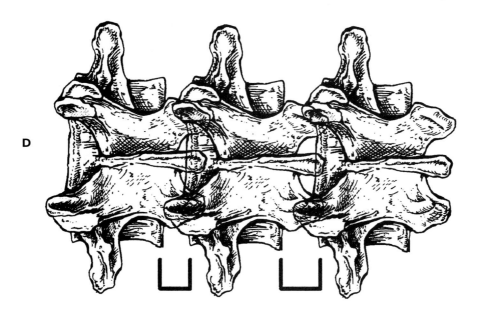

Fig. 6-22, D Diagrammatic representation of intersegmental separation developed by distraction of the pelvic section against the contact provided by the clinician, which is thought to make other movements (rotation, lateral flexion, flexion, extension) more easily accomplished.

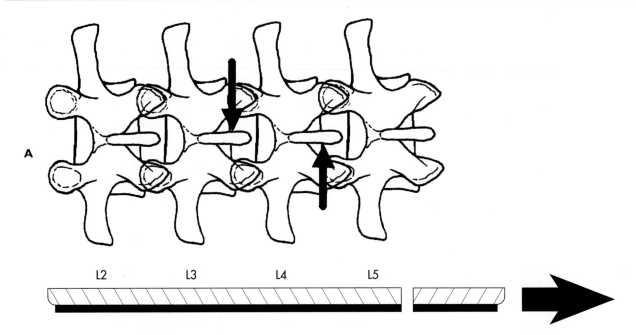

Fig. 6-23, *A* Diagrammatic representation of segmental contact points against each side of the spinous processes of the involved vertebrae (right side of SP L3, left side of SP L4) to produce rotation.

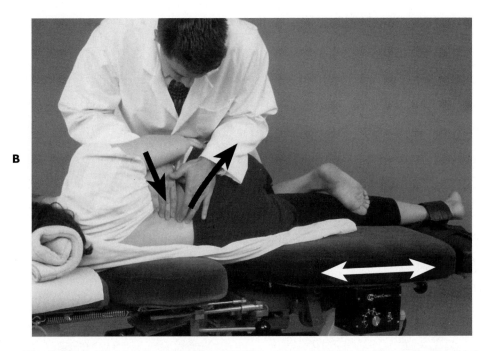

Fig. 6-23, *B* Clinician demonstrating MATT for intersegmental rotation (left rotated L3-4 [PR; LP], right rotation restriction L3-4).

PP: Patient in side-posture position, with lower leg strapped to footpiece (on left side).

DP: Clinician standing at side of table, facing the patient at right angles; caudal foot off the floor, with an anterior knee-to-knee, thigh-to-thigh contact.

CH: Caudal-hand digital contact pulling against the spinous process of the lower vertebra (e.g., left digital contact, left side SP L4).

IH: Cephalad hand establishes a digital contact, pushing against the spinous process of the upper vertebra (e.g., right digital contact, right side SP L3).

LOD: Counterrotation developed (left to right L4, right to left L3).

P: With the pelvic section providing long axis distraction at a rate of 10 to 15 cpm, remove slack with CH, IH, and thigh; CH and IH thrust in opposite directions against both SPs, creating rotation between the two vertebrae.

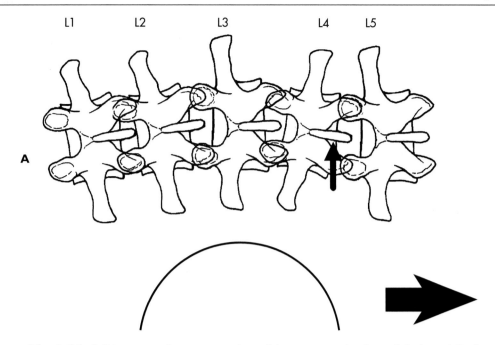

Fig. 6-24, *A* Diagrammatic representation of the contact point for a right lateral flexion malposition L4-5, left lateral flexion restriction L4-5.

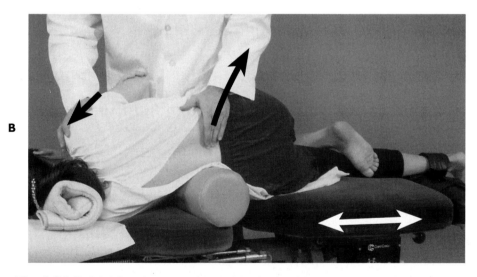

Fig. 6-24 *B* Clinician demonstrating MATT for intersegmental lateral flexion dysfunction (right lateral flexion malposition L4-5, left lateral flexion restriction L4-5).

PP: Patient in side-posture position over foam roll (Dutchman's roll), with lower leg strapped to footpiece (on left side).

DP: Clinician standing at side of table, facing the patient at right angles; caudal foot off the floor, with a lateral knee-to-knee, thigh-to-thigh contact or an anterior leg-to-thigh contact ("kick start").

CH: Caudal-hand digital contact, pulling against the lateral aspect of the spinous process of the upper vertebra (e.g., left digital contact, left side SP L4).

IH: Cephalad hand grasps the lateral aspect of the upper humerus over the deltoid tubercle (e.g., right hand, patient's right humerus).

LOD: Lateral-to-medial (left-to-right).

P: With the pelvic section distracting in the long axis at a rate of 10 to 15 cpm, remove slack with CH, IH, and thigh; IH stabilizes in cephalad direction against the distraction provided by the pelvic section, CH develops a pulling thrust on the SP, lateral-to-medial (left-to-right) at the peak of distraction.

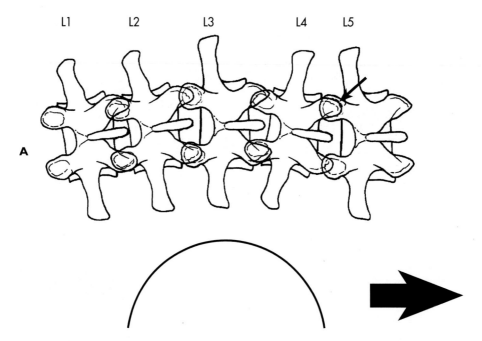

Fig. 6-25, A Diagrammatic representation of the contact point for an intersegmental rotation combined with lateral flexion (left rotational malposition L4-5, right rotational restriction L4-5; right lateral flexion malposition L4-5, left lateral flexion restriction L4-5).

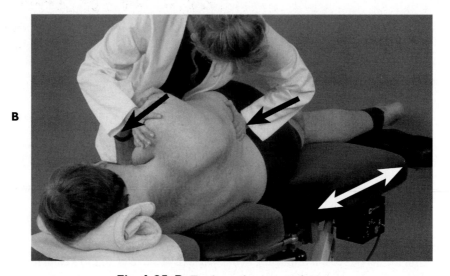

Fig. 6-25, B For legend see opposite page.

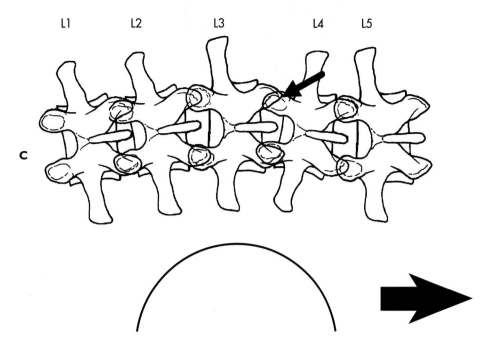

Fig. 6-25, C Diagramatic representation of the contact point for lateral flexion malposition (right lateral flexion malposition, left lateral flexion restriction L4-5) using the mammillary process. The direction of thrust is more inferior to superior than when rotation is involved.

Fig. 6-25, B Clinician demonstrating MATT for intersegmental rotation combined with lateral flexion (left rotational malposition L4-5, right rotational restriction L4-5; right lateral flexion malposition L4-5, left lateral flexion restriction L4-5).

PP: Patient in side-posture position, with lower leg strapped to footpiece (on left side).

DP: Clinician standing at side of table, facing the patient at right angles; caudal foot off the floor, with a lateral knee-to-knee, thigh-to-thigh contact.

CH: Caudal-hand pisiform contact against the mammillary process of the vertebra (e.g., left pisiform contact, right MP L5).

IH: Cephalad hand grasps the lateral aspect of the upper humerus over the deltoid tubercle (e.g., right hand, patient's right humerus).

LOD: Posterior-to-anterior, inferior-to-superior.

P: With the pelvic section distracting in the long axis at a rate of 10 to 15 cpm, remove slack with CH, IH, and thigh; IH stabilizes in cephalad direction against the distraction provided by the pelvic section, CH develops a pushing thrust on the MP, posterior-to-anterior and inferior-to-superior at the peak of distraction.

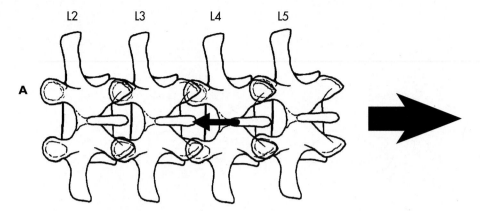

Fig. 6-26, A Diagrammatic representation of the contact point for an extension malposition, flexion restriction of L3-4, indicating the assistance of pelvic distraction; this procedure can be performed with the patient in the prone or side-posture position.

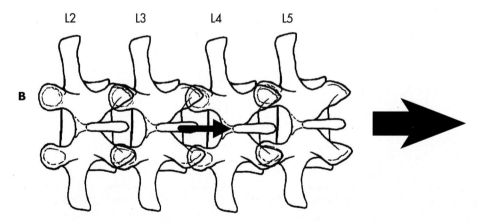

Fig. 6-26, B Diagrammatic representation of the contact point for a flexion malposition, extension restriction of L4-5, indicating the assistance of pelvic distraction; this procedure can be performed with the patient in the prone or side-posture position.

manipulated (Fig. 6-27). Again, with facet joint and disc space separation produced by the prestress of the table, movement of the joint in rotation, lateral flexion, or flexion-extension should be more easily accomplished. Motion-assisted techniques can therefore be performed to influence thoracic intersegmental rotation and lateral flexion (Fig. 6-28). Intersegmental flexion and extension movements can also be accomplished using MATT (Fig. 6-29, *A*), with the patient in the prone position or the supine position, as in the traditional anterior thoracic procedure (Fig. 6-29, *B*).

CERVICAL SPINE

Motion-assisted manipulation for the cervical spine is performed with the patient in the supine or prone posi-

tion, using contacts and thrust directions in the same fashion as in typical high-velocity, low-amplitude thrust techniques for the cervical spine. The addition of the long axis distraction (y-axis translation) developed by the moving pelvic piece (β section) provides separation between the vertebrae to be manipulated. Facet joint and disc space separation can occur with the prestress of the table, making movement of the joint in rotation, lateral flexion or flexion-extension more easily accomplished. Motion-assisted techniques can be performed to influence cervical intersegmental rotation and lateral flexion individually or in combination (Figs. 6-30 through 6-32). Intersegmental long axis distraction movements can also be accomplished using MATT (Fig. 6-33), with the patient in the supine position.

Text continued on p. 228

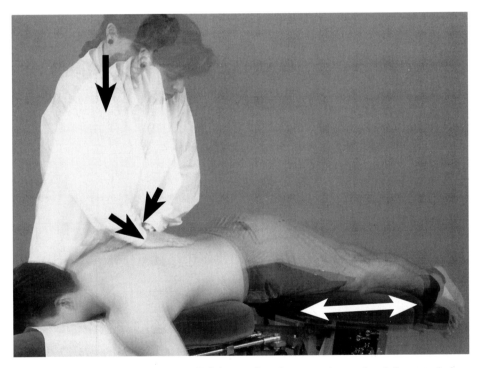

Fig. 6-27 Multiple exposure of a clinician performing a motion-assisted thrust technique (MATT), using a pushing posterior-to-anterior thrust applied to transverse processes in the thoracic spine, with the assistance of the moving pelvic piece providing long axis distraction.

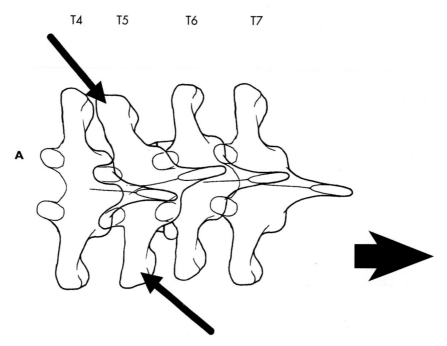

Fig. 6-28, A Diagrammatic representation of the contact point for an intersegmental rotation combined with lateral flexion in the thoracic spine (right rotation, left lateral flexion malposition and/or left rotational, right lateral flexion restriction T5-6).

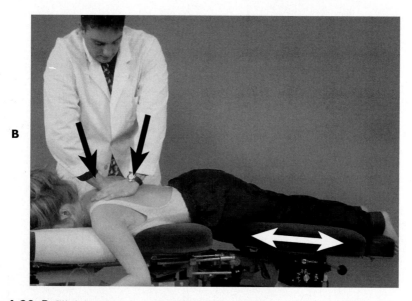

Fig. 6-28, B Clinician demonstrating MATT for the procedure for a right rotation, left lateral flexion malposition and/or left rotational, right lateral flexion restriction T5-6.

PP: Patient lying in the prone position, with feet strapped to footrest.

DP: Clinician standing at side of table, facing the patient at right angles (e.g., right rotated, left laterally flexed T5-6 [PLI-T, RPS], left rotational, right lateral flexion restriction T5-6: stand on right side).

CH: Cephalad-hand pisiform contact over transverse process of upper vertebra (e.g., right pisiform, right TP T5).

IH: Caudal-hand pisiform or thenar contact over transverse process of upper vertebra (e.g., left pisiform, left TP T5).

LOD: Posterior-to-anterior, clockwise torque.

P: With the pelvic section distracting in the long axis at a rate of 10 to 15 cpm, remove slack with CH and IH against the distraction provided by the pelvic section; both hands develop a pushing thrust on the TPs, posterior-to-anterior at the peak of distraction.

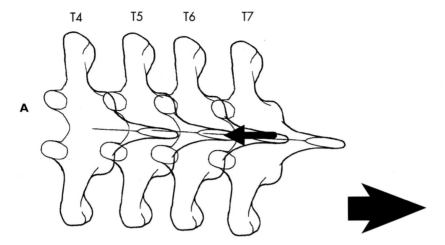

Fig. 6-29, *A* Diagrammatic representation of the contact point for an intersegmental extension malposition, flexion restriction of T5-6 performed with the patient in the prone position, with the pelvic section providing distraction.

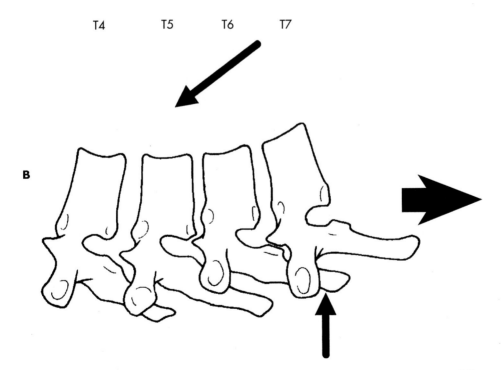

Fig. 6-29, *B* Diagrammatic representation of the contact point for an intersegmental flexion malposition, extension restriction of T5-6 performed with the patient in the supine position, with the pelvic section providing distraction.

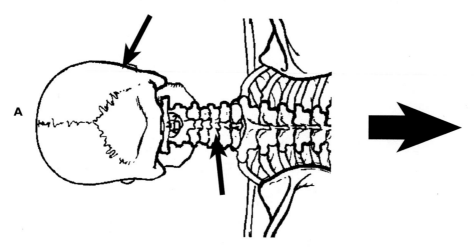

Fig. 6-30, A Diagrammatic representation of the contact point for an intersegmental left rotation, right lateral flexion malposition and/or right rotational, left lateral flexion restriction C5-6.

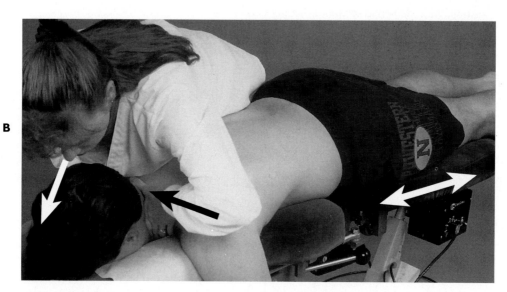

Fig. 6-30, B Clinician demonstrating MATT for a left rotation, right lateral flexion malposition and/or right rotational, left lateral flexion restriction C5-6.

PP: Patient lying in the prone position, with feet strapped to footrest.

DP: Clinician standing at side of table, facing headward (e.g., left rotated, right laterally flexed C5-6 [PRI-L, LPS], right rotational, left lateral flexion restriction C5-6: stand on right side). Alternatively, stance can be on other side.

CH: Caudal-hand index (metacarpophalangeal joint) contact over posterior aspect of articular pillar (e.g., left index, left AP C5).

IH: Cephalad-hand thumb contact under base of occiput, palmar and finger contact on side face and head (e.g., right hand, right side of head).

LOD: Posterior-to-anterior, lateral-to-medial (left-to-right).

P: With the pelvic section distracting in the long axis at a rate of 10 to 15 cpm, remove slack with CH and IH against the distraction provided by the pelvic section; CH develops a pushing thrust posterior-to-anterior on the AP at the peak of distraction, while the IH opposes the caudal distraction and applies rotational and lateral flexion prestress.

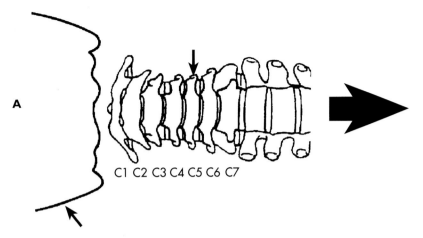

Fig. 6-31, A Diagrammatic representation of the contact point for an intersegmental right lateral flexion malposition and/or left lateral flexion restriction C5-6.

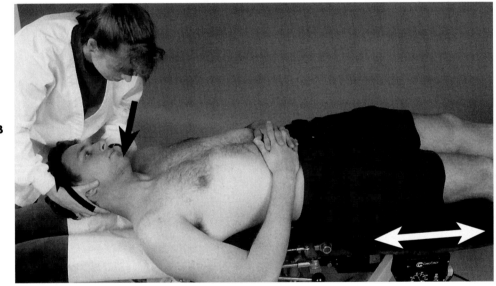

Fig. 6-31, B Clinician demonstrating MATT for a right lateral flexion malposition and/or left lateral flexion restriction C5-6.

PP: Patient lying in the supine position, with feet strapped to footrest.

DP: Clinician standing at side of table, facing the patient (e.g., right laterally flexed C5-6, left lateral flexion restriction C5-6: stand on left side).

CH: Caudal-hand index (metacarpophalangeal joint) contact over lateral aspect of articular pillar (e.g., right index, right AP C5).

IH: Cephalad hand index and middle finger straddle the SCM, ring finger and little finger wrap around the base of the occiput (e.g., left hand, left side of neck).

LOD: Lateral-to-medial (left-to-right).

P: With the pelvic section distracting in the long axis at a rate of 10 to 15 cpm, remove slack with CH and IH against the distraction provided by the pelvic section; CH develops a pushing thrust lateral-to-medial on the AP at the peak of distraction, while the IH opposes the caudal distraction and applies lateral flexion prestress.

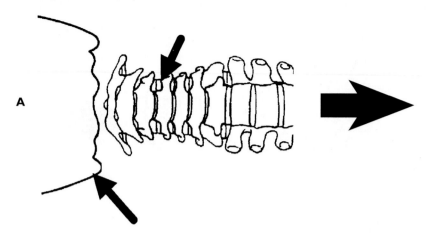

Fig. 6-32, A Diagrammatic representation of the contact point for an intersegmental left rotation malposition and/or right rotational restriction C5-6.

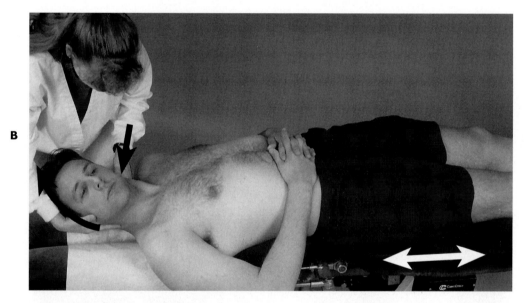

Fig. 6-32, B Clinician demonstrating MATT for a left rotation malposition and/or right rotational restriction C5-6.

PP: Patient lying in the supine position, with feet strapped to footrest.

DP: Clinician standing at side of table, facing the patient (e.g., left rotated C5-6 [PR, RL], right rotational restriction C5-6: stand on the left side).

CH: Caudal-hand index (metacarpophalangeal joint) contact over posterior aspect of articular pillar (e.g., left index, left AP C5).

IH: Cephalad hand index and middle finger straddle the SCM, ring finger and little finger wrap around the base of the occiput (e.g., right hand, right side of neck).

LOD: Posterior-to-anterior.

P: With the pelvic section distracting in the long axis at a rate of 10 to 15 cpm, remove slack with CH and IH against the distraction provided by the pelvic section; CH develops a pushing thrust posterior-to-anterior on the AP at the peak of distraction, while the IH opposes the caudal distraction and applies rotational prestress.

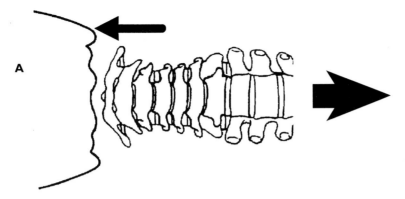

Fig. 6-33, *A* Diagrammatic representation of the contact point for a loss of long axis distraction C0-1 and rotational and lateral flexion dysfunction in the atlantooccipital articulation.

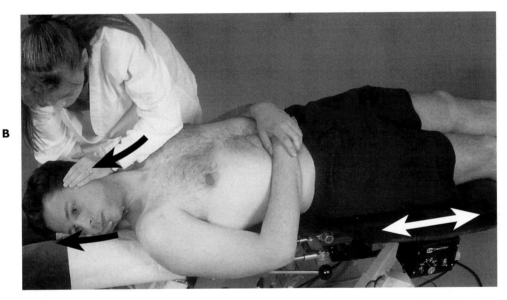

Fig. 6-33, *B* Clinician demonstrating MATT for a loss of long axis distraction C0-1 and rotational and lateral flexion dysfunction in the atlantooccipital articulation.

PP: Patient lying in the supine position, with feet strapped to footrest.

DP: Clinician standing at side of table, facing the patient (e.g., left rotation, right lateral flexion malposition; right rotation, left lateral flexion restriction C0-1: stand on left side; stand on either side for long axis distraction).

CH: Caudal-hand pisiform contact over posterior aspect (for rotation) or inferior aspect (for lateral flexion or long axis distraction) of the mastoid process (e.g., left pisiform, left mastoid).

IH: Cephalad hand index and middle finger straddle the chin (e.g., right hand, right side of chin).

LOD: Inferior-to-superior.

P: With the pelvic section distracting in long axis at a rate of 10 to 15 cpm, remove slack with CH and IH against the distraction provided by the pelvic section; CH develops a pushing thrust inferior-to-superior on the mastoid process at the peak of distraction, while the IH opposes the caudal distraction and applies rotational and lateral flexion prestress. This procedure can also be used on the cervical segments to C4-5 by contacting the artioular pillars.

CONCLUSION

This chapter presents the concepts of motion-assisted thrust technique (MATT). Although drop section procedures have been described and used for many years, very little evidence exists to support their use. Anecdotes do exist, and they have withstood the so-called test of time. Furthermore, the principles on which they are based are sound.

Also introduced in this chapter are techniques that may be enhanced by the use of linear distraction provided by a motorized pelvic section. These procedures represent fairly new technology, and, again, there are no clinical trials to support their effectiveness and efficiency. The principles on which they are based do seem to be sound, also.

Both drop-piece mechanical assistance techniques and motorized mechanical assistance have the potential to augment the clinician's ability to apply a thrust to dysfunctional joints.

REFERENCES

1. Lawrence, DJ. General overview of the chiropractic profession. In: Bergmann TB, Peterson DH, Lawrence DJ, eds. *Chiropractic Technique: Principles and Procedures.* New York: Churchill Livingstone; 1993.
2. Gillette RG. A speculative argument for the coactivation of diverse somatic receptor populations by forceful chiropractic adjustments: a review of the neurophysiologic literature. *Manual Med.* 1987;3:1-14.
3. Haas M. The physics of spinal manipulation, IV: a theoretical consideration of the physician impact force and energy requirements needed to produce synovial joint cavitation. *J Manipulative Physiol Ther.* 1990;13:378-383.
4. Haas M. The physics of spinal manipulation, II: a theoretical consideration of the adjustive force. *J Manipulative Physiol Ther.* 1990;13:253-256.
5. Herzog W. The physics of spinal manipulation. *J Manipulative Physiol Ther.* 1992;15(6):402-405.
6. Herzog W. The physics of spinal manipulation: work-energy and impulse-momentum principles. *J Manipulative Physiol Ther.* 1993;16(1):51-54.
7. Heilig D. The thrust technique. *J Am Osteopath Assoc.* 1981;81(4):244-48.

8. Haas M. The physics of spinal manipulation, III: some characteristics of adjusting that facilitate joint distraction. *J Manipulative Physiol Ther.* 1990;13:305-308.

9. Sandoz R. Some physical mechanisms and effects of spinal adjustments. *Ann Swiss Chiropr Assoc.* 1976;6:91-141.

10. Wood J, Adams AA. Comparison of forces used in selected adjustments of the low back by experienced chiropractors and chiropractic students with no clinical experience: a preliminary study. *Palmer Coll Chiropr Res Forum.* 1984;1:16-23.

11. Hessel BW, Herzog W, Conway P, McEwen MC. Experimental measurement of the force exerted during spinal manipulation using Thompson technique. *J Manipulative Physiol Ther.* 1990;13:448-453.

12. Jackson, RD. Thompson terminal point technique. *Today's Chiropr.* 73-75.

13. Grice AS. A biomechanical approach to cervical and dorsal adjusting. In: Haldeman S, ed. *Modern Developments in the Principles and Practice of Chiropractic.* New York: Appleton-Century-Crofts; 1980.

14. Bergmann TF. Manual force, mechanically assisted articular chiropractic technique using long and/or short levers: a literature review. *J Manipulative Physiol Ther.* 1993:16:33-36.

15. Cooperstein R. Thompson technique. *Chiropr Tech.* 1995;7(2):60-63.

16. Thompson JC. *Thompson Technique Reference Manual.* Elgin, Ill: Williams Manufacturing; 1984.

17. Mennell JM. *The Musculoskeletal System: Differential Diagnosis From Symptoms and Physical Signs.* Gaithersburg, Md: Aspen; 1992.

18. Kaltenborn FM. *Mobilization of the Extremity Joints.* Oslo Norway: Olaf Norlis Bokhandel; 1980.

19. Mennell JM. *Joint Pain.* Boston: Little, Brown; 1964.

20. Frank C, Akeson WH, Woo S et al. Physiology and therapeutic value of passive joint motion. *Clin Orthop.* 1984;185:113-125.

21. Salter RB. The biologic concept of continuous passive motion of synovial joints. *Clin Orthop.* 1989;242:12-25.

22. Davis PT. GAIT (Gravity-assisted intermittent traction): a motion-assisted form of distractive manipulation. *Chiropr Tech.* 1995;7(4):125-130.

23. Bergmann TF, Peterson DH, Lawrence DJ. *Chiropractic Technique.* New York: Churchill Livingstone; 1993.

7

Adjunctive Approaches to Traction

Several devices that apply traction to the spine do not require the use of the operator's hands in the treatment process. With these devices the operator only places and attaches the patient and switches the machine on and off. Some of these devices, including a computer-monitored medical device for the application of controlled traction for the low back, are described in the following paragraphs. Only a few of the devices have undergone extensive testing for safety and effectiveness; therefore the clinician must rely on promotional rather than scientific literature. It is important to maintain a critical mind and observe carefully the potential effects of each therapeutic modality.

THE SPINALATOR

The Spinalator table has been available for many years and has been used by chiropractors to provide intersegmental traction to patients. The traction is intersegmental only, and the force is provided through the action of molded rubber rollers that pass back and forth under the patient, mobilizing bony joints and massaging muscles. Through this movement the rollers lift the spinal segments, causing mobilization. It should be noted that the rollers, rather than the table, move. The patient is placed supine on the device, and the level of the rollers and the speed of the intersegmental traction are regulated. The treatment time is controlled by a timer. There is no harness for the patient, and the intersegmental traction is applied to the full spine. (Fig. 7-1.)

The purpose of the intersegmental traction device is to induce movement at each vertebral level, causing slight motion of the vertebral segment with reference to the one above and the one below. Several of these devices are presently on the market. Jaskoviak[1] notes that, "It applies a series of stretches interspersed with periods of relaxation." The intended effect is to provide motion to each vertebra and accompanying facet joints that are treated. This provides a general introduction of movement to several vertebral segments at a time and may be used either before or following the specific segmental adjustment. Each segment is lifted as the roller passes under the vertebrae. This treatment aids in joint motion and provides a stretching of adjacent musculature.

Although this kind of movement can be beneficial in generating and reinforcing motion, certain caveats (indications and contraindications) should be observed. Indications include tissue conditions such as hypertonic muscles and hypomobile joints. Contraindications include osteoporosis, acute inflammatory or infectious conditions of the joints or muscles, unstable joints, certain arthritic conditions and neoplastic conditions, and other conditions noted in works discussing traction and tractive methods.[1]

THE ANATAMOTOR

The Anatamotor is designed to provide intersegmental traction and long axis traction using a harness. The traction can be applied to both the lumbar spine and cervical spine. The top of this table is mobile, with rollers protruding through slots in the table (set at a specific height for patient comfort). The patient lies supine on the top, and the spine passes over the rollers as the table top moves back and forth. The speed of the pass is controlled by the operator, and the table has an integral timer for controlling the length of the traction session.[2] (Fig. 7-2.)

Additional traction is provided by thoracic and pelvic harnesses. A harness for the cervical spine allows the application of cervical traction as the table moves through its long axis trajectory. The cervical traction force is controlled by a complex tractioning mechanism at the head of the table.

The expected effect of this unit includes improved motion of the spinal joints, including the facets. Muscle kneading is also an expected effect of the action and is

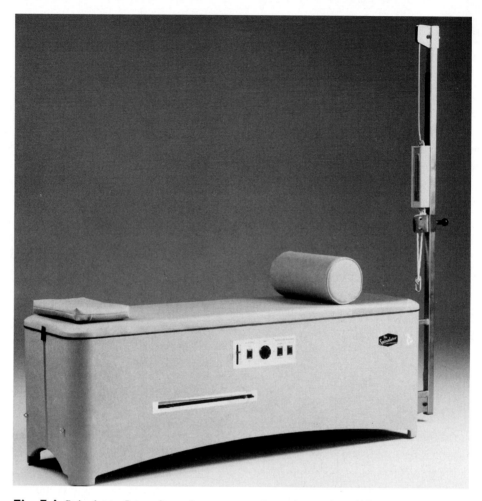

Fig. 7-1 Spinalator: Intermittent intersegmental traction and mobilization applied with table only.

- The patient is positioned supine.
- The surface is smooth and is upholstered in a plastic cover.
- Formed rubber rollers pass back and forth under the patient, mobilizing bony joints and massaging muscles.
- Patient is positioned on the table for a specified time controlled by a timer.
- This is an unattended therapy. *(Courtesy Chatanooga Corp., Hixon, Tenn.)*

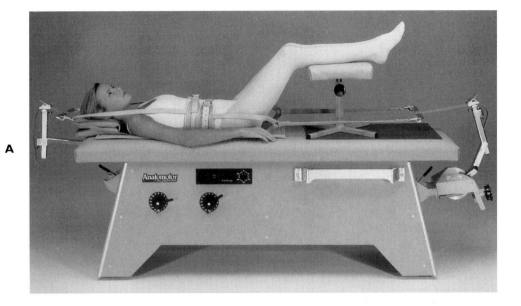

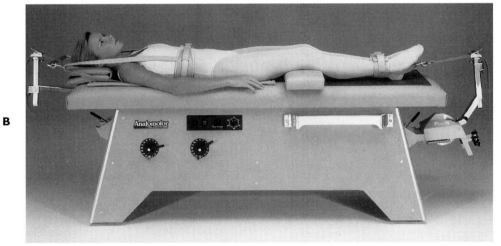

Fig. 7-2 Anatamotor: **A**, Traction harnesses around the thoracic cage and lumbar spine. **B**, Traction harnesses around thoracic cage and ankles.
- The surface of the table moves in a linear manner.
- Patient is placed supine on the table, with the head on the appropriate end.
- Round rubber rollers are located under the table top; as the top (and patient) passes over the rollers, intersegmental motion takes place.
- The table includes a speed control, a timer, and a depth setting for the rollers.
- Some tables are also equipped with vibration and heating capabilities.
- An optional feature is a cervical traction unit. *(Courtesy Hill Laboratories, Frazer, Pa.)*

thought to aid in relaxation of the spine and its musculature. The usual indications and contraindications for the use of traction to the cervical, thoracic, and lumbar spine apply to the Anatamotor.

AUTOTRACTION

Autotraction is another method of traction in which the therapist or operator is only indirectly involved. This process was developed by Lind in 1974 and improved by Natchev in 1984. Autotraction requires a specially designed traction table that employs a manipulable bed with upper and lower sections. The angle of the bed (flexion-extension and lateral flexion) and the degree of position are controlled by the therapist, using the device's internal motors. The patient is connected to the table with a pelvic harness that is attached to the table by a chain. The position of the patient is either side-lying, prone, or supine, depending on patient comfort and desired effect.[3] (Fig. 7-3.)

The force is provided by the patient and can include either traction or compression by pulling or pushing. The patient can pull with the hands on the bar at the head of the table to provide a tractive force or can push with the feet on the bar at the foot of the table to provide a compressive force.

The patient should push or pull to comfort level, with the clinician adjusting the position of the sections or upper and lower positions of the bed to patient comfort. The section is angled by the table motors (in Lind's original table, the whole device was fully manual). The patient then pushes with the feet or pulls with the hands to achieve sufficient traction or compression to relieve symptoms. The therapist gradually repositions the sections, approximating the position at which the patient originally felt pain. If pain is felt, the table is repositioned to a point at which no pain is felt. By placing the feet on a bar at the foot of the table while in a supine position, the patient can flatten the lordosis of the lumbar spine. The patient then pulls vigorously on the upper bar for 3 to 6 seconds. The pulling and pushing activity may be alternated according to patient comfort. The patient rests for approximately 1 minute, then repeats the procedure for the remainder of the 30- to 60-minute treatment period.

The distraction, rotation, and bending forces are

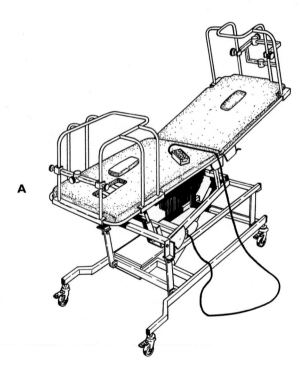

A

Fig. 7-3, A The Autotraction table.
- Note the control on a remote. One end of the unit is elevated.
- Note the cutout on either end for the face.
- This unit is manufactured by the Chattanooga Group. (*Courtesy Chatanooga Group, Hixon, Tenn.*)

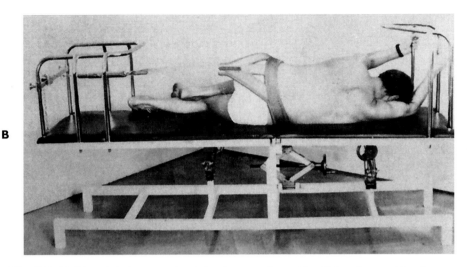

B

Fig. 7-3, B Historial photograph of the Autotraction table: Using feet and hands to provide traction.
- Patient is in a side-lying position, with the table in neutral (0) position.
- Patient's feet are in contact with the caudal frame, and the hands are in contact with the frame on the cephalad end.
- The harness is attached to the patient's waist, with an orientation toward the left side.
- Patient pushes with the foot while the hands pull the patient, tractioning the lower back as the two forces interact in opposite directions. *(Lind G. Autotraction treatment of low back pain and sciatica: an electromyographic, radiographic, and clinical study. Linköping, Sweden; 1974, Thesis.)*

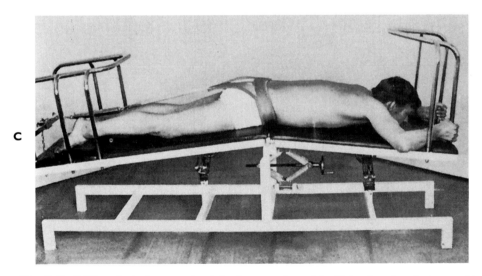

C

Fig. 7-3, C Historical photograph of the Autotraction table: Using hands only to provide traction.
- Patient is positioned prone on the table.
- Clinician positions the α and β sections downward-bent (flexed).
- Traction is provided by the hands pulling on the frame at the α end while the harness tractions the low back. *(From Lind G. Autotraction treatment of low back pain and sciatica: an electromyographic, radiographic, and clinical study. Linköping, Sweden; 1974, Thesis.)*

applied to help restore mobility to the lumbar spine without causing pain to the patient. The number of treatments and length of treatment time varies with the speed of improvement. Autotraction provides strong rhythmic contractions of the lumbar paraspinal muscles. A study of the results of treatment with autotraction compared with treatment with passive traction was conducted by Tesio and Merlo in Milan, Italy, in the early 1990s. Tesio and Merlo[3] state that "Autotraction is a safe and effective conservative approach to chronic low back pain syndrome with or without lumbar disc herniation and there are few contraindications." This study suggests that autotraction is much more effective than passive traction. Three months after treatment, 63% of the respondents in the study still reported relief from pain.

A study on autotraction conducted in Sweden in 1985 reports that after treatment with autotraction, there was no difference on myelographic examination in either size or location of a herniation. However, patients did demonstrate clinical changes not reflected on the myelographic evaluation.[4]

In a study on height changes as a result of autotraction, Pope and Klingenstierna[5] conclude that autotraction and recumbent rest with no traction will provide approximately the same change in height in the human body. They note that there is an increase in overall height with overnight recumbency, and the body tends to get shorter during the daytime with upright posture. The traction appears to produce its effect through creep or deformation over time, until a new equilibrium is reached in the osmotic pressure in the disc. A side issue is the apparent disagreement Pope and Klingenstierna[5] found in the literature regarding the potential for increase or decrease of intradiscal pressure under traction.

THE VAX-D TABLE

Surgical procedures using conventional and microsurgical procedures have established the merits of decompression of intravertebral disc spaces in the management of low-back pain syndrome associated with lumbar disc herniation. According to the developer of the VAX-D table, surgery continues to play an important role in the treatment of patients with low back pain and sciatica associated with herniated discs and degenerative disc

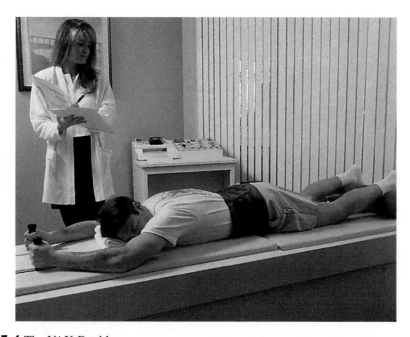

Fig. 7-4 The VAX-D table.
- Patient is placed on the table in a prone position.
- The harness is attached to the patient's lower body.
- Patient holds onto hand grips, creating resistance for the traction procedure.
- The table achieves its tractive force through a mechanical distraction controlled by an operator and computer located next to the traction device.
- The force and timing of the distraction are monitored and controlled. *(Courtesy VAX-D Medical Technologies, L.C., Palm Harbor, Fla.)*

problems.[6] However, for patients who are not candidates for surgery, there is a need to establish a conservative approach that offers an effective means of returning the patient to a functional level of activity.

The VAX-D (vertebral axial decompression) traction table is a relatively new device for treatment of back-related problems. In a study by Ramos and Martin[7] on the effects of the device, the VAX-D traction table was tested as a conservative method of treatment and as an alternative to back surgery. The basic premise for the device is its manner of applying traction therapy with a specific force for a specific period. The measurements are recorded by the integrated computer that provides the program and records the forces applied. The results indicate that it is possible to lower pressure in the nucleus pulposus of herniated lumbar discs to levels significantly below 0 mm Hg when distraction tension is applied according to the protocol described for vertebral axial decompression therapy. (Fig. 7-4.)

Traction is applied through the use of a harness connected to the patient's waist (the pelvis) while the patient lies prone on the VAX-D table. Traction is calculated in the computer, and traction is applied at a given force for a specified time. A rest period provided between traction sessions allows the patient to recover. The lower section of the table moves as the tractive force is applied, with the patient's hands providing the resistance as the table generates traction to the spine. If the patient experiences pain during the traction, relaxing the grip will reduce or stop the force.

The treatment concept is based on research demonstrating that the nucleus of the disc is affected by a negative pressure created by the traction generated by a given level of force for a specific period. In the study noted previously by Ramos and Martin[7] a catheter was inserted into the nucleus of a disc of a person scheduled for surgery. While the catheter was in the nucleus, the table was used to provide traction to the low back. Ramos and Martin[7] found that the normally positive intradiscal pressures were reduced to negative levels when tensions in the therapeutic range were applied by the VAX-D table (these were in the range of -100 to 160 mm Hg).

The authors of the VAX-D literature note that changes in intradiscal pressure appeared to be insignificant until a certain level of traction tension was achieved. When this point was reached, then intradiscal pressure was observed to decrease to a level greater than 200 mm Hg below the positive pressure encountered before the traction began.[7] The manufacturer suggests that this will occur when traction is applied according to the recommended protocol.

OTHER DEVICES USED FOR TRACTION

Several other devices are used in the traction process, many of which are used without the effect of motion. These devices could be considered static traction. Some, however, are used by the patient, with some motion on the part of the patient, and one can even be worn while the patient is ambulatory. The following review is a selective sample of the devices that are available. This sampling includes the Back Bubble, the LTX 3000, and two cervical traction devices, as well as others.

THE BACK BUBBLE
The Back Bubble is designed for traction of the low back, to relieve pain in the lumbar spine. This device is an air-inflated bladder that is suspended from above by a strap attached to a spring. The inflatable bladder resembles an inner tube from a truck tire suspended above the device. The patient is seated, with the device around the body and above the waist, with the bubble under the arms. As the patient assumes the seated position with knees flexed and feet flat on the floor the lower back is suspended, creating traction. The objective is to minimize the weight borne by the spine, thus reducing compression on this area and creating traction on the lower back with the weight of the pelvis. This position is termed the *upright Back Bubble traction* position. (Fig. 7-5.)

An alternative position places the patient suspended, with the bubble below the hips, the upper body lying flat on the floor, and the feet vertical along the suspension strap. This position creates traction in another manner, by suspending the pelvis and hanging the low back. The approach is termed *low inverted Bubble traction*. This device provides considerable traction to the low back with a minimal investment in equipment.

A study was conducted on eleven subjects, drawn from a chiropractic college, who suffered from mild and moderate mechanical low back pain. Results of the study show that a 2-minute use of the Back Bubble is able to reduce mechanical back pain.[8]

THE LTX 3000
The LTX 3000 is a device for creating traction in the low back of a patient in a sitting position. It is promoted as a

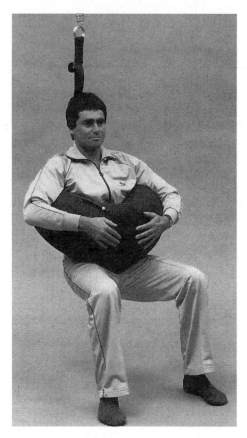

Fig. 7-5 The Back Bubble.
- Patient secures the device around the waist and under the arms.
- Patient assumes a seated posture while suspended in the device.
- Patient maintains seated posture and maintains the position of knees flexed, with feet flat on the floor, creating traction on the lower back. (*Courtesy Back Bubble, Inc., Solana Beach, Calif.*)

portable gravity-dependent, self-operated traction device for use in either a clinical or home setting. The unit consists of two upright members, adjustable for height and width. The upper section of the unit contains a sling seat, with arm rests further toward the top of the unit. These arm rests include a padded structure that, when fully engaged, rests against the lower rib cage. This support is important because it provides support for the body as it sits suspended, with the pelvis creating the weight for tractioning the lower back. (Figs. 7-6 through 7-12.)

The initial purpose for the unit was to create traction for the lower back. The LTX 3000 has evolved, however, and is now used extensively in the rehabilitation process, with exercises and stretching positions developed for use with the unit. A recent study by the University of Minnesota tested the capability of the device to produce spinal unloading. Fourteen subjects used the device for a series of sessions lasting 4 weeks.

Radiographic images taken at various times during the unloading process show a considerable increase in intervertebral spaces. The results of the study led researchers to determine that 10 minutes of this traction appears to be the optimum time for maximal lumbar lengthening. The study also reports that nearly all subjects demonstrated a dramatic reduction in lumbar curvature.[9]

The results expected from use of the LTX 3000 include increasing the intradiscal area by providing traction on the lumbar spine and unloading the spine, thereby reducing low back pain. Sitting in the position required by the LTX 3000 allows the patient to perform certain rehabilitation exercises to stretch and strengthen the low back. This device also allows the clinician to perform mobilizing manipulation.

THE GRAVITY LUMBAR TRACTION FRAME

The Gravity Lumbar Traction Frame was used prominently and written about by Charles Burton, M.D. This device was used frequently at the Sister Kenny Institute in Minneapolis, Minnesota, since the mid 1970s, when the program of low back treatment known as the Gravity Lumbar Reduction Therapy Program (GLRTP) was introduced. As noted by Burton,[10] the protocol for use of the device was to gradually load the lower body in traction by increasing the tilt of the frame over several days. This allowed the patient to acclimate to the traction and allowed the force to be applied gradually. (Fig. 7-13.)

This device is used on both chronic and acute patients with low back pain and is coupled with a course of exercises and toughening, or hardening, activities. This treatment has become generally an outpatient activity, and the Low Back Club was formed for ambulatory patients at the Sister Kenny Institute. The objective is to return the injured worker to work as soon as possible, before compensation issues arise.

INVERSION: THE BACK-A-TRACTION AND GRAVITY GUIDING SYSTEM

The Back-A-Traction is a Swedish-designed form of inversion therapy performed on a table. Most inversion devices are related to the early gravity boots or Gravity Guiding System that were used in the past but have since fallen from favor because they allow little control by the patient. The Gravity Guiding System required the use of special foot and ankle supports that snapped into place. Each support had a hook on the front that allowed a temporary connection to an overhead bar, which had to be installed by the patient. The inverted mounting of the bar by the patient proved difficult or impossible for most patients. (Fig. 7-14)

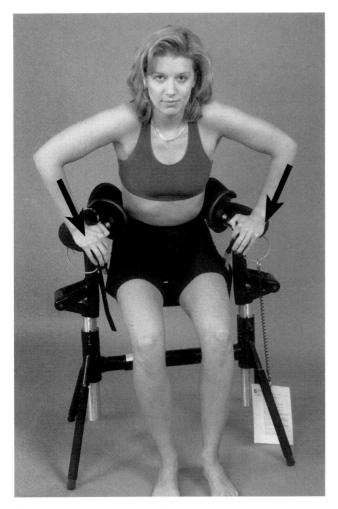

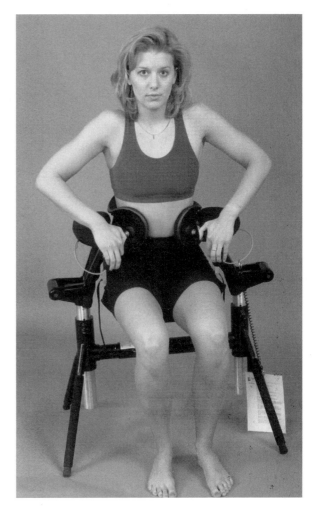

Fig. 7-6 Patient entering LTX 3000 lumbar traction device.
- The LTX 3000 is adjusted for patient height and size, ensuring that the device is correctly adjusted for patient comfort and safety.
- To enter, the patient grasps the lock releases with the fingers of each hand while assuming a sitting position on the sling located under the buttocks.
- The full weight is not borne by the sling but is partially supported by the patient's hands. With release of the locks, the torso pads move toward the body to support the torso and allow traction to the lower spine.
- Note that the knees are flexed and help support the weight of the patient as seating is completed. The torso is to maintain a near vertical position as the device is adjusted.
- Note the white rectangular sheet to the left of the device; this is the instruction sheet for the operator and the patient. *(Courtesy Spinal Designs, Minneapolis, Minn.)*

Fig. 7-7 Patient assuming a seated position in LTX 3000 traction device.
- Patient is fully seated, and the feet are relocated, with a right angle bend of the knees. The full weight is borne by the seat, and the torso pads press against the body.
- After a few seconds in this position, the torso pads are released to create an improved position against the body and the seat sling is released about 1 inch, increasing the traction on the lower spine.
- This process of increased release of the sling coupled with adjustment of the torso pads can be repeated 2 or 3 times, until the appropriate traction in the lower spine is achieved.
- All the adjustments should initially be performed by the operator.
- With supervision, the patient can become proficient in making most of the adjustments. *(Courtesy Spinal Designs, Minneapolis, Minn.)*

The Back-A-Traction inversion device incorporates high quality and heavy-duty construction. The patient is fastened into the foot clamps, which then allow control of the inversion process through stages. When the table tilts backward and the patient is positioned, the first stop is at full parallel to the ground. A release of this position must be initiated by the patient, and the second and third positions are accessed. The greatest inversion of this device is approximately 15 degrees below horizontal, and stops are automatic at each subsequent position toward the maximum inversion. Release from the position is initiated with the handle that is held constantly by the patient. (Fig. 7-15.)

Text continued on p. 244

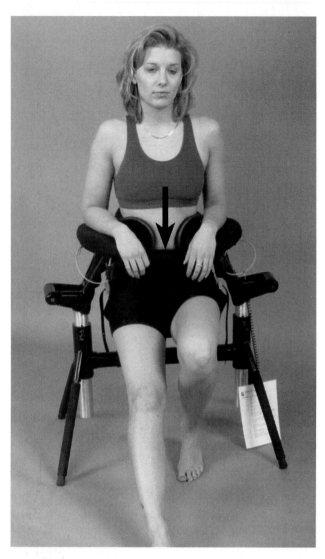

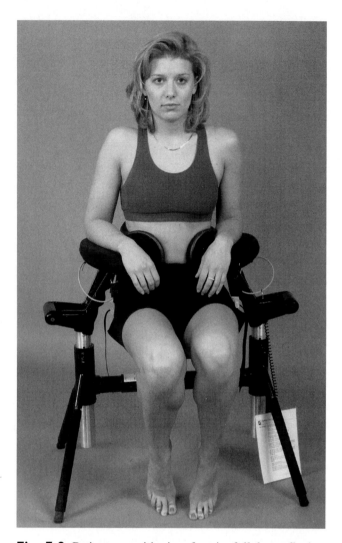

Fig. 7-8 Patient repositioning feet for exercise in LTX 3000 traction device.

- Patient is seated comfortably and correctly in the LTX 3000, with the sling tension partially released, so that more of the body weight is borne by the torso pads and the lower back is in traction.
- Exercises can be performed while the patient is in the traction position; proper positioning of the feet can facilitate the exercise process.
- This illustration demonstrates the way in which the pelvis can be rocked forward and backward (extension-flexion).
- The patient's arms can rest on the padded rests adjacent to the torso. *(Courtesy Spinal Designs, Minneapolis, Minn.)*

Fig. 7-9 Patient repositioning feet in full knee flexion under LTX 3000.

- Patient is seated correctly in the LTX 3000, with the knees in full flexion under the device, in preparation for pelvic tilting and rotation of the pelvis right and left. *(Courtesy Spinal Designs, Minneapolis, Minn.)*

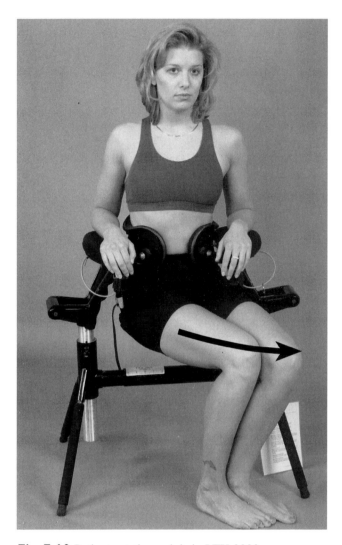

Fig. 7-10 Patient rotating pelvis in LTX 3000.
- Patient with feet positioned so that knees are near right angles and rotated to the left.
- This is another exercise position for the device. Other exercises can be performed on the LTX 3000 by acute, chronic, or rehabilitating patients. *(Courtesy Spinal Designs, Minneapolis, Minn.)*

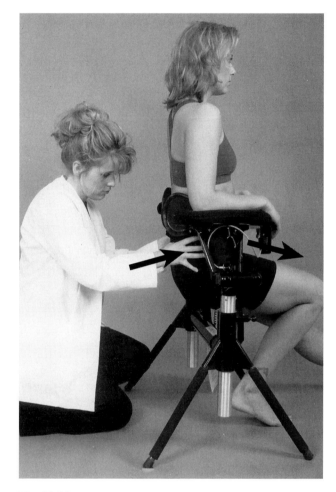

Fig. 7-11 Clinician positioned for posterior adjustment of patient on LTX 3000.
- Patient is positioned on the LTX 3000, with the arms at rest and traction on the lower back resulting from the seated position.
- One leg is fully extended; the other leg is flexed, with the knee less than 90 degrees; and the lower back relaxed.
- Clinician is positioned behind the patient, kneeling with a stable squatting stance to create sufficient leverage on the patient.
- With this position, the right ilium is flexed slightly. This facilitates the clinician performing a mobilizing repeated thrust into the right ilium, creating movement in the right sacroiliac joint. *(Courtesy Spinal Designs, Minneapolis, Minn.)*

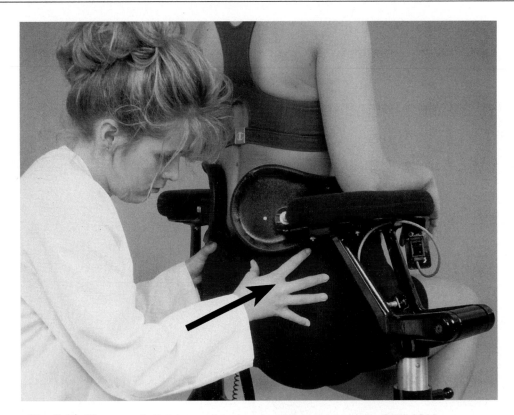

Fig. 7-12 Close-up of clinician performing posterior adjustment on LTX 3000.
- Patient is positioned on the LTX 3000, with traction on the lower back.
- Clinician is positioned kneeling behind the patient, mobilizing the ilium.
- This is being performed while the patient is in seated traction, with the spine unloaded. *(Courtesy Spinal Designs, Minneapolis, Minn.)*

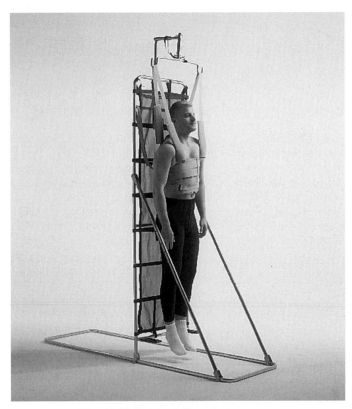

Fig. 7-13 See legend opposite page.

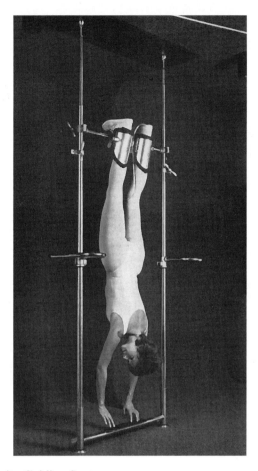

Fig. 7-14 The Gravity Guiding System
- The gravity boots are fitted to the patient's ankles and strapped on.
- Patient is assisted or climbs into an inverted position, clipping the boots onto the hanging rod.
- Patient then hangs suspended for a period ranging from 2 minutes to 30 minutes. *(From Martin RM. The Gravity Guiding System: Turning the Aging Process Upside Down. Pasadena, Calif: Gravity Guidance, Inc; 1975.)*

Fig. 7-13 The Gravity Lumbar Traction Frame.
- Patient ready to receive traction in a near-upright position.
- Patient is harnessed into the frame, with the harness connected to the upper body.
- The frame is gradually positioned upright to increase the pull of gravity on the low back. *(Courtesy Sammons Preston, Bolingbrook, Ill.)*

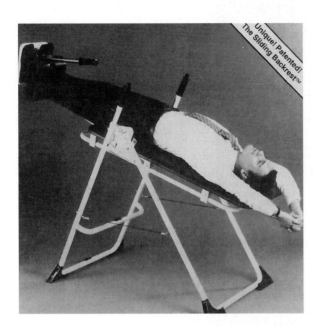
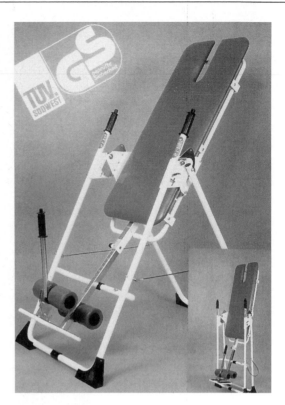

Fig. 7-15 Advertisement for the Swedish Back-A-Traction.
- Patient is fastened into the device at the ankles.
- The bed is adjusted for patient height.
- The release is manually controlled by the patient and can be set for a comfortable angle.
- As each level of inversion is attempted, the table (bed) stops at predetermined angles and must be released by the patient to continue the tilt toward full inversion. *(Courtesy Swedish Back Care System, St. Augustine, Fla.)*

Once the desired inversion is reached, the patient may initiate a mild exercise by flexing and straightening the knees, allowing the bed on which the patient is lying to slide back and forth a few inches. This process is controlled completely by the patient and can be used to enhance the condition of the back. Earlier versions of this device produced full inversion, and some patients incurred problems. In some hypertensive individuals, full inversion has the potential for increasing intraoccular pressure, leading to possible damaging effects on blood vessels in the eyes.[11-13] The inversion produced by the modern table is much less than with earlier similar products, therefore decreasing the possibility of damaging effects.[14]

The concept of inversion therapy is to provide for unloading of the lower back, reducing pressure and discomfort. These devices can be used at home and are considered to be adjunctive therapy for the patient.

Certain contraindications for use of this therapy must be considered, and some precautions must be taken during the course of the therapy protocol. Patients must be selected carefully, with consideration given to the patient's cardiovascular health (possible hypertension) and the condition of the spine (osteoporosis or arthritic condition).

CERVICAL TRACTION DEVICES:
THE PRONEX AND THE PNEU-TRAC

Two of the cervical traction devices available use a pneumatic traction mechanism to create the desired traction. Glacier Cross makes the Pronex, which is used with the patient in a supine position on a bed or other flat surface. The traction is provided by an expandable section over the cervical spine that is inflated by compressing a bulb similar to that on a sphygmomanometer. A headband binds the head into a contoured section designed to pre-

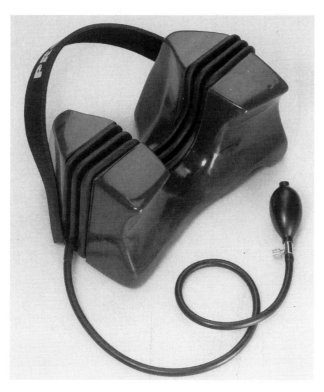

Fig. 7-16 Pronex cervical traction device.
- The unit consists of a contoured device made to fit the cervical spine, with an expanding bellows that creates traction.
- A strap for the forehead and a pump bulb for creating the air pressure are included. *(Courtesy Glacier Cross, Inc., Kalispell, Mont.)*

serve the cervical lordosis. After the section is inflated, the patient rests on the device for a few minutes, then the unit is deflated and the headband is removed. This device is also accompanied by a list of contraindications that includes severe rheumatoid arthritis, infections and inflammatory disease, fractures, extruded disc fragmentation, spreading or aggravation of patient's symptoms, serious pathology or disease, malignancy, and spinal cord compression.[15] (Figs. 7-16 and 7-17.)

The second such pneumatic device is the Pneu-trac, made by Zinco Industries. This unit can be worn while the patient is ambulatory. It consists of a stiff collar that is attached to the standing or sitting patient and fastened with Velcro closures. As with the Pronex, a hand bulb is used to inflate the device, which has an air bladder at the base of the collar. The bulb is pumped repeatedly, inflating the bladder and raising the collar against the chin and the base of the occiput. The literature for this device

makes no mention of maintaining the cervical lordosis. When the traction session is completed, the release valve is turned and the air released.[16] (Fig. 7-18.)

The expected effect of these devices is traction of the cervical spine, with the objective of separating the spinal joints and stretching the cervical paraspinal musculature. One of the units can be worn for extended periods while the patient is ambulatory; the other purports to enhance the cervical spine lordosis, but can only be worn while lying supine.

THE VERTETRAC AMBULATORY LUMBAR TRACTION DEVICE

The Vertetrac is an ambulatory traction device that can be worn by the patient with a lumbar problem that could respond to traction. The advantage is that it allows the patient to move around during the therapy. The unit is a pair of U-shaped padded frames equipped with a belt

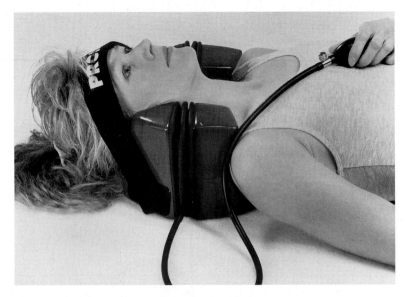

Fig. 7-17 Pronex cervical traction device on a patient.
- Patient lies supine on the device, placing it beneath the cervical spine and placing headband over forehead.
- Patient pumps the device to achieve cervical traction, but also maintains cervical lordosis.
- Traction can be maintained for several minutes, gradually increasing the time from 3 to 20 or more minutes at a session.
- Patient comfort should be maintained.
- Air can be introduced by the pump and then increased after 2 minutes, according to patient comfort. Air pressure should be released in the same way: gradually decreasing the air pressure in the device and thus reducing the cervical traction.
- Patient should take care when arising from the supine position, allowing the body to adapt to the upright position. *(Courtesy Glacier Cross, Inc., Kalispell, Mont.)*

assembly by which it is strapped to the patient. A leverage system allows the patient to adjust the tensioning device that spreads the two belts apart and creates the traction. A movable knob maintains or increases the lordosis in the lumbar spine.

The patient is fitted with the Vertetrac while in a standing position; the two belts are attached, fitting the U-shaped rings to the body. The two rings are ratcheted apart until the skin is very tight and the appropriate traction applied (approximately 20 kilograms on each side). The patient is instructed to walk around wearing the device or may, if necessary, be seated on a stool. The initial wearing time is approximately 15 to 20 minutes. It is suggested that the patient build up to wearing the device for 30 minutes at least once a day for about 10 days and on consecutive days if possible.[17] (Fig. 7-19.)

The developers claim that the device brings relief to the patient suffering from a disc problem, relieving pain and allowing the patient to be ambulatory. It is also sug-

gested that the Vertetrac is appropriate for treatment of other conditons that include facet syndrome.

CERVICAL EXTENSION TRACTION (CET-1) AND PAYNE TRACTION

The CET-1 was developed to provide traction for the cervical spine in either a seated position or lying supine on a table. The device is purported to aid in restoring the normal cervical lordosis. It is designed to be used in conjunction with a foam fulcrum placed under the neck, creating a longitudinal traction in the cervical spine. The pull of the traction device is provided by weight in an accompanying bag filled with lead shot. The shape and size of the fulcrum can be changed to provide a variation in the fulcrum under the neck. The device is attached to the chin and forehead with a strap.

An alternative to the CET-1 is the Payne traction device, which has a harnessing attachment for the head that does not put any compression forces on the temporo-

Fig. 7-18 Pneu-trac cervical traction device.
- Patient places the device on the cervical spine and fastens it in place.
- Patient pumps the device to achieve cervical spine traction.
- Patient wears the traction device for several minutes while ambulatory, several times per day.
- The device is gradually deflated, and the cervical spine adapts to a nontraction state. *(Courtesy Zinco Industries, Inc., Pasadena, Calif.)*

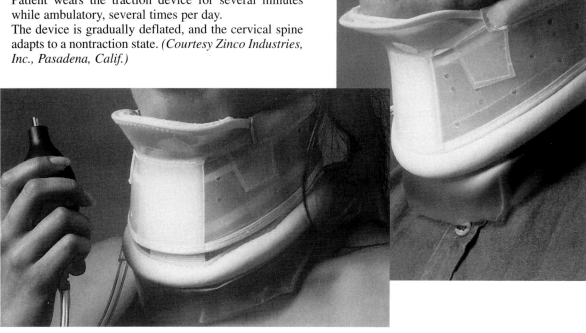

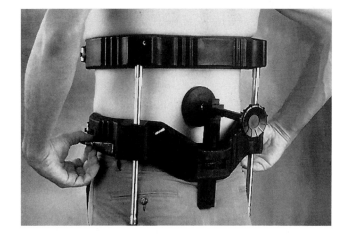

Fig. 7-19 Vertetrac ambulatory lumbar traction apparatus.
- Patient attaches the device to body using the belts and frames.
- The tensioning device is adjusted by the patient to achieve the desired amount of traction.
- The lumbar knob is adjusted to enhance the lordosis in the lumbar spine.
- Patient is instructed to gradually increase the wearing time to 30 minutes.
- The device should be worn for approximately 10 days consecutively.
- Patient may be seated on a stool. *(Courtesy Meditrac, Palm Desert, Calif.)*

mandibular joint (TMJ). The weight mechanism is the same as in the CET-1.[18] Further explanation of the theory and contraindications of extension traction is given elsewhere.[19] (Fig. 7-20.)

The rationale for this form of traction is explained by Harrison,[19] who emphasizes lateral spinal curve harmonics as being of primary concern to the clinician. These include several categories of abnormal configurations of the cervical spine and methods for providing correction that include various cervical spine positions of traction. For a hypolordosis of the cervical spine, the foam block is placed under the lower part of the cervical spine, the neck is "draped" over it, and traction applied. The same treatment is recommended to correct a military, or very straight, neck. The approach for treatment of a kyphotic cervical spine is to place the fulcrum opposite or slightly below what is described as the *stress vertebra.* In the case of an S-curve kyphotic neck, the fulcrum of the foam block is placed under the upper cervical spine. In the case of an S-curve lordotic neck, the fulcrum is placed under the lower cervical spine.[20,21]

THE FIVE POINT TRACTION SYSTEM

An example of traction carried to the extreme is another off-shoot of the Harrison model. This is a static traction system that supports the entire body in traction inside a frame, with harnesses attached to adjustable tensioning pulleys. The system derives its name, the *Five Point Traction System,* from the five points of subject control: the pelvis, the thoracolumbar area, the shoulders, the cervical area, and the head, or skull. According to the system's developer, Steve Foster, it is a method of postural remodeling, which he claims is critical to the application of the technique he advocates.[22] (Fig. 7-21.)

THE INVERTABOD: TRACTION, INVERSION, AND EXERCISE DEVICE

The Invertabod is a variation on the inversion table, which positions the patient in an inverted kneeling position, with the torso hanging from a stabilizer at the knees. The patient is positioned with the knees secured behind a foam-covered stabilizer. The patient then leans forward, causing the support base beneath the pelvis to

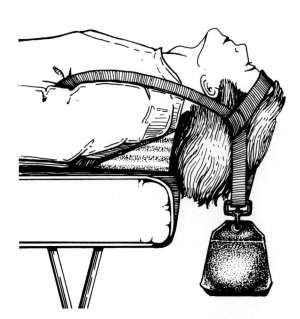

Fig. 7-20 CET-1 traction device.
- Patient is placed on a flat therapy table, with the foam block placed according to the specified location, under the cervical spine and extending the neck.
- The traction straps are placed over the forehead and/or chin, depending on the type device.
- Traction in extension is maintained for a specified period. *(Courtesy Matlin Mfg., Inc., Hartselle, Ala.)*

tilt. This position places the person so that the torso hangs downward, creating a traction and resultant unloading of the lumbar spine. The person is encouraged to exercise in this position by extending the trunk and, in some instances, rotating the trunk right and left. This device is similar to inversion devices, although the whole body is not extended fully and hung by the ankles as with other units.[23] (Fig. 7-22.)

CTD MARK I: WRIST TRACTION

The CTD Mark I is a traction unit designed for treating carpal tunnel syndrome (CTS) and possibly other cumulative trauma disorders (CTD). The unit is designed around the concept that reapproximation of the radius and the ulna in the forearm is necessary in treatment of CTS. According to this hypothesis, the appropriate repositioning of these bones will affect the volume of the carpal tunnel in the hand and relieve the symptoms. The manufacturer recommends that the clinician perform an examination of the patient, including orthopedic and neurologic tests, radiographs of the wrist and the cervi-

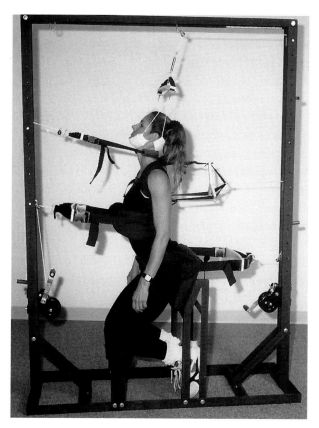

Fig. 7-21 Foster's Five Point Traction System.
- Patient is fastened into the traction system, with the cords attached to the various specified connecting points on the body.
- The tensioning pulleys are adjusted to achieve the desired traction on the specified areas. *(Courtesy Steve Foster, DC.)*

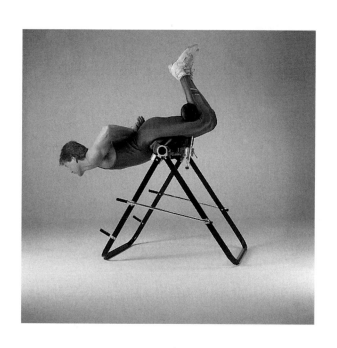

Fig. 7-22 Invertabod.
- Patient is positioned upright, with the knees in the knee pad.
- Patient tilts the device forward and assumes a position perpendicular to the plane of the floor.
- Patient can perform certain exercises from this position or can simply allow gravity inversion to the spine.
- Patient arises to an upright position following inverted traction. *(Courtesy Brilhante Co., Inc., West Los Angeles, Calif.)*

cothoracic spine, and, possibly, electrodiagnostic evaluation of the area, before beginning treatment. This unit, developed by Para Tech Industries, provides a cradle for positioning the elbow, securing it to act as a base for the traction process. The upper arm is also secured as part of the base for traction. The wrist is secured in a wrap that is tethered to a pneumatically activated post.

The manufacturer lists several contraindications, including "severe rheumatoid arthritis, circulatory disease, patient taking blood thinners, vasculitis, fractures of the wrist, and wrist lesions."[24] The protocol for use of the CTD Mark I suggests 30 distractions in a sequence of 10. The T bar is then relocated by tilting it either to the right or to the left; this positioning is determined by a muscle test, and the muscles' relative strength or weakness characteristics are determined at that time.[24]

The mechanism for the operation of the device is enclosed in a frame and housing that contains the compressor for the pneumatic mechanism. The controls for the unit are on the front of the machine and reflect the capability of creating and controlling air pressure and of setting the sequence of the traction cycles and the rests between. The hand and wrist may be positioned for a variable angle of traction. Treatment on the CTD Mark I requires several cycles through wrist traction, with rests between traction and repositioning of the wrist at a different angle, while the elbow and upper arm are securely tethered to the elbow cradle.[24]

With this traction treatment, the expected effect is that the symptoms of numbness and tingling in the fingers will be relieved and function in the hand will improve. (Figs. 7-23 through 7-25.)

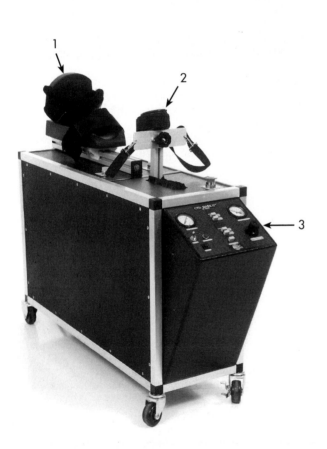

Fig. 7-23 CTD Mark I.
- The unit with the (1) elbow cradle, (2) wrist attachment, and (3) controls.
- The unit can be placed adjacent to a chair and can be used from either the right or left side. *(Courtesy Para Tech Industries/Therasys, Dayton, Ohio.)*

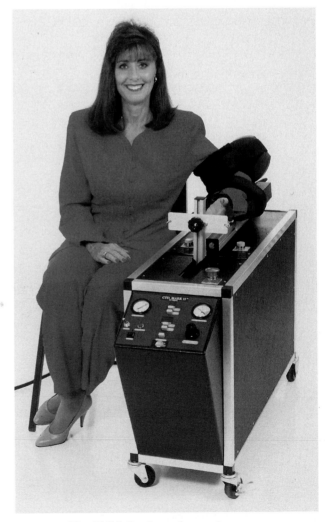

Fig. 7-24 See legend opposite page.

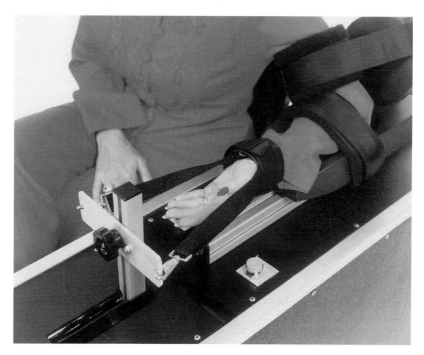

Fig. 7-25 CTD Mark I: Close-up view.
- Note the position of the elbow in the cradle, with the restraining strap attached.
- Note the wrist in the first position of traction.
- The elbow and wrist straps are attached to the patient with Velcro.
- The wrist can be repositioned, using the knob to change the angle of the wrist positioner.
- The emergency stop button is located next to the patient's left hand. *(Courtesy Para Tech Industries/Therasys, Dayton, Ohio.)*

Fig. 7-24 CTD Mark I: Patient positioning.
- The patient is seated adjacent to the tractioning unit, positioned according to the wrist to be treated.
- The elbow is placed in a cradle and secured with a strap.
- The wrist is positioned and the tractioning strap is attached appropriately.
- The device is set by the controls for appropriate timing of the traction sequence.
- The traction is initiated and progresses through the traction/rest cycle and the wrist is repositioned and traction begins again.
- The device is set by the operator for a specific traction force, timing, and repetitions. *(Courtesy Para Tech Industries/Therasys, Dayton, Ohio.)*

REFERENCES

1. Jaskoviak PA, Schafer RC. *Applied Physiotherapy: Practical Applications with Emphasis on the Management of Pain and Related Syndromes.* Arlington, Va: ACA; 1986.
2. Anatamotor traction device brochure. Malvern, Pa: Hill Laboratories.
3. Tesio L, Merlo A. Autotraction versus passive traction: an open controlled study in lumbar disc herniation. *Arch Phys Med Rehabil.* 1993;74:871.
4. Gillstrom P, Erickson K, Hindmarsh T. Autotraction in lumbar disc herniation: a myelographic study before and after treatment. *Arch Orthop Trauma Surg.* 1985;104:207-210.
5. Pope MH, Klingenstierna U. Height changes due to autotraction. *Clin Biomechan.* 1986;1:191-195.
6. Dyer A. VAX-D Table brochure. Allandale, Fla: National Spine Institute, Inc.
7. Ramos G, Martin W. Effects of vertebral axial decompression on intradiscal pressure. *J Neurosurg.* 1994;81:350-353.
8. Hubka MJ, Black D. The immediate effect of Back Bubble traction on mechanical low back pain: a pilot study. *Chiropr Tech.* 1995;7(1)18-21.
9. Janke AW, Kerkow TA, Griffiths HJ, Sparrow EA, Iaizzo PA. The biomechanics of gravity-dependent traction of the lumbar spine. *Spine.* 1996;22(3):253-260.
10. Burton CV. Low back care: the gravity of the situation. In: Kirkaldy-Willis WH, Burton CV, eds. *Managing Low Back Pain.* New York: Churchill Livingstone; 1992.
11. Friberg TR, Weinreb RN. Ocular manifestations of gravity inversion. *JAMA.* 1985;253(12):1755-1757.
12. Sanborn GE, Friberg TR, Allen R. Optic nerve dysfunction during gravity inversion: visual field abnormalities. *Arch Opthalmol.* 1987;105(6):774-776.
13. Vehrs PR, Plowman SA, Fernhall B. Exercise during gravity inversion: acute and chronic effects. *Arch Phys Med Rehabil.* 1988;69(11):950-954.
14. Norell P. Back-A-Traction brochure. St. Augustine, Fla: Swedish Back Care, Inc.
15. Pronex sales brochure. Kalispell, Mont: Glacier Cross, Inc.
16. Pneu-trac brochure. Pasadena, Calif: Zinco Industries.
17. Tucker JH. Ambulatory traction technique for low back pain. *Chiropr Econ.* 1993;36(3):70-71.
18. Professional Chiropractic Products, Catalog 3. Cet-1: Payne Traction. Hartselle, Ala: Matlin Mfg., Inc.
19. Harrison DD, ed. *Biomechanics, Physiology and Applications to Chiropractic.* (privately published, 1992).
20. Garde R. Cervical traction: the neurophysiology of lordosis and the rheological characteristics of cervical curve rehabilitation. In: Harrison DD, ed. *Biomechanics, Physiology and Applications to Chiropractic.* (privately published, 1992).
21. Harrison DD, Jackson BL, Troyanovich S, Robertson G, DeGeorge D, Barker W. The efficacy of cervical extension-compression traction combined with diversified manipulation and drop table adjustments in the rehabilitation of cervical lordosis: a pilot study. *J Manipulative Physiol Ther.* 1994;17(7) 454-464.
22. Foster S. The Five Point Traction System: a step toward full spine postural traction. *Am J Clin Chiropr.* 1996;6(1):2.
23. Invertabod brochure. West Los Angeles, Calif: Brilhante Co., Inc.
24. CTD Mark I instruction manual. Dayton, Ohio: Para Tech Industries.
25. Fulk P. CTD Mark I Pneumatic Traction Device brochure. Dayton, Ohio: Para Tech Industries, Inc.

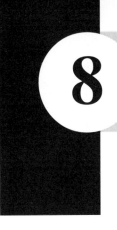

Outcome Measures, Research Directions, and Case Reports

Clinicians must have a perceptive assessment strategy for managing patients with joint pain and dysfunction, which is one of the most complex areas in health care and carries a weight of responsibility. Treatment of joint pain and dysfunction is complex because mechanical causes are hard to differentiate in many patients. The responsibility issue springs from the fact that a pathologic spine or a condition beyond the scope of conservative manual methods should not be treated, and appropriate referral should be made.

In addition, health care is in the midst of major change. Health care providers must stay abreast of the current literature and keep pace with advances in diagnostic and therapeutic sophistication while still making decisions on what is best for their patients. Furthermore, the effectiveness and efficiency of health care services are coming under close scrutiny. There is great haste from both the public and private sectors for developing standards of care, outcome measures, and quality assessments. It is clear that if the health care profession does not move forward proactively into standard setting and quality measurement, these tasks will certainly be handled by another party (whose motivation may not be in the best interest of the patient nor the provider). The ultimate goal is to find out systematically what treatments produce the best results and then put that knowledge into guidelines or standards that clinicians can use in daily practice. This has the potential to affect the quality of care primarily and the cost of care secondarily.

This chapter discusses the use of outcome measures generally and how they are applied to the use of mechanically assisted manipulative therapy. Research directions for the application of manipulative therapy in general and mechanically assisted and motion-assisted techniques specifically also are addressed. Case reports are presented to demonstrate the clinical use of mechanical-

ly assisted and motion-assisted techniques that suggest the need for further investigation.

OUTCOME MEASURES

Measurement of outcomes helps to assess the efficiency and effectiveness of a specific modality of care.[1,2] Joint dysfunction pain syndromes have the primary impact of affecting the patient's ability to function; fortunately, these syndromes are not life-threatening. Because chronicity and recurrence are likely, a cure of these conditions seldom occurs. Instead, improvement in the functional status for performing activities necessary for daily living is an important and attainable goal. Functional status is a term used to indicate measures of joint mobility, muscle strength, employment status, and other indicators. In some settings, instruments that primarily assess patient functioning have been called *health status* or *quality of life* indexes.[3,4] The term *functional status measures* is used to denote questionnaires or other instruments that assess a patient's limitations in performing the usual tasks of living.

Functional status measures have been considered a subjective evaluation and hence less desirable than physical measures that are deemed objective. However, many of the objective tests are influenced by the patient's motivation, effort, and psychologic state.[5] Thus measures of flexibility, strength, or timed activities may often reflect nonphysical, highly subjective states, as well as actual physical capabilities. For example, the straight leg raising test relies on the patient report of pain, which adds considerable subjectivity to an objective test.

The chiropractic profession has stumbled over the concept of outcome measures, favoring leg length inequality, line drawings on radiographs, resistive muscle strength, and other physical assessments. These measures are used to identify the presence of the subluxation, which is the lesion treatable with chiropractic methods. However, ignoring other components of health (or lack of health [illness]), such as pain and disability, greatly decreases the ability to address clinical effectiveness and efficiency.[6]

Useful outcome measures are available that generally relate to the patient's relative capacity to be mobile, undertake self-care, and function with minimal pain.[7] Self-reporting instruments generally take the form of questionnaires that are used to quantify the degree of pain or the severity of disability as a result of impairment. The Oswestry Disability Questionnaire for low back pain and the Neck Disability Index for neck pain are supported in the literature as being valid and reliable to a sufficient degree to be clinically useful.[8,9] Pain scales such as the visual analog scale (VAS) to rate pain have also been determined to be reliable and valid. Other instruments include the Roland-Morris, Sickness Impact Profile, SF 36, and COOP Charts.

Outcome measures such as these do not generally provide information about the diagnosis. Instead, these tools answer questions about the patients' perception of their quality of life in comparison with the state before the illness. Outcome measures that evaluate functional status typically allow the assessment of multiple dimensions of patient functioning (e.g., physical and psychosocial), have well-demonstrated reliability and validity, and will stand as an appropriate index, monitoring patient response in clinical practice. As such, they can be used by the clinician to decide if a specific approach to dealing with patient complaints is effective and efficient compared with other approaches. The use of reliable and valid outcome measures in clinical studies and practices will help quell the critical echoes of unscientific claims.

RESEARCH DIRECTIONS

Intensifying scrutiny by the public, the need for cost containment, and the demands of third-party payment groups makes it imperative that practitioners of manipulative therapy be prepared to defend, with rational and scientific evidence, the effectiveness of the discipline's practices and procedures.[10] The clinical practice of manipulative therapy should be based on experimentation and testing of clinical methods. It is important to identify and eliminate ineffective treatment procedures and inaccurate diagnostic procedures while preserving those tests and treatment procedures that provide clinical benefits as compared with costs and risks. The focus must be on principle issues such as the identification of parameters, relation to known information, and published research. Without this support, clinicians cannot be sure what really does help patients or what is useless or potentially harmful.

The science of chiropractic is now beginning to investigate the art of chiropractic. The profession now has a body of credible research to document some of what it claims, it supports several fine scientific journals, and it has an increasing number of high-quality textbooks. Because of this complex of available knowledge, chiropractic is rapidly gaining acceptance. More research will further this process.

A major area of concern is that various forms of manual therapy exist that affect different aspects of joint function.[11] Although the goals of manual therapy include a combination of mechanical effects, soft tissue effects, neurologic effects, and psychologic effects, the way in which these goals are met can vary greatly. All procedures referred to as adjustments are not equivalent. The majority of chiropractic technique systems were started by interested and probing doctors who noticed a pattern in their results and began to ask why those results occurred. The impetus to gain new knowledge and then disseminate it was largely self-driven. Many of these approaches developed into somewhat dogmatic systems of diagnosis and treatment (system techniques).

A challenge for the future is to classify and place all forms of chiropractic technique and all other manual procedures into a framework that allows researchers to determine whether any of the techniques are based in fact. The profession can then begin to weed out unacceptable procedures that are promoted largely on the personality of the system's founder. To allow those systems to flourish solely because of the effort of those individuals who devise and promote their system is a grave disservice to those who come after. Serious investigation into some of these approaches is underway, but more must be done. It is the responsibility of the developers and followers of a specific technique to establish efficacy, not through anecdotes and testimonials but through properly documented case reports followed by clinical trials. Despite chiropractors' claims that their form of spinal manipulative therapy-centered health care is superior, the profession has yet to experimentally substantiate the clinical value of any uniquely chiropractic method of health care.[12] However, the rejection of a therapeutic procedure because it is untested is just as wrong as the acceptance of the same procedure in the absence of convincing evidence. At this time it has not been established that any adjustive or evaluative procedure is more or less effective than any other for any condition. Studies comparing effectiveness and efficiency of technique systems are long overdue.

It is time to begin the process of validating manual therapies, specifically those unique to the chiropractic profession. The ultimate purpose of validating clinical procedures is to provide a means to examine and explain the process by which clinicians can test and improve treatment procedures. Validity has been defined as *the extent to which measurements are useful for making decisions relative to a given purpose*.[13] Questions of validity are first and foremost questions of logic and rationality.

Manipulative therapy requires validation through randomized, controlled clinical trials that meet the skepticism of its critics. However, it is likely that even if such studies were done and manipulative therapy was found to be successful, very little notice would be taken by the critics. In most instances the randomized clinical trial (RCT) is the design most suited for answering questions concerning effectiveness. The RCT is a method by which a new therapy can be compared with a placebo or an accepted procedure, a therapy currently in use can be shown to be ineffective, or a combination of treatment approaches is demonstrated to be of greater benefit than a single therapy. Although there are other ways in which the outcome of a therapy can be investigated, none are as credible or as necessary as the RCT.

A reasonable argument can be made that virtually anything of interest to chiropractic practitioners could be the subject of credible research. For example, there would clearly be a benefit from investigations providing evidence that the spinal subluxation complex is indeed responsible for pathophysiologic sequelae that can be mitigated by spinal adjustment and manipulation. Other basic research questions are equally important, as are investigations that form a foundation for the development of new chiropractic examination and therapy procedures.

However, in the current climate of accountability, health care financing reform, and demands on all health professions for evidence, consideration by the profession of fundamental clinical questions may be more important and timely. Relman[14] states that health care has begun an era in which the excesses of both the providers (overutilization and overcharging) and those paying for the services (arbitrary denial of coverage) are restrained, and both are asked to account for their actions. There are, of course, many uncertainties as to how this will finally resolve, particularly regarding the chiropractic profession. There is, however, one certainty: the single most important factor in shaping health care policy will be reliable data on the effectiveness of diagnostic and therapeutic procedures. The lack of these data on chiropractic care will limit the growth and maturation of the chiropractic profession or result in a decline of the profession.

A recent case has been made in the chiropractic literature for the urgency of research on contemporary health care questions.[15,16] Answers to the following questions are particularly relevant to the profession:

- Which procedures are ineffective, and which tests and treatments currently being used are unnecessary or redundant?
- Does treatment produce meaningful clinical outcomes (e.g., ability to work or function) or improvements in clinical indicators (e.g., range of motion or measurements of spinal mechanics)?
- Are the results of care sustained or temporary?
- How much care should be provided and for how long?
- What are the relative clinical and economic advantages compared with other alternatives?
- Under what circumstances is care appropriate?
- Which procedures, services, and techniques promote improved health status more quickly and at a lower cost?
- What are the important elements related to quality of health care?
- Which practitioners, clinics, and interventions do patients believe would meet community needs?

One difficulty in studying manipulative therapy is that the detection of joint dysfunction is not an exact science; therefore any examination procedure used to detect subluxations may produce false positive, false negative, or equivocal results. Although the appropriateness of manipulative therapy for treating back pain has been demonstrated and patient satisfaction well established, the reliability and validity of some procedures used to detect joint subluxation and dysfunction has not been fully confirmed.[17-41] Based on the present data, it would seem prudent to refrain from drawing any firm conclusion on the independent reliability of many of the procedures commonly applied in the assessment of joint dysfunction. Definitive statements await further professional investigation.

Only a few examination procedures used to detect joint dysfunction have been subjected to sufficient validity testing, making this an area ripe for evaluation. However, chiropractic is not the only health care profession lagging in reliability and validity assessment. Other core health disciplines also suffer from variations in the application of diagnostic tests, and many lack experimental evaluation and confirmation.[42-47] Further assessment and study will lead to the refinement, exclusion, and addition of physical examination procedures used in the detection of joint dysfunction and subluxation. Although many of the physical examination procedures commonly applied in clinical practice lack experimental evaluation and confirmation, they still contribute greatly to the formation of a clinical impression and the relationship between practitioner and patient. The chiropractic practitioner must be aware of the limits of joint assessment procedures but must also constructively use the physical evaluation to help gain the patient's confidence and compliance. Within this context, undue reliance should not be placed on any one procedure. A combination of diagnostic procedures should be used, and the weight of evidence allowed to build a clinical impression of the patient's problem.

With the evolution of chiropractic, many techniques of manipulation/adjustment have emerged. Some of these are based on sound principles of anatomy and physiology; others are not so soundly based. Attention within the scientific community to date has been based primarily on determining the effectiveness of thrusting forms of manipulation in the treatment of low back pain. Some of the approaches that have been tested include those of manual medicine in allopathy and physical therapy. As scientific research focuses on the way in which manipulation is performed, it is now time for evaluation of the methods of treatment used in chiropractic.

This new focus on the details of treatment using manipulation/adjustments, referred to internationally as *manual therapy,* will mean that categories of treatment such as force vs. non-force, instrument vs. noninstrument, and soft tissue vs. bony joint treatment must undergo close evaluation by scientific methods, with rigorous analysis. It means, for example, that Gonstead's method of adjustment in the pelvis, in which a high-velocity, low-amplitude thrust is applied to the sacroiliac joint to achieve an improved and alleged correct posi-

tion, has to be compared with a technique such as the Thompson high-velocity, drop-piece adjustment that is used to achieve the same goal. Comparisons such as these will allow the determination of which technique is more effective. Likewise, traction-distraction techniques must be compared with other techniques to determine which is most effective in treating conditions of chiropractic concern. Even within technique types, evaluation is necessary. For example, a comparison can be made of the various forms of distraction, from the mechanically-assisted, with its manual application of therapy (Cox), to the motion-assisted techniques, including those of Hill and Leander.

Which is the best technique for any given problem? This is not presently known. No research on the comparison of chiropractic techniques exists that would withstand the scrutiny of peer review nor are there any clinical trials involving specific technique testing. Research for the future should address this concern that, with the advent of managed care, is indeed an important question for all chiropractors. When the techniques are analyzed, it is likely that some will be found to be ineffective or, at least, some will be shown to be more effective than others. The techniques shown to be more effective will become a standard for the clinician. Others that do not show like merit must fall by the wayside. Should the chiropractor continue to use ineffective or irrational techniques, the all-too-familiar term *quackery* would indeed be justified.

Along with effectiveness of the technique itself, other factors must be considered. These factors include safety and liability issues for the patient and ergonomic considerations for the clinician. The technique should be effective for the treatment of problems and should also be the safest option for the patient, with the least likelihood of causing harm. Anecdotal evidence on the relative effectiveness of various techniques abounds within the profession; however, there is no definitive answer to the question of which techniques are the most effective and also safest. Is the directive to "do no harm" possible with the technique of choice?

Another factor for consideration relates to the clinician. Failure to comply with the best ergonomic principles may result in injury to the clinician. Some techniques require a powerful thrust into the area of concern, whereas others allow for a more incremental approach to manipulation. Some techniques and their required equipment allow the clinician to exert less physical force. This means that the clinician can use less physical energy during a given period, thus preserving some physical well-being for the "long haul" of a lifetime of practice. Some practitioners become partially disabled in their lifetime through injury or illness and thus do not have full capacity to treat with the unassisted techniques. An alternative may be a welcome respite, allowing the clinician to continue in practice rather than terminating for health reasons.

Women are entering the field in record number. All of the techniques commonly in use were developed by and for men. Many of these require the exertion of much physical force to accomplish the objective of the move. The smaller person or the woman with less upper body strength and mass is forced to try to emulate the thrust of the major techniques. Alternative procedures with mechanical or motion-assists could be beneficial. Therefore new and modified techniques should be developed and tested to rectify this shortcoming. Many female clinicians are very successful in the use of high-velocity, low-amplitude thrust techniques; however, there appears to be a need for new developments in the approach to performing chiropractic manipulation/adjustments.

Specific recommendations can be made for a clinical trial of known techniques (particularly distraction techniques) to include a comparison between a given distraction approach performed with motion-assisted distraction (MAD) and with mechanically assisted distraction (MEAD). This may be compared with a thrust technique and a possible third treatment that involves a medication, such as a nonsteroidal antiinflammatory drug (NSAID). The focus may be on a clinical condition, such as a radiculopathy in the lumbar spine. The treatment must take into account some standard for determining the presence of the condition, such as MRI of the lumbar spine or an EMG of the lower extremity. The study should include outcomes instruments to measure patient satisfaction with the treatment and the patient's evaluation of function before and after treatment. The appropriate power calculations would determine the size of the population to be studied. The location for the trial would be determined by the availability of facilities with an experienced professional staff and the potential for attracting the necessary subjects.

Although many more details must be considered in such a study, the funding to undertake such a clinical trial is a major factor. The profession must be willing to make the necessary sacrifices to provide the research to establish the efficacy of the techniques that are in use. It cannot be assumed that the federal government or some other agency will fund the research. The responsibility for proving the effectiveness of the treatments and providing the funds for the necessary research belongs to the chiropractic profession and specifically to the developers/promoters of a technique system.

Research efforts, therefore, should be directed toward the basic sciences, reliability studies, and controlled clinical trials. Basic science research is necessary to gain knowledge of the physiologic and anatomic foundations of the clinical process.[6] The anatomic, physiologic, and pathophysiologic mechanisms of the manipulable lesion (subluxation, somatic dysfunction, osteopathic lesion, and so on), whether structural or functional, must be identified. The effects of this lesion on the body locally and globally must be determined. Reliability studies are necessary to demonstrate that a procedure can produce similar results when applied more than once to the same subject or when applied to a series of subjects with similar qualities. Reliability tests are commonly used to evaluate specific evaluative procedures. Interrater reliability is established when several examiners are able to locate the same finding. Intrarater reliability is established when the same clinician is able to find the same finding on multiple tries. Both are important characteristics necessary for reproducibility of clinical procedures. Finally, but most importantly, is the need for controlled clinical trials. It is essential to determine which techniques are the most effective treatment for which problems and under what circumstances. With this information, standards of care can be developed that best serve patients with problems of neuromusculoskeletal origin.

A model for evaluation of manipulative procedures, including both assessment and technique application has been proposed by Kaminski et al.[48,49] Although the primary purpose of this model is to establish the status of a procedure through the use of experts and scientific evidence, it is also valuable in creating questions for further research. At this time, no technique systems have been able to fulfill all necessary requirements for full acceptance. Most have not attempted it. The mechanically assisted forms of technique are no exception. It is important that they be submitted to this scrutiny.

CASE REPORTS

The case report represents a general approach to controlled observation and therefore is the most simplistic form of nominal descriptive research. It is appropriate to ask more specific questions when sufficient information is not known about a topic. Conclusions cannot be drawn from case reports because many biases and variables exist and the strength of evidence is not adequate. However, the case report does offer support for or against further study of a particular subject and establish the direction for future research. Presented here are a series of cases from the authors' practices, representing several clinical problems that were treated with forms of mechanically assisted and motion-assisted manipulative therapies.

CASE 1

A 48-year-old female consulted for pain in the low back area and left leg. The patient had been in good health until 6 days previous, when she began experiencing difficulty walking and standing in an upright position. There was no reported or remembered traumatic incident. She reported pain and numbness in her left leg and lower back region. The pain became worse as the day progressed, and by early afternoon she could not walk, sit, or lie down without severe pain in the left leg and hip area. On a pain drawing, she localized the pain to the left lumbosacral area, traversing the left buttock, and down the posterolateral thigh and calf to the dorsum of the foot. Using a visual analog scale (0-100) to rate the pain, she indicated the pain to be a constant 82/100 and with any activity a 100/100. She completed an Oswestry Pain Questionnaire with a score of 86%. This indicates a severe disability as a result of pain. The patient denied any bladder or bowel changes. She also

reported subjective numbness and weakness of her left foot and toes.

Assessment procedures revealed diminished ranges of lumbar movement as a result of pain. Quantitative measurements with an inclinometer were not attempted at the initial evaluation because of the amount of pain. The patient was using a walker to achieve an upright and ambulatory posture. Muscle stretch reflexes of the lower extremities were equal and graded as 2+. Sensory to pin evaluation revealed a decrease in sensation over the dorsum of the left foot and toes. Motor evaluation of the lower limb revealed a weakness of the left extensor hallucis longus muscle, graded as 4/5. Straight leg raising produced low back pain but no leg pain to 70 degrees. The well leg raise produced left leg pain when the right leg was raised to 30 degrees. Sciatic notch tenderness was present, and palpation of the sciatic nerve along its posterior course produced pain to the knee. Palpatory tenderness was noted over the left sacroiliac joint, gluteus maximus muscle, and left lower lumbar paraspinal muscles. Intrathecal pressure tests were negative. Spinal examination revealed joint dysfunction and palpatory pain at the L4-5 functional unit and left sacroiliac articulation. A computed tomography (CT) scan was obtained (Fig. 8-1), which demonstrated radiographic evidence of a small and apparently contained focal disc herniation into the left subarticular and lateral recess, causing possible compromise of the left L5 nerve root.

The findings were reviewed with the patient, and a diagnosis of mechanical dysfunction at the L4-5 functional unit, including posterior joint dysfunction and disc disruption, was discussed. With the evidence of L5 nerve root compression demonstrating sensory and motor deficit, the

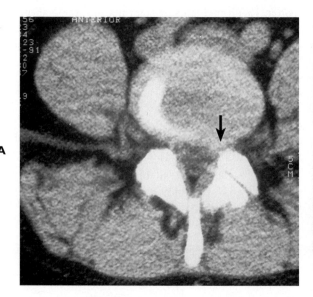
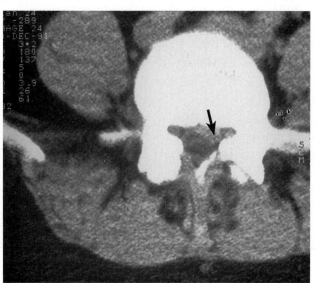

Fig. 8-1 Computerized tomograms (CT) through the L4-5 segment demonstrating a moderate disc herniation of the L4 disc, with possible compression of L5 nerve root in the lateral recess.

patient was advised that a surgical consult should be considered. She chose instead to undergo a trial of manipulative treatment.

Ice was applied to the lower back for 5 minutes, followed by flexion-distraction mobilization performed by placing a hand contact over the L4 spinous process and using the pelvic section of the table to distract and flex the lumbar spine between the L4-5 segment. This procedure was repeated 3 times, with each distractive process being held for 20 seconds. The patient was told to lie on her back at home whenever possible, with her hips flexed to 90 degrees and knees flexed to 90 degrees, and to use ice for 5 minutes every hour. She was to get up only to go to the bathroom. She was seen again 2 days later and reported improvement in the pain, which was evidenced by her ability to walk nearly upright without support. However, her posture and gait were still quite guarded. Sensation to pin was nearly equal over the dorsum of both feet and toes. Extensor hallucis longus weakness persisted. Treatment consisted again of ice and flexion-distraction. Included with this session was long axis distraction applied to the left lower extremity in the supine position, with a towel wrapped around the ankle to serve as a "handle" to apply the distraction. Soft tissue massage was also applied to the paraspinal and gluteal muscles. She was seen for a third visit, 3 days later, and again reported improvement, demonstrating improved ability to walk and stand. Sensory evaluation to pin was equal, and the extensor hallucis longus muscle again tested 4/5. Lumbar flexion-distraction was again applied. The patient was instructed to resume daily activities but not sit for long periods. She returned for treatment 1 week later and reported that the pain in her low back was minimal and only twinges of pain occurred into her left leg. Sensation to pin was still symmetric; however, a slight disparity in strength of the extensor hallucis longus muscle continued. Palpatory tenderness over the osseous and soft tissue structures of her low back was also greatly reduced. Sciatic notch tenderness was no longer apparent.

One week later she reported that her low back pain was nearly gone, and the leg pain no longer bothered her. She stated that she was still cautious with activities but was able to do most things without problem. Sensation to pin remained symmetric, and extensor hallucis longus strength was nearly symmetric. Only minimal palpatory tenderness was noted over the L4 spinous process. Ice was discontinued and heat begun, applied in the form of hydroculator packs. Treatment again consisted of lumbar flexion-distraction and long axis distraction of the left lower extremity, but side-posture rotary manipulation was added. This consisted of a high-velocity, low-amplitude thrust applied to the L4 segment, with the patient lying on her right side. She was seen 4 more times over the course of the next 6 weeks and reported an occasional sense of lower back pain and activity-related aching pain in her leg. These events, however, did not eventuate into any major problem. She was last seen for this complaint 3 months after the onset and was asymptomatic. She completed another Oswestry Pain Questionnaire, with a score of 7%, demonstrating a marked improvement over the original 86%. In a 2-year follow-up phone call, the patient reported no recurrence of low back or leg pain. A total of nine treatments was provided over the course of 3 months. This case demonstrates the use of different forms of manual therapy as the condition and patient's tolerance allow, specifically here for a lumbar disc herniation with neurologic deficit.

CASE 2

A male, age 39, presented with a complaint of low back pain in the area of L5-S1, apparently as a result of a work-related injury. He reported that he lifted a roll of carpet and pulled it through a door that he held open with his foot. When he lifted the carpet, he felt something release in his low back and experienced a gradual onset of acute pain. He localized the pain to the L5-S1 level, primarily on the left but also with some pain on the right. He noted that the pain was relatively sharp, and he was observed to have a slightly forward-leaning antalgic posture. Using a visual analog scale (0-100) to rate the pain, he indicated the pain to be 74/100. He completed an Oswestry Pain Questionnaire, with a score of 52%. This indicated a severe disability as a result of pain. He denied any bladder or bowel changes. He noted that he awakened at approximately 3:00 AM that night with severe low back pain. He had to arise from his bed, with some difficulty, at that time to move around. He reported that during the day, after he experienced the strain, he tried to keep his back straight and work more carefully but still experienced some severe discomfort in his low back. He denied other injuries but did report that he had been taking aspirin as needed. This individual had been a patient in the past for a similar problem and was treated successfully with chiropractic manipulation.

The patient had very limited range of motion in the lumbar spine in all directions because of pain. He was antalgic forward and had both knees slightly flexed. He was able to move slightly in all directions but was limited by pain in the low back. Deep tendon reflexes in the lower limbs demonstrated a left patellar at 1+, a right patellar at 2+, and the Achilles at 2+ bilaterally. Percussion over L3-5 was negative. Valsalva's and Bechterew's tests produced left low back pain. Straight leg raising produced low back pain bilaterally, with the left at 60 degrees and the right at 70 degrees but with no radiation of pain. Milgram's test could not be performed because the patient could not lift his feet off the table without experiencing pain. Ely's, Nachlas', Yeoman's, Kemp's, and Gaenslen's tests were all negative. Digital palpation over the left quadratus lumborum revealed hypertonicity and produced a pain response. Evaluation of the lower limb musculature for strength revealed symmetry, with no apparent weakness. Sensory evaluation to pin and light touch over the lower limbs was within normal limits. Standard anterior-to-posterior (APLP) and lateral (LLS) projections of the lumbar spine and pelvis were obtained (Fig. 8-2).

The findings were reviewed with the patient, and a diagnosis of mechanical dysfunction at the L5-S1 functional unit, including posterior joint dysfunction with capsular sprain and quadratus lumborum, lumbar paraspinal muscle strain, was discussed. This patient underwent a short trial of therapy with linear axial distraction while lying prone on the Hill Intertrac table, contacting the L5 spinous process. Deep muscle massage therapy was also used over the lumbar paraspinal and quadratus lumborum muscles while the motorized pelvic section applied linear distraction. Interferential current was applied following the treatment. The patient was taken off work for 3 days and then returned with limited physical responsibilities. He was treated a total of 10 times over 6 weeks. His VAS went to 10/100 and the Oswestry score was 18%. This case demonstrates the use of motorized mechanical assistance to produce intersegmental

and soft tissue distraction to the lumbar spine for an uncomplicated sprain/strain.

CASE 3

This 34-year-old female was seen for evaluation and treatment of right shoulder pain, headache, neck pain, and tightness of the cervical musculature. The patient related the onset to an incident that occurred while checking into a hotel. A 15-foot pole fell from the ceiling and hit her on the head, knocking her unconscious. When she regained consciousness, she could not see, although she was aware of people talking about her. The patient reports that her behavior was described as similar to a petit mal seizure. She was transported to the hospital, where the laceration on the left side of her head was stitched. She reported a headache on the right side of her head. She stated that no diagnosis was made nor given to her at that time, and she was not given any medication or other treatment options. She experienced difficulties sleeping and had nausea accompanied by occa-

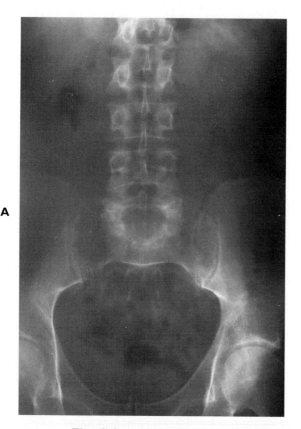
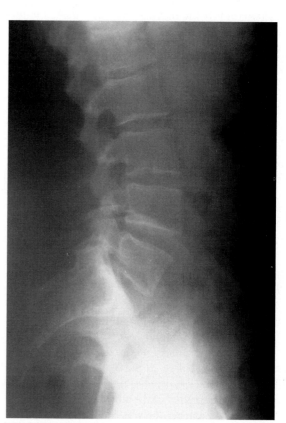

Fig. 8-2 A, Anterior-to-posterior and **B,** lateral lumbopelvic plain film radiographs demonstrating mild pelvic unleveling, low on the right; a minimal left lumbar convexity; mild increased lumbar lordosis; moderately increased sacral base angle; mild disc space narrowing, with spondylosis at L3-4; facet asymmetry at L3-4; minimal degenerative change in the upper aspect of the right sacroiliac articulation. Also noted are some possible prostatic calculi.

sional vomiting with the severe headaches. She continued to have headaches for which no treatment was provided. The patient's main symptoms at the time of examination were headache and right arm numbness. She stated that her headaches came without warning and were located temporally and behind the right ear. The headaches were quite severe but only lasted for a short time in the severe state and then slowly resolved. The head pain was described as throbbing, and she reported having approximately two of these severe headaches per week. The head pain was quite severe, causing her to stop whatever she was doing at the moment. As the pain subsided, she could resume her daily activities. She reported that the sensations in her arm felt as though her "funny bone" was being continually irritated. She also related that in certain positions her hands would "fall asleep," although she denied having these symptoms at night, stating that her sleep was "fairly good."

On examination, the patient's vital signs were as follows: blood pressure, 110/80 mm Hg; pulse rate, 60; respiratory rate, 20; height, 5 ft 5 in; and weight, 180 lb. Muscle stretch reflexes of the upper extremity were equal and graded as 2+. Sensory evaluation to pin and light touch revealed an increase in sensation over the right C6 and C8 dermatomes. Motor evaluation of the upper limb was essentially normal, with the exception of her right deltoid, which was slightly weak and graded as 4/5. Evaluation of cranial nerves II to XII was essentially normal; however, there was a hypersensitivity and some proprioceptive changes in the form of deep pressure loss to the left side of her tongue. Palpation of the soft tissues of her neck and upper back demonstrated tenderness and increased tone in her right trapezius muscle. Also noted was pain and hypertonicity of her right scalene muscle, with pain in the right pectoralis minor muscle. Pressure applied over the coracoid process reproduced the tingling sensation into her forearm and hand. Evaluation of her temporomandibular joints was noncontributory. Specific spinal examination revealed pain, misalignment, and loss of movement at the C5-6 functional unit and the atlantooccipital articulation. Radiographs were obtained (Fig. 8-3), revealing some degenerative change in

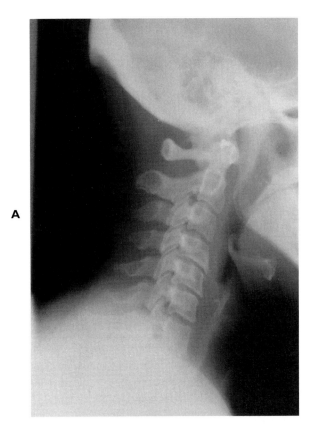
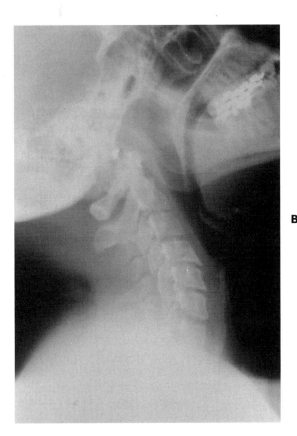

Fig. 8-3 Lateral cervical views in the **A**, neutral, **B**, extended, and **C**, flexed positions demonstrating an alordotic cervical spine with minimal kyphotic reversal, overall diminished flexion and extension movement, degenerative disc disease at C4-5 and C5-6, and uncovertebral arthrosis at C5-6.

Continued

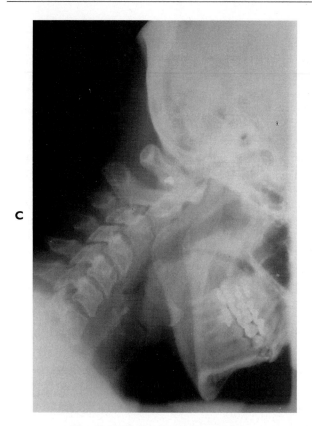

Fig. 8-3 C, For legend see p. 261.

the uncovertebral joints and spondylosis of the intervertebral disc of the C5-6 functional unit. Diminished segmental movement in flexion and extension was also observed. Review of the patient's records indicated that a CT scan of her head and an MRI of her cervical spine had been performed, both of which were read as normal. An EMG study had also been performed and was interpreted as normal.

The findings were reviewed with the patient. She sustained a traumatic blow to her head that possibly resulted in a posttraumatic headache, creating some evidence of a post traumatic hyperirritability syndrome. This is a poorly understood and difficult to manage condition. Individuals with this syndrome have incurred a major impact to the body and/or head, in which consciousness was disrupted. This inflicts damage to the sensory pathways of the central nervous system, and patients experience constant pain that is augmented by normally inconsequential sensory stimuli, such as loud noises, vibration, prolonged physical activity, and emotional stress. Evidence also supported the presence of a coracoid pressure syndrome, characterized by arm pain and clinical symptoms and signs of compression or irritation of the brachial plexus. Pressure applied over the coracoid process reproduced the radiation of pain down the arm. Also of note, but quite possibly of no great clinical importance, is an apparent neck-tongue syndrome, characterized

by the change in sensation over the left side of her tongue. This involves the posterior primary division of second and third cervical nerves as they intermix with the lingual nerve in the ansa cervicalis.[50]

A course of manipulative therapy was deemed appropriate in this case. The patient was treated using long axis distraction applied to the cervical spine in the supine position on the Hill Intertrac table. Contacts were established under the posterior aspect (base) of the occiput. Soft tissue manipulation, moist heat, and ultrasound were applied to muscles of the neck and shoulder. She tolerated treatment well but complied poorly with treatment and home exercise recommendations. She received a total of 15 treatments, reaching objective and subjective resolution in 1 ½ years. This case illustrates the use of motorized mechanical assistance to produce distraction and mobilization to the cervical spine and supportive soft tissues for an unusual array of clinical problems.

CASE 4

The patient presented for an evaluation and possible treatment for a history of low back pain. He reported that he had experienced some mild episodes of low back pain with minimal leg pain during the past 2 months. He had experienced recurrent bouts of low back pain for many years and reported that the discomfort at the time of this evaluation was fairly minimal compared with his previous experiences. He denied any accident, injury, or illness, stating that he had been performing his normal activities of daily living. He did note that one change in his household was the birth of a new child. This required him to do some lifting of the child, which perhaps put additional stress on his back.

On examination, the patient was an adult male, and his vital signs were as follows: blood pressure, 120/75 mm Hg; pulse, 64; height, 5 ft 8 in; and weight, 184 lb. Lumbar range of motion was adequately accomplished within normal limits. Motor, sensory, and reflex evaluation of the lower extremity was symmetric, with no deficits elicited. Ely's, Yeoman's, SLR, Milgram's, Valsalva's, and Bechterew's tests were negative. Digital palpation of the right SI joint produced slight pain, rated as 20/100. Slight tenderness was reproduced through digital palpation of the lumbar spinous processes and paraspinal muscles, that was also rated at 20/100. He reported that the pain was more intense with sitting. Plain film radiographs of his low back had been obtained previously (Fig. 8-4), and, with no new trauma, additional radiographs were not deemed indicated.

This patient was likely suffering from a slight exacerbation of his previous lumbar strain/sprain, with probable sacroiliac involvement and without neurologic deficit. The findings were discussed with the patient, and it was recommended that he be treated for this minimally acute episode and then be treated as often as once per month to maintain his comfort level. He was advised to continue his exercise routine, which he notes doing relatively faithfully. The

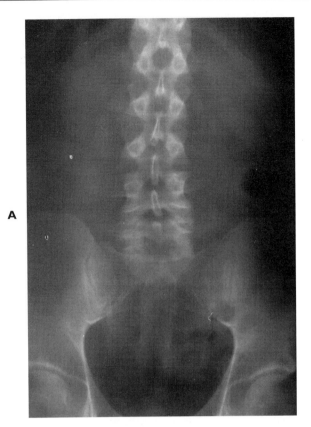 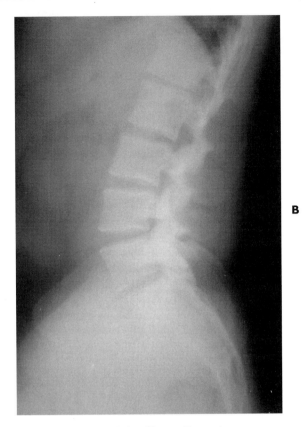

Fig. 8-4 A, Anterior-to-posterior and **B**, lateral lumbopelvic plain film radiographs demonstrating minimal pelvic unleveling low on the right and minimal degenerative disc disease L4-5 and L5-S1.

patient was treated with deep muscle massage over the lumbar paraspinals and the gluteal muscles bilaterally. Long axis distraction, with the patient prone on the Hill Intertrac table, was applied to the lumbar spine while in slight flexion and lateral flexion to both sides alternately to emphasize distraction of the SI joints bilaterally. The patient was able to rise from the table with comfort and appeared to have a normal stance and gait after the treatment. The patient was advised to continue to exercise and to seek chiropractic treatment perhaps as often as once per month to minimize the effects of any possible exacerbation of the low back problem. He was treated a total of 4 times, with resolution of the complaint. This case demonstrates the use of motorized mechanical assistance to influence sacroiliac joint function.

CASE 5

This patient was a male, age 54, who presented with a complaint of low back pain on the right side, with right-sided pain in the groin that he described as a "catch." He also reported some left leg pain, with occasional numbness and tingling in his leg. He noted having had an episode of low

back pain as far back as 4 years previous. At that time, he was examined medically, including radiographs and CT scans, with subsequent recommendations of NSAIDs for treatment. He reported that this occurrence of low back pain was constant and localized to the right side, rated at 40/100. The pain also disturbed his sleep. The groin pain was present only when he was lifting and tended to be on the right side, rated at 60/100. The patient reported a history of colon cancer, with surgery 20 years previously and also claimed to have some apparent prostate problems but had difficulty with the treatments. On further examination, a colon tumor was found. A prophylactic radiation series was performed following the surgery (approximately 15 years ago), and the patient experienced some subsequent colon "lockups." He had a partial resection of the colon to correct this, and his medical doctor noted at that time that he may experience some effects of the radiation as late as 20 years after the treatment was administered. The patient was therefore concerned whether the current problem might be a result of the radiation. He noted that several years ago he was lifting and wrenched his lower back, creating a low back problem for which he received medical treatment at the time. He noted minimal history of low back problems before that time. The patient was employed as a business consultant, which caused him a high level of stress and required him to sit for long periods.

On examination, the patient's vital signs were as follows: blood pressure, 120/78 mm Hg; height, 6 ft 0 in; and weight, 195 lb. His mastoid process was lower on the left, as was the crest of the ilium. His stance appeared somewhat distorted because he had a right low shoulder and high hip, suggestive of a scoliosis. He had a normal-appearing gait and, when viewed laterally, appeared to be basically normal. Dorsolumbar motion was within normal limits, with no pain accompanying movement. Heel walk, toe walk, and supported Adam's test were negative; however, Kemp's test to the left produced some discomfort at L3-4. SI motion was within normal limits bilaterally. Motor and sensory evaluation of the lower limb was symmetric and essentially normal. Muscle stretch reflexes of the lower limb revealed the left patellar at 1+, the right patellar at 3+, and the Achilles at 2+ bilaterally; no Babinski's response was noted. Bechterew's test produced

pain in the anterior thigh and lumbar spine. Valsalva's test produced slight pain in the lumbar area, but the pain was there constantly. Also noted was a short leg on the left (approximately $1/2$ in) that is slightly reactive to stimulation at the hip.

Weight-bearing lumbar radiographs were obtained and compared with previous studies (Fig. 8-5). The series of plain film radiographs show progression of the scoliosis, which gradually increases from 13 to 40 degrees over a 20-year period.

The patient appears to have chronic ongoing low back pain, perhaps complicated by degenerative changes associated with a left convex, marked progressive scoliosis between T12 and L5. He now has increased back pain and left leg pain, numbness, and tingling, that is likely a result of the development of a lateral spinal stenosis producing nerve compression. This is sometimes referred to as a *lumbar claudication syndrome*. The patient was treated using linear distraction in the prone position on the Hill Intertrac table. A contact was established over the L5 spinous process

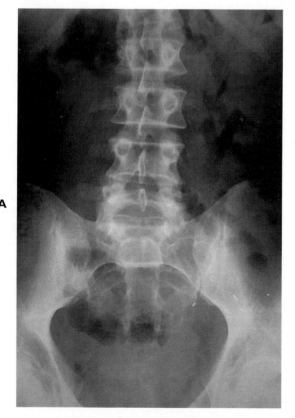

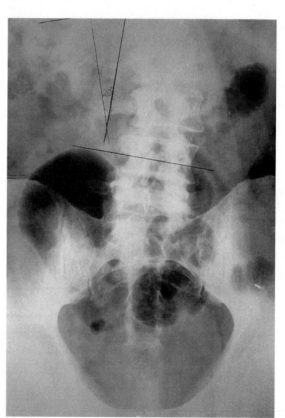

Fig. 8-5 Anterior-to-posterior lumbopelvic radiographs demonstrating a progressive rotatory scoliosis spanning 20 years. **A,** The earliest film shows a mild right convexity of about 10 degrees; **B,** a film taken 18 years later shows progression of the curve to 20 degrees.

initially. Some flexion and lateral flexion was added to applied separation to the concave portion of the scoliosis. Twenty treatments were administered. The patient also participated in a comprehensive 5-day supervised rehabilitation program that included education, instruction in spinal unloading, stabilization exercises, and stretching in consultation with a neurosurgeon and rehabilitation center. On completing the program, he was instructed to begin a daily independent low-back health maintenance regimen. The goal was to relieve his symptoms and begin to reverse the progression of the scoliosis. However this type of program likely would have been most valuable approximately 10 years previously. Because he had to do a lot of sitting in front of a computer, the use of an LTX 3000 unloading device (Fig. 7-7) was recommended. The subjective results of this comanagement treatment plan were encouraging. The patient reported much less pain, allowing him to do activities that were impossible previously. It is too soon to determine whether the progression of the scoliosis has slowed, however. This case does demonstrate the use of

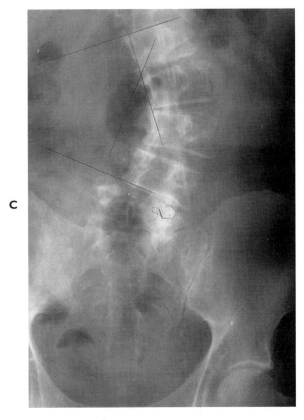

Fig. 8-5 C, a film taken 2 years after the second film shows progression to 40 degrees; also noted is progressive degenerative changes to the disc and facets of L3-4, L4-5, and L5-S1.

motorized mechanical assistance and sustained mechanical traction in the treatment of degenerative scoliosis and lateral recess stenosis.

CASE 6

The patient is a female, age 46, who presented with a complaint of diffuse pain in the legs, low back, face, and top of head, with occasional forearm pain. She noted that this was diagnosed medically within the last 6 months as fibromyalgia. She indicated that she tends to be stiffer in the morning, and that this affects her back and legs. The patient experiences difficulty climbing stairs, and walking tends to make the problem worse after only 10 to 15 minutes. She noted that hot packs or a hot bath make the areas feel better but not very much nor for very long. She reported a traumatic event 1 ½ years ago, in which she fell down stairs and hit a wall. She stated that following this event, the pains started and have gradually gotten worse over time. A month after the fall, she had a second fall but does not know what caused it. She fell on the street and hit her knee and subsequently suffered increased pain. She was originally diagnosed with lupus, but that has since been superseded by the fibromyalgia. She has great difficulty sleeping, partly because of the pain. The pain, in her estimation, seems to be spreading over her body. She denies illness of importance, fractures, or injuries in the past. She had a weight gain over the past 5 years of approximately 50 pounds.

On examination, the patient's vital signs were as follows: blood pressure, 130/100 mm Hg in the first reading and 130/94 mm Hg in the second reading; pulse rate, 74; respiration rate, 20; oral temperature, 98.0° F; height, 5 ft 2 in; and weight, 186 lb. A postural elevation was noted at the right mastoid, the left shoulder, and the right iliac crest. The patient had an apparent flattened left longitudinal arch of the foot. Cervicothoracic and lumbar curves were increased. Cervical and lumbar range of motion were adequately accomplished, with no restriction or increase in pain. All movements were performed in both active and passive ranges of motion. Sensory evaluation for light touch and pin of the upper and lower extremity was within normal limits. Motor function tests of the upper and lower extremity were evaluated, with all muscles graded at 5/5, with the exception of weak wrist flexors, graded at 3/5. The reflexes of the upper and lower extremity were brisk and symmetric, although the Achilles reflex was absent bilaterally. Heel and toe walk was performed within normal limits. Orthopedic tests were performed with no important findings, although Patrick's (fabere) test could not be performed on the right because of pain in the pelvis and Milgram's test produced pain to the top of the head. Algometer readings were taken at several locations on her body, and the findings noted in the record (Fig. 8-6).

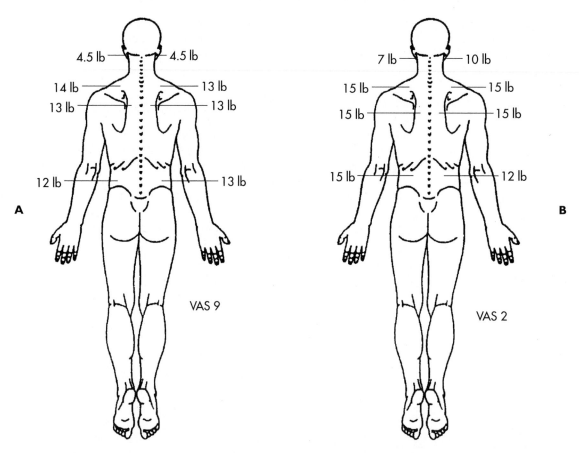

Fig. 8-6 Pain drawings indicating algometer readings and visual analog scales ratings from the **A**, initial and **B**, subsequent evaluation, demonstrating a marked change in perceived pain in the soft tissues.

The patient appeared to show sufficiently diverse pain sites with additional characteristics to conclude that she could indeed have the fibromyalgia complex. She was placed on a treatment program to produce an increase in range of motion and strengthening, with relaxation of her musculature. She underwent a trial period of therapy for approximately 2 weeks. This included full spine long axis distraction applied with the patient in the prone position on the Hill Intertrac table. Long axis distraction was also applied to the knees, with the patient in the supine position on the Hill Intertrac table. Paraspinal soft tissue massage was performed, and she began an aquatics course to facilitate her exercise routine. She was treated 50 times over 2 years and she demonstrated considerable improvement. She experienced periods of increased symptoms but responded favorably to a short course of treatment as needed. This case illustrates the use of motorized mechanical assistance applied to a primary soft tissue condition. These conditions are difficult to manage and tend to recur.

CASE 7

The patient was a 24-year-old female, seen at the request of another chiropractor for evaluation and treatment of low back and leg pain, apparently the result of an automobile accident nearly 2 years previous. The patient reported that she was stopped at a stop sign when her vehicle was hit on the front left side, causing the car to be pushed sideways. She felt immediate back and neck pain; however, this pain became more intense the next day. She consulted a chiropractor, who began treatment to her neck and low back. This treatment helped considerably with the neck pain; however, the low back and leg pain persisted. She felt that the leg pain was becoming more intense and disabling. The pain awakened her, and she had difficulty sitting at work. She needed to stand or even lie on the floor for a while to enable her to remain at work. Lying down, however, no longer relieved the leg pain. She described the leg problem as a numbness sensation, with tingling all over her leg and,

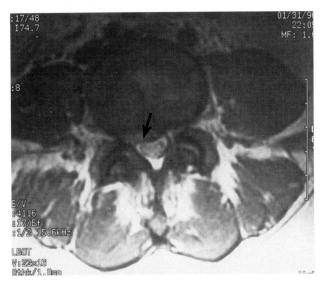

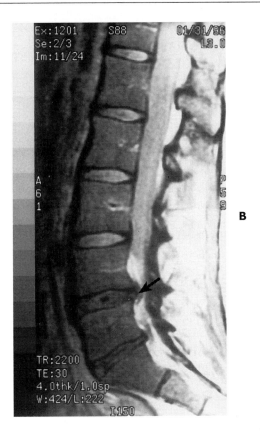

Fig. 8-7 Magnetic resonance imaging (MRI) examination demonstrating two-level degenerative disc disease of L4-5 and L5-S1, with a moderately large right-sided extruded disc herniation at L4-5, with moderately severe subarticular compression on the L5 nerve root, as seen in the **A**, axial sections and **B**, sagittal sections.

specifically, sharp pains in the heel and between the last two toes of the right foot. This pain description suggested a radicular quality because it shot down the back of the leg from the pelvis, over the gluteals, and down the posterior thigh. She also described a cramping type of pain in her calf. The patient was questioned regarding past health and any history of serious or contributory illness. Of note was that she had temporomandibular joint surgery 3 months before to the accident. Although this did not contribute to the trauma to her neck and low back, the experience she had with surgery was a negative one, creating a sense of fear of surgery for her low back. Secondarily, she also reported some residual discomfort in the neck and shoulder area.

On examination the patient demonstrated the following vital signs: blood pressure, 110/78 mm Hg; pulse rate, 84; and respiratory rate, 16. She was adequately able to toe walk and heel walk, although with weight bearing there was an increase in leg pain and calf ache. Kemp's test on the right produced low back pain and radicular pain into the right heel and last two toes. Lumbar ranges of motion, as measured with an inclinometer were as follows: flexion, 30 degrees; extension, 30 degrees; lateral flexion, 35 degrees bilaterally; and rotation, 30 degrees bilaterally. Flexion was significantly limited because of pain rated at 80/100. Although the other ranges of motion were adequately

accomplished, pain was produced in the right sacroiliac area during all movements. The seated straight leg raise test (Bechterew's test) reproduced right radicular leg pain. The supine straight leg raising test (Laségue's) produced right leg pain at 30 degrees on the right and 70 degrees on the left. Gaenslen's and Patrick's (fabere) tests produced right calf and right low back pain. Evaluation of muscle strength of the lower extremity revealed equal muscle strength bilaterally, with all muscles graded at 5/5. On subsequent evaluation, however, the extensor hallucis longus muscle began to demonstrate a slight motor weakness on the right, graded 4/5. Sensory evaluation to pin and light touch was essentially normal, and muscle stretch reflexes of the lower extremity were brisk and equal, with the patellar graded as 3+ and the Achilles graded as 2+. Palpatory pain was produced over the L4 and L5 spinous processes. Radiographs of the lumbar spine and pelvis were obtained. Because of the severe and progressive nature of the leg pain, the patient was referred for an MRI (Fig. 8-7).

Based on the examination and imaging findings, it was concluded that this patient sustained a traumatic injury to her low back, resulting in a disc herniation at the L4-5 level that produced compression of the right L5 nerve root. This was complicated by the traumatic effects of a sprain to the capsular ligaments and a strain to the paraspinal musculature.

The patient began a course of manipulative therapy that included long axis distraction techniques performed on the patient in the prone position on the Hill Intertrac table to separate the lumbar intervertebral segments to facilitate alignment and allow for diminished effect of the mass lesion on the nerve root. Interferential current was also applied to reduce pain and irritability to the facilitated nerve roots. Soft tissue massage and trigger point therapy was applied to the surrounding musculature to aid in balancing the tone of the muscles across the lumbar spine. The patient was also seen in a rehabilitation center and given a course of exercises. Initially the exercises were performed in a pool to diminish the gravitational effect on her spine, allowing some activity without gravitational loading. She was also given extension exercises, because this was the range of motion that was most easily accomplished with no peripheralization of pain. This rehabilitative program was designed to increase joint mobility, promote lengthening of the shortened supporting tissues, and increase endurance to the supporting musculature.

The patient was seen 43 times. She showed some moderate improvement in low back pain but only minimal improvement in leg pain. She has been able to continue to work and can do so without having to lie down as often. She was also able to reduce the amount of pain medication. However, there was continued pain, with probable permanency, related to this injury. The patient would not consider surgery and has disregarded repeated recommendation for a surgical consult. Nearly 3 years after the injury, the condition has had more than enough time to resolve with conservative measures. There is suggestion that over time the body may be able to resorb portions of the disc herniation, which could lessen pain; however, this is no longer likely in this case. The patient remained unable to do any physical activities that required lifting or added compressive loads to her lumbar spine. Her employment activities do not require these kinds of physical stresses. However, sitting for long periods was an aggravating factor, and this is part of her job. Before the accident she had been actively pursuing very specific forms of vigorous and demanding exercise, including body building and weight lifting, that were no longer possible. Walking more than 15 to 20 minutes caused considerable leg pain. The patient decided not to explore a surgical solution because she had a previous negative experience with surgery. However, surgery cannot be ruled out for her in the future. This case demonstrates the use of motorized mechanical assistance unsuccessfully applied for a disc herniation with radiculopathy in the lumbar spine. Furthermore, high-velocity, low-amplitude thrust techniques had been previously applied with no benefit. There of course is no panacea in the treatment of joint conditions.

CONCLUSION

Chiropractic practitioners are similar to medical physicians in the way they must make clinical decisions. Prior experience and clinical intuition; proficiency with diagnostic and treatment interventions; and an applied knowledge of anatomy, physiology, and biomechanics are factors brought to bear when care is provided to patients.

However, all practitioners will increasingly be expected to base their clinical decisions on an examination of evidence from clinical research. The revolutions described by Relman[14] are primarily political, sociologic, and economic in nature. A parallel scientific revolution has taken place within the health care community. This is the emergence of evidence-based health care, which seeks to overcome the inherent unreliability of traditional clinical decision making. Until recently there has been an overreliance on unsystematic clinical observations, experience, common sense, and understanding of basic mechanisms of disease. Procedures and clinical guidelines based on these principles have commonly been shown to be of questionable benefit or even harmful to patients. By contrast, evidence-based health care emphasizes the importance of outcomes-based clinical research, of regularly consulting original, current literature, and of understanding certain rules of evidence that apply in evaluating that literature.

One of the postulates of evidence-based health care is that it matters a great deal what type of scientific research is carried out and not just that research is done. Of particular interest is the distinction between research into disease (pathophysiology) mechanisms and research directed at actual patient outcomes. Although not an either/or proposition, the principles of evidence-based health care establish a clear hierarchy that places outcomes-based clinical research ahead of basic, mechanism-based research. The evidence-based medicine working group reports[51]: "The rationales for diagnosis and treatment which follow from basic pathophysiologic principles, may in fact be incorrect." This leaves all of us a monumental but not impossible task ahead. If the question to be answered concerns the effectiveness or relative effectiveness of chiropractic assessment and management, there is no alternative but to conduct the highest levels of clinical, outcomes-based research (preferably RCTs). Ultimately, a clinical decision must be informed by clinical evidence.[52]

There are irreducible uncertainties that accompany all health care decisions, which no amount of research can eradicate. However, the health care industry will be required to reduce those uncertainties to a minimum, and professions that fail to do so will be at a distinct competitive disadvantage.

The science of chiropractic is now beginning to investigate the art of chiropractic. In this manner, the profession will better be able to define itself for the coming debate on managed care and national health insurance. The nation has become increasingly cost conscious, and many decisions regarding health care no longer rest with those involved in delivering that care. Instead, these decisions rest with insurance company executives, politicians, and government agencies. These groups are not likely to support methods of health care that lack scientific credibility. The need to continue scientific research is paramount to maintaining the status quo chiropractic practice rights.

The fact that clinical research is finally taking place in the field of spinal manipulation is promising. The intended purpose of this research is improvement in the standard of care of patients treated by all health professionals. The chiropractic profession must embrace the need for research. The profession's credibility depends on it, the quality of care will be enhanced by it, and it is, most importantly, what the patients deserve. Furthermore and finally, all chiropractic practitioners must develop and maintain a higher level of clinical scholarship by regularly and consistently diverting a small amount of time to the reading of the profession's accomplishments, to the ultimate benefit of those we serve.

REFERENCES

1. Hansen DT. Chiropractic outcome measures. *Impulse CNS Newsletter.* September/October 1990.
2. Hansen DT. Searching for the common authority in validation and standardization of chiropractic methods. *J Chiropr Tech.* 1990;2(3):72-73.
3. Deyo RA. Measuring the functional status of patients with low back pain. *Arch Phys Med Rehabil.* 1988;69:1044-1053.
4. Deyo RA. Measuring the functional status of patients with low back pain. *J Chiropr Tech.* 1990;2(3):127-137.
5. Pope MH, Rosen JC, Wilder DG, Frymoyer JW. Relation between biomechanical and psychological factors in patients with low back pain. *Spine.* 1980;5:173-178.
6. Triano JJ. The subluxation complex: outcome measure of chiropractic diagnosis and treatment. *Chiropr Tech.* 1990;2:114.
7. Vernon HT. Applying research-based assessments of pain and loss of function to the issue of developing standards of care in chiropractic. *J Chiropr Tech.* 1990;2(3):121-126.
8. Fairbank JCT, Couper J, Davies JB, O'Brien JP. The Oswestry Low Back Pain Disability Questionnaire. *Physiotherapy.* 1980;66:271.
9. Vernon H. The neck disability index: a study of reliability and validity. *J Manipulative Physiol Ther.* 1991;14(7):409.
10. Bergmann TF. Introduction and opening statement, Consensus Conference on Validation of Chiropractic Methods. *Chiropr Tech.* 1990;2(3):71,160.
11. Bergmann TF. Various forms of chiropractic technique. *Chiropr Tech.* 1993;5(2):53-55.
12. Keating JC. Traditional barriers to standards of knowledge production in chiropractic. *Chiropr Tech.* 1990;2(3):78-85.
13. Payton OD. *Research: The Validation of Clinical Practice.* Philadelphia: FA Davis; 1979.
14. Relman AS. Assessment and accountability: the third revolution in medical care. *N Engl J Med.* 1988;319:1220-1222.
15. Hansen DT, Mootz RD. Formal procedures in health care technology assessment: a primer for the chiropractic profession. *Top Clin Chiropr.* 1996;3:71-83.

16. Mannello DM, Lawrence DJ, Mootz RD. The evolution of chiropractic research: a foundation for technology assessment. *Top Clin Chiropr.* 1996;3:52-64.

17. Shekelle PG, Adams AH. *The Appropriateness of Spinal Manipulation for Low-Back Pain: Project Overview and Literature Review.* Monterey, Calif: RAND Corp; 1991.

18. American Chiropractic Association. *Comparison of Chiropractic and Medical Treatment of Nonoperative Back and Neck Injuries, 1976-1977.* Des Moines: American Chiropractic Assoc; 1978.

19. Brunarski DJ. Clinical trials of spinal manipulation: a critical appraisal and review of the literature. *J Manipulative Physiol Ther.* 1984;7:243-249.

20. Nyiendo J. Chiropractic effectiveness, I. Oregon Chiropractic Physicians Association legislative newsletter. April 1991.

21. Anderson R, Meeker WC, Wirick BE et al. A meta-analysis of clinical trials of spinal manipulation. *J Manipulative Physiol Ther.* 1992; 15(3):181-194.

22. Waagen GN, Haldeman S, Cook G. Short-term trial of chiropractic adjustments for the relief of chronic low back pain. *Manual Med.* 1986;2:63-67.

23. Meade TW, Dyer SD, Brown W. Low back pain of mechanical origin: randomized comparison of chiropractic and hospital outpatient treatment. *Br Med J.* 1990; 300:1431-1437.

24. Kane RL, Olsen D, Leymaster C et al. Manipulating the patient: a comparison of the effectiveness of physician and chiropractor care. *Lancet.* 1974;1:1333-1336.

25. Cherkin DC, MacCornack FA. Health care delivery. Patient evaluations of low back pain care from family physicians and chiropractors. *West J Med.* 1989;150(3):351-355.

26. Cherkin DC, MacCornack FA, Berg AO. The management of low back pain: a comparison of the beliefs and behaviors of family physicians and chiropractors. *West J Med.* 1988;149:475-480.

27. Russell R. Diagnostic palpation of the spine: a review of procedures and assessment of their reliability. *J Manipulative Physiol Ther.* 1983;6(4):181-183.

28. Keating J. Inter-examiner reliability of motion palpation of the lumbar spine: a review of quantitative literature. *Am J Chiropr Med.* 1989;2(3):107-110.

29. Keating JC, Bergmann TF, Jacob G et al. Interexaminer reliability of eight evaluative dimensions of lumbar segmental abnormality. *J Manipulative Physiol Ther.* 1990;13(8):463-470.

30. Mior SA, King RS, McGregor M, Bernard M. Intra- and inter-examiner reliability of motion palpation of the cervical spine. *J Can Chiropr Assoc.* 1985;29(4):195-198.

31. Brunarski DJ. Chiropractic biomechanical evaluations: validity in myofascial low back pain. *J Manipulative Physiol Ther.* 1982;7:243-249.

32. Addington ER. Reliability and objectivity of the Anatometer, supine leg length test, Thermoscribe ll, and the Derm-therm-o-graph measurements. *Upper Cervical Monographs.* 1983;3:8-1134.

33. Deyo R, McNiesh LM, Cone RD et al. Observer variability in the interpretation of lumbar spine radiographs. *Arthritis Rheum.* 1985;28(9):1066-1070.

34. Antos JC, Robinson K, Keating JC, Jacobs GE. Interrater reliability of fluoroscopic detection of fixation in the mid-cervical spine. *Chiropr Tech.* 1990;2(2)53-55.

35. Fuhr AW, Osterbauer PJ. Interexaminer reliability of relative leg-length evaluations in the prone, extended position. *Chiropr Tech.* 1989;1:13-18.

36. Haas M. The reliability of reliability. *J Manipulative Physiol Ther.* 1991;14(3):199-208.

37. Keating J. Several strategies for evaluating the objectivity of measurements in clinical research and practice. *J Can Chiropr Assoc.* 1988; 32(3):133-138.

38. Boline P, Keating J, Brist J et al. Interexaminer reliability of palpatory evaluations of the lumbar spine. *Am J Chiropr Med.* 1988; 1(1):5-11.

39. Johnston W, Allan BR. Interexaminer study of palpation in detecting location of spinal segmental dysfunction. *J Am Osteopath Assoc.* 1983; 82(11):839-845.

40. Panzer DM. Lumbar motion palpation: a literature review. In: *Proceedings of the sixth annual conference on research and education.* Arlington, Va: Foundation for Chiropractic Education and Research; June 1991.

41. Panzer DM. The reliability of lumbar motion palpation. *J Manipulative Physiol Ther.* 1992;15(8):518-524.

42. Koran LM. The reliability of clinical methods, data, and judgments. *N Engl J Med.* 1975;293:642-646.

43. Nelson MA, Allen P, Clamp SE et al. Reliability and reproducibility of clinical findings in low back pain. *Spine.* 1979;4:97-101.

44. Alley RJ. The clinical value of motion palpation as a diagnostic tool. *J Can Chiropr Assoc.* 1983;27:91-100.

45. Waddell G, Main CJ, Morris EW et al. Normality and reliability in the clinical assessment of backache. *Br Med J.* 1982;284:1519-1523.

46. Shekelle PG. Current status of standards of care. *J Chiropr Tech.* 1990;2(3):86-89.

47. Adams AH. Determining the usefulness of diagnostic procedures and tests. *Chiropr Tech.* 1990;2(3):90-93.

48. Kaminski M, Boal R, Gillette RG et al. A model for the evaluation of chiropractic methods. *J Manipulative Physiol Ther.* 1987;10(2):61-64.

49. Kaminski M. Research models for validation of chiropractic methods. *Chiropr Tech.* 1990;2(3):107-113.

50. Terrett A. The neck-tongue syndrome. In: Vernon H, ed. Upper Cervical Syndrome. Baltimore: Williams & Wilkins; 1988.

51. Evidence Based Medicine Working Group. Evidence-based medicine: a new approach to teaching the practice of medicine. *JAMA.* 1992; 2420-2425.

52. Sawyer C, Haas M, Nelson C, Elkington W. Clinical research within the chiropractic profession. In: *Proceedings of the National Workshop to Develop the Chiropractic Research Agenda.* Washington, DC: US Dept of Health and Human Services. 1996.

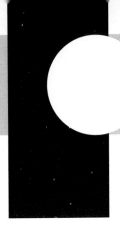

Appendix

List of Manufacturers with Addresses

Zenith-Cox
Williams Health Care Systems
158 N. Edison
Elgin, IL 60123
(800) 441-4967

Leander
Leander Health Technologies Corp.
12300 S.W. Sidney Rd.
Port Orchard, WA 98366
(800) 635-8188

Chattanooga Ergostyle (and Ergotrak)
Chattanooga Group, Inc.
4717 Adams Rd.
Hixon, TN 37343
(800) 592-1451

Back Specialist Flexion Table
Health Care Manufacturing, Inc.
2146 E. Pythian St.
Springfield, MO 65802
(800) 641-4107

Hill Air-Flex
Hill Laboratories Company
445 Lincoln Highway
Malvern, PA 19355
(610) 644-2867

Titan
Titan Technology International
300 Ozark Trail Dr., No. 212C
Ellisville, MO 63011
(800) 688-4826

Galaxy McManis
Lloyd Table Company
102-122 W. Main St.
Lisbon, IA 52253
(800) 553-7297

Spinalight
Spinalight, Inc.
320 A Bell Park Dr.
Woodstock, GA 30188-166
(800) 4-TABLES

Jensen
Annova Enterprises, Inc.
3405 Dakota St.
Alexandria, MN 56308
(800) 826-6082

Index